20+9
1-19

UNDERSTANDING CELIAC DISEASE

Also by Naheed Ali

Understanding Lung Cancer: An Introduction for Patients and Caregivers
Understanding Parkinson's Disease: An Introduction for Patients and Caregivers
Arthritis and You: A Comprehensive Digest for Patients and Caregivers
Understanding Alzheimer's: An Introduction for Patients and Caregivers
The Obesity Reality: A Comprehensive Approach to a Growing Problem
Diabetes and You: A Comprehensive, Holistic Approach

UNDERSTANDING CELIAC DISEASE

An Introduction for Patients and Caregivers

Naheed Ali, MD

ROWMAN & LITTLEFIELD
Lanham • Boulder • New York • London

Published by Rowman & Littlefield
A wholly owned subsidiary of The Rowman & Littlefield Publishing Group, Inc.
4501 Forbes Boulevard, Suite 200, Lanham, Maryland 20706
www.rowman.com

16 Carlisle Street, London W1D 3BT, United Kingdom

British Library Cataloguing in Publication Information Available

Library of Congress Cataloging-in-Publication Data

Ali, Naheed, 1981– author.
Understanding celiac disease : an introduction for patients and caregivers / Naheed Ali.
p. ; cm.
Includes bibliographical references and index.
ISBN 978-1-4422-2655-5 (cloth : alk. paper) — ISBN 978-1-4422-2656-2 (electronic)
I. Title.
[DNLM: 1. Celiac Disease. WD 175]
RC862.C44
616.3'99—dc23
2014016086

♾™ The paper used in this publication meets the minimum requirements of
American National Standard for Information Sciences Permanence of Paper for
Printed Library Materials, ANSI/NISO Z39.48-1992.

Printed in the United States of America

Understanding Celiac Disease is dedicated to my readers, to celiac disease sufferers, and to all who have provided encouragement and support for my research.

CONTENTS

PREFACE

Celiac disease, also known as *gluten-sensitive enteropathy* or *celiac sprue*, is a common disease that occurs in a person's digestive system. Patients with this condition have adverse reactions to foods containing gluten. Gluten is a type of protein found in certain types of cereals such as wheat, rye, and barley. It also can be found in foods such as bread, pasta, and biscuits. In the case of celiac disease, the immune system of the body treats one of the substances that makes gluten, *gliadin*, as a threat and responds negatively to it. The immune system produces antibodies to fight off the supposedly harmful substance.

These antibodies can cause the surface of the intestine to become inflamed, disrupting the ability of the celiac disease patient's body to absorb the nutrient from the food, leading to malnourishment in people suffering from celiac disease. If the disease happens to an infant or toddler, it will make them fail to thrive in terms of weight and height. One in every 100–200 people in the United States has this disease, while in the United Kingdom it affects one out of every 100 individuals. [1] The number might be higher because some milder cases may go undiagnosed or misdiagnosed and treated as other disorders. The disease may affect people at any age. Women are two to three times more susceptible to celiac disease than men from all the cases that were reported. [2]

The symptoms have a high probability of taking place during early childhood—between eight and twelve months of age—and usually it takes several months before a correct diagnosis is made. [3] Before going further, the reader should understand that there is no exact science as to the specific conditions that can lead to celiac disease. The risk is approximately 10 percent with family history, compared to 1 percent in those without any close relative who has this disease.[4] In identical twins, the risk can be up to 85 percent if the other twin is also a celiac disease patient.[5]

READING THIS BOOK

One reason to read about celiac disease is to learn about who the most commonly targeted people to have this disorder are. The history, anatomy, physiology, and disorders associated with the disease will be covered. Moreover, there are several works of research concerning the causes or reasons and the diagnoses needed to heal the effects of celiac disease. Reading *Understanding Celiac Disease* will lead to the proper management of the symptoms, both naturally and conventionally, as well as how to promote intestinal healing. Moreover, this writing uses several evidence-based sources, such as journals and medical books that tackle the topic. Advanced research and medical studies have been performed around the world, as this particular disease is affecting an increasing number of populations.[6]

As the saying goes, "You are what you eat, or at least what you take in; you are basically what lives inside of you." This adage pertains to both mental and physical aspects, and while a distinctive feature of *Understanding Celiac Disease* is a hearty chapter devoted to the often-overlooked psychological side, the book intends to emphasize a well-rounded understanding of celiac disease as a whole.

SIGNIFICANCE OF A COMPREHENSIVE REVIEW

Given that celiac disease, or "coeliac disease," can lead to malnutrition and several organ malfunctions, knowing about the disease comprehensively is still the best measure for having a healthy lifestyle. A person reported to have acquired the disease could have a mental breakdown, thus having a difficult time with acceptance if they do not know how to thoroughly deal with the problem or know whether it is already in its late stages. It is very important to be knowledgeable about a disease to avoid further issues that will occur in response to having it. People with celiac disease, for instance, need to be able to cope with and adapt to a newly prescribed antigluten diet.

In due time, the management of celiac disease will get easier, especially with a deeper understanding of the gluten-free diet and gastrointestinal systems. Most doctors and psychologists can help patients gain insights on how to improve their health, and comprehensive information about celiac disease certainly helps that whole process. Forums and other support outlets can give celiac disease patients the ability to gain confidence and possibly learn some coping strategies or techniques from other sufferers, dietitians, and other clutches of professionals around the world. Simply put, a comprehensive review of the disorder better prepares the patient for all sorts of support groups.

As the reader may already know, just about every epidemic has been researched by professionals in the medical field; some require decades of research before medical authorities come up with solid conclusions. These are the same individuals who have found treatments and cures for so many other serious disorders. Therefore, all readers, regardless of whether they have absorbed information on celiac disease comprehensively, who believe they are suffering from the disease are highly encouraged to go to their doctor for an examination.

As I compiled the information presented in *Understanding Celiac Disease*, I looked to expand the scope of my own knowledge about the disease, and I later decided to put into writing every bit of reliable information to offer readers a firsthand feel of what it is like to be a celiac disease patient or caregiver. It has been a long road for medical institutions to do research and finally come up with feasible methods that would help long-term sufferers to finally ease all the pain and *still* be confident enough to enjoy the rest of their lives as they battle celiac disease.

Part I

Groundwork

I

HISTORY OF CELIAC DISEASE

An extensive look into the history of celiac disease requires one to consider the history of digestive system disorders in general. There have been drastic changes in medical technology for the past few years, and in desiring to find effective diagnosis and treatment of digestive disorders, many patients' lives were saved and their overall health improved.

HISTORY OF DIGESTIVE DISORDERS

Some may be wondering how early humans survived stomach flu, constipation, and diarrhea, as well as how forms of treatment evolved from the past millennia until today. It is fascinating that ancient peoples such as the Egyptians, Romans, and Babylonians had their own methods of dealing with digestive problems. Since formal caregivers such as physicians were not too common "back in the old days," and families had to travel great distances to see one, the Chinese and the Indians relied on herbal remedies to cure digestive disorders. Manuals containing careful descriptions of diseases were even available for common households so they could diagnose the ailment and treat it without the presence of a doctor.[1] This made it easier (if not bearable) for them to deal with different diseases such as those of the digestive organs, and to alleviate pain immediately.

References tracing back to as far as the reign of the ancient Egyptians point to the digestive system and the common ailments connected to it. Numerous ancient Egyptian papyri discovered during archaeological excavations contain references to how practicing physicians back then demonstrated significant knowledge in treating *peptic* ailments with the use of herbs and oils. One of the early discoveries that helped in the identification and treatment of today's common digestive disorders is that of Claudius Galen, who lived circa 130–200 AD. His time was after that of Hippocrates and ancient Greek doctors, whose teachings he studied carefully and understood. He was then able to come up with the theory that the human stomach is an independent structure in the body—in fact, he even believed that it almost had a brain of its own. Even his conclusion that the stomach has four faculties was widely accepted by medical doctors until the early seventeenth century.[2]

It was in 1780 when Lazzaro Spallanzani, an Italian physician, conducted different experiments to understand the role of gastric juice in the digestive system and how it breaks down food.[3] This was followed by the development of the *lichtleiter* in the early 1800s by Philipp Bozzini, which was then used for examining the rectum, urinary tract, and the pharynx.[4] In short, this was the period when endoscopy was first practiced.[5]

Who could even believe that swords would be a stepping-stone in the medical breakthroughs of digestive disorders? Adolf Kussmaul, a German physician, was able to develop a diagnostic process for digestive disorders in 1868 with the help of a sword swallower.[6] In the early 1970s, Hiromi Shinya was the first general surgeon to present a report on the colonoscopy procedure to an audience of the New York Surgical Society. The following year, he delivered the same report to the American Society for Gastrointestinal Endoscopy (ASGE). Through this, more medical professionals gained additional knowledge on digestive disorders, as well as how such procedures can help in treating affected patients.[7]

HISTORY OF AUTOIMMUNE DISORDERS

Celiac disease is an autoimmune disorder, among other medical maladies. Consideration of the autoimmune system of the human body failed to arrive until 1900, when Paul Ehrlich formulated the doctrine of horror autotoxicus,[8] which was then interpreted and understood as if autoimmunity did not exist and cannot happen. Four years after the doctrine was published, a description on *autohemolysin*'s antibody nature, which is responsible for the development of *cold hemoglobinuria*, came about and was confirmed the same year. Despite its confirmation, there were neither claims nor proof pointing to autoimmunization as one of the causes of the disease, due in part to the influence of Ehrlich's theories, and also because there were no advances in understanding immunology or how the body responds to autologous substances. There were countless discoveries relating to kidney, brain, and other diseases that were made from 1915 to 1945, but there were no feasible concepts presented on autoimmunity disorders. However, studies were conducted after World War II that in some way related to proving autoimmunization in the body. This is demonstrated with the introduction of the rheumatoid factor by Eric Waaler and H. M. Rose, Robin Coombs's antiglobulin reaction, and Malcolm Hargraves's lupus erythematosus (LE) cell, to name a few. In the 1960s, resistance to autoimmunization and autoimmune diseases weakened, and more medical journals on the topic were published by 1965.[9]

Digging Deeper

The clinical manifestations of autoimmune disorders have already been known for years, but the knowledge that the immune system is responsible for such was not clearly established until the 1960s. Experimental evidence then became reproducible for confirmation, making it easier for doctors, physicians, and scientists to find ways to defend against the destructive effects of autoimmune diseases. The year 1965 was significant for the immunological industry because the autoantibodies that can fight against diseased organs caused by *Sjögren's syndrome* were then discovered.[10] Using animal models, scientists also discovered the correlation with some types of anemias of antibodies forming against red blood cells.[11] Clinical observations were also conducted in the 1960s to show the connections between autoimmune diseases—namely, hemolytic anemia and viral infections.[12]

A decade later, autoimmune diseases were described in molecular detail to show diagnostic correlations among molecular markers and local inflammation caused by Sjögren's syndrome. This served as a possible diagnosis through identification of specific molecules that cause autoimmune disease development in the body.[13] Theories on the connection between autoimmunity and aging were also discovered, as well as the link of autoimmune heart disease with the α-hemolytic streptococcus.[14] Indeed, the 1970s served as a historical leap for the medical field to further comprehend the root cause of autoimmune disorders and its correlation with specific biological markers.

HISTORY OF CELIAC DISEASE

Before the Iron Age or the Industrial Revolution, humans survived through hunting and gathering food for their groups and families. The usual diet consisted of nuts and fruits, and, if hunting went well, a feast of meat for everyone. Before fire was "discovered," the meat was eaten raw, as, luckily, the early human's digestive system was able to accept and process such. As time went on, they learned to cultivate grains and plants, and pretty soon, the agricultural revolution that is known today began. Their way of life evolved from hunting to the domestication of animals and meat. [15]

Time Line

People used to gather and hunt for food, but as the Neolithic period approached and agricultural development ensued, cultivated grains and wheat then became a part of their everyday diet. This became a problem for the digestive system that had developed and evolved for the past two million years. It was used to taking in and processing antigens included in raw meat and harvested greens. So how did the human gut react to the new antigens introduced together with the new diet? The Neolithic period's agricultural revolution also brought in strange antigens unknown to the human body, such as unwanted proteins from goat's and cow's milk as well as those coming from harvested eggs and grains. While there were individuals who were able to adapt to this new diet, there were also some whose digestive systems were unable to tolerate this newly introduced antigen—hence, the birth of celiac disease.

It was not until after the second century AD that celiac disease was formally named and identified. Aretaeus of Cappadocia wrote *The Co-eliac Affection*. [16] Koiliakos was first termed by Aretaeus as a cause for diarrhea and abdominal pain in patients with celiac problems. During the early nineteenth century, Matthew Baillie published a medical journal on how adults suffered from chronic diarrheal disorder that causes malnutrition and which was often described and characterized by bloating or an abdomen that is gas distended. Baillie even suggested a dietetic treatment and described some patients living entirely on rice. Unfortunately for him, his observations and findings were largely unnoticed, which became an advantage for Samuel Gee, an English doctor who took full credit for the modern medical description of celiac disease, 75 years after Baillie published his journal. The former gave the first lecture on celiac affliction to his medical students, which became a milestone for the diagnosis and treatment of celiac disease today. As with what Dr. Baillie suggested, Gee believed that celiac patients could be cured through therapeutic dieting. He also added that the amount of *farinaceous food* included in the diet should be small. With this, Dr. Gee documented a study on the introduction of a gluten-free diet and a relapse after gluten was reintroduced in the diet. In 1888, Gee published a modern description of koiliakos. He suggested that the condition is initially associated with diet.

During the 1920s, different diets were introduced, which also included pure carbohydrate and all-banana diets to help relieve the painful symptoms brought about by celiac disease.[17] The banana diet was considered an effective therapy against celiac disease back then. Sidney Haas claimed he successfully treated eight children diagnosed with celiac disease through this new nutrition method, which he based on his previous studies treating anorexic patients with bananas. In 1924, he was able to publish ten cases in which eight patients were successfully or clinically cured of celiac disease, while the two patients who did not undergo the banana diet died. The medical world and the public accepted his study with enthusiasm, and the diet enjoyed its share of popularity for decades. The banana diet proved to be beneficial to many celiac children and may even have helped prevent untimely deaths due to the disease. What actually makes this diet effective is its exclusion of crackers, potatoes, bread, and cereals. Basically, its complete elimination of grains containing gluten helped to cure celiac disease in patients.

Despite other well-documented viewpoints, Haas was resistant to them and remained proud of his belief that carbohydrates caused the painful symptoms of the disease. Forty years later, a Dutch pediatrician, Willem Dicke, discovered that wheat protein, and not starch, was the real culprit. Haas remained firm in his banana diet theory and insisted that people can be cured, without relapse, through specific diets. The shortage of bread in the Netherlands during World War II nevertheless proved

Dicke's discovery to be true. The number of children suffering from the disease decreased and only rose when relief soldiers provided bread again. Together with his group, Dicke published a series of medical journals documenting the major role of gluten found in rye and wheat in celiac disease.

In 1940 Dicke recommended wheat-free diets for patients suffering from celiac disease. Due to the bread shortages during World War II, it was discovered that occurrences of celiac disease declined but climbed back when the war was over and when the Allied forces dropped bread from planes for starving populations. In 1952, Dicke, along with his colleagues, studied human waste, and in doing so, they were able to identify gluten as one of the major triggers for the disease. This then started the gluten-free diet as the standard "treatment" for celiac disease.

There was a major breakthrough in celiac disease after World War II. Margot Shiner was successful in reaching the distal duodenum and performing a biopsy in it. The biopsy together with the development of a less bulky capsule allowed doctors to link celiac disease with a recognizable and specific damage pattern to the small intestinal mucosa of the digestive system. Shiner, then a gastroenterologist based in London, developed definitive ways on diagnosing celiac disease in the 1950s. The diagnosis, based on the biopsy on the specific damage pattern to the small intestine's fingerlike *villi*, makes it easier for a physician to identify patients suffering from the disease so that the recommended gluten-free diet can be administered.

Historically, there were three major elements in celiac disease identification and treatment in the 1960s: (1) the knowledge that the major culprit and triggering agent for the disease is gluten; (2) the easily identifiable and remarkable lesion in the proximal small intestinal mucosa; (3) and the availability of the biopsy instrument that can help unravel the ever-enigmatic *pathogenesis* of celiac disease.

By the 1960s, doctors were able to routinely diagnose the disease using a jejunal biopsy instrument that could show the weakening of the villi. Due care, however, was observed, since there could be other causes for the lesion and a celiac disease confirmation could only be given if mucosal deterioration could be specifically pointed out to gluten. The steps for diagnosis included the complete clinical remission after a specific time period of adhering to a gluten-free diet, which was then followed by the proper documentation of lesion normalization, and finally the re-currence of the lesion after gluten was reintroduced into the patient's diet.

The criteria mentioned were then formalized in the late 1960s by the European Society for Pediatric Gastroenterology, Hepatology, and Nutri-tion (ESPGHAN), which consisted of a panel of experts in autoimmune disease. This served as the "Interlaken" criteria, which was globally ac-cepted as the diagnostic standard for celiac disease. Unfortunately, ex-perts were unable to consider a very important discovery on the disease made a number of years prior: that antibodies were present—which ap-parently was due to gluten ingestion—in the blood of children diagnosed with celiac disease. [18]

In the 1980s, pieces of medical evidence proved that celiac disease is also associated with other autoimmune disorders such as diabetes mellit-us, as well as with genetic conditions such as Down syndrome. Decades after its formal discovery, the disease evolved and became less of a diges-tive matter and showed more *extraintestinal* signs and symptoms. In 1989, two versions of the *histocompatibility leukocyte antigen (HLA)* molecule were discovered by Ludvig Sollid's group of immunologists from Oslo. While this molecule was identified as celiac disease's major genetic risk, *transglutaminase*, another molecule (enzyme) that is re-leased by the intestine once gluten passes through the mucosal layer, was determined to be impaired in patients suffering from celiac disease. A doctor from Berlin discovered the enzyme. [19] With it, he was able to find a way to use blood-screening tests for uncovering celiac disease.

During the 1990s, more and more doctors and the medical world in general considered celiac disease as an autoimmune disease. With thorough research and study, it was then discovered that the disease is associated with the DQ2/DQ8 genes, and the enzyme transglutaminase was finally identified as the missing autoantigen. [20]

In 2000, a researcher at the University of Maryland discovered zonu-lin, a molecule that he believed has (1) a potential of increasing the permeability of the intestines, and (2) vulnerability against celiac dis-ease. [21]

In 2010 nondietary therapies were heavily undergoing clinical trials to make the lives of people suffering from celiac disease easier. Instead of undergoing drastic lifestyle and dietary changes, patients would be able to choose therapies proven to reduce the permeability of the intestines, thereby reducing the occurrence of celiac disease among them. [22]

History of the Name

Celiac disease has been around since the agricultural revolution, but no one really knew how to accurately describe or name the said disease. Aretaeus believed that the pain associated with what is today called celiac disease is due to the lack of heat in the patient's abdominal area, which in turn causes disruption in the stomach's digestive enzymes. Since there were no tools for internal observations of the body, Aretaeus was, of course, unaware of the full complexity of the abdomen and the intricacies of the immune system, let alone autoimmune disorders. Interestingly enough, the Greek physician even believed that celiac disease could be blamed on the frequent drinking of cold water.[23]

In 1856, the work of Aretaeus was translated and presented at the Sydenham Society by Francis Adams, which caught the attention of many notable experts in Western medicine. The patient in Aretaeus's work was described as suffering from stomach pain and was incapable of doing his work. Diarrhea was also present, and the disease was said to return periodically and was too stubborn to be cured.[24]

In 1888, pediatrician Samuel Gee gave another modern-day description of the disease. He kept the Greek term *coeliac*, which was coined by Aretaeus—hence the name *celiac disease*. In his study, he claimed that a change in daily diet is the only way to treat the disease, which then seemed prevalent in children. Those who were suffering from celiac disease had a low tolerance for milk and starched foods, which Gee recommended avoiding at all costs.[25]

FAME AND CELIAC DISEASE

Like other digestive disorders, celiac disease does not *choose* its victims, and even celebrities are known to change their diets because of the disease. Listed below are stars and athletes who are known to be coeliacs or are intolerant to gluten.

Drew Brees is a National Football League (NFL) star quarterback whose rise to fame is attributed to his uncanny ability to throw a football more than 5,000 yards in a single season. Despite his energy-demanding sport, all the energy he burns during training and games does not come from gluten (since he suffers from celiac disease), and he experiences gluten intolerance when eating wheat and other grains.[26]

Justin Morneau, the first baseman of the Minnesota Twins, suffered numerous injuries in 2012, including two concussions. To keep himself fit and in good health, he visited different doctors during his off-season in 2012. That was when he found out about his gluten allergy, and, in fact, his condition may be the leading cause of his game injuries. When he ingests gluten, he develops tissue and intestinal inflammation, which the body prioritizes to fight off rather than the injury-induced inflammation.[27]

Chelsea Clinton, former U.S. president Bill Clinton's daughter, follows and enjoys a strict vegetarian diet due to gluten allergy issues. Her New York wedding was catered with gluten-free and vegetarian foods so she would not have to suffer from the negative, if not painful, side effects of gluten consumption.[28]

Zooey Deschanel, who played the female protagonist in *(500) Days of Summer* and is now known for her role in *New Girl*, is an active promoter of the gluten-free diet due to her sensitivity to the substance. She has appeared in different cooking shows to share gluten-free recipes with other celiac disease patients to enjoy as well.[29]

Novak Djokovic is a renowned tennis player who practices a gluten-free diet because of his intolerance to the substance. The famous tennis player even claims that doing so has helped him improve his game since there are no longer serious symptoms associated with gluten. Apparently this even led to his winning streak against fellow tennis megastar Rafael Nadal in 2011.[30]

Jessica Simpson has problems with digesting wheat products. Before she discovered her allergic reaction to gluten, she suffered bouts of ulcers due to the severe inflammation in her intestines and stomach when trying to digest wheat products. Apparently her gluten-free diet has helped her maintain a superfit body after childbirth.[31]

Unlike other bodybuilders, *Ryan Phillippe* refuses to rely on carbohydrates to "bulk up." He has appeared on the front cover of *Men's Health* magazine and has shared his diet secrets on maintaining physical fitness. Despite his gluten allergy, he has managed to change his eating habits to those that still allow him to hold on to great health.[32]

Rachel Weisz is a famous actress who has appeared in many films, including *The Mummy* and *Constantine*, as the wife of an archaeologist and a detective, respectively. The actress suffers from intolerance to gluten found in wheat and grains, and in order to avoid digestive issues and painful stomach inflammation, she avoids wheat products at all costs.[33]

Keith Olbermann is currently a sports broadcaster and has been diagnosed with celiac disease. He completely avoids gluten-containing products because of this. He considers gluten poison and advises other celiac disease sufferers to be aware and well informed of the effects and dangers caused by gluten consumption.[34]

Cedric Benson is an NFL running back who was diagnosed with celiac disease. This has pushed him to have a lifestyle change and follow a gluten-free diet. Instead of seeing his diagnosis as a cause of failure, he used it to change his attitude toward life and to improve his performance on the field.[35]

Elisabeth Hasselbeck shared how she has accepted and consistently deals with celiac disease as part of her daily life. The former *View* star offers tips on avoiding the negative allergic reactions caused by gluten-containing substances. She helps other celiac disease sufferers by providing gluten-free recipes and discussing how they can enjoy the diet despite the drastic change in lifestyle that the disease causes them. Hasselbeck cited her condition on the show every now and then, and she proved to others that living without gluten is possible and even easy.[36]

ANALYSIS

The majority of today's known digestive disorders such as celiac disease are not new, and in fact, their history and roots can be traced back to ancient civilization. With the basic understanding of how medicines historically were administered to alleviate pain, ancient doctors treated their patients regardless of the limited understanding of the human body and its digestive tract in particular.

2

ANATOMY AND PHYSIOLOGY
OF CELIAC DISEASE

When people with celiac disease ingest gluten, their immune system responds in a way that impairs the villi of the small intestine.[1] Villi are tiny, fingerlike projections involved in the absorption of nutrients from food into the bloodstream. This trauma to the gastrointestinal tract results in a number of complications to major organ systems, and failure of patients to strictly observe a gluten-free diet may lead to serious health conditions such as osteoporosis, anemia, cancer, or even death.[2]

AFFECTED STRUCTURES

Main Target

Celiac disease primarily targets the *gastrointestinal tract*, and to better understand this sometimes-genetic disease, it is useful to be able to grasp how food absorption takes place in the body as well as the essential organs and structures involved in its fundamental process. The digestive organs are divided into the upper and lower gastrointestinal tract. The human gastrointestinal tract commonly only refers to its two major organs, which are the stomach and the intestines. However, in some cases it can refer to all structures involved in food processing, starting from the mouth all the way to the anus.[3] Anatomically, the upper gastrointestinal tract comprises the stomach, esophagus, and duodenum while the lower gastrointestinal tract consists of most of the small intestine and all of the large intestine.

WHERE DIGESTION REALLY TAKES PLACE

Upon the ingestion of food, mechanical digestion begins in the mouth through the grinding and chewing of the teeth, a process clinically termed *mastication*. This mechanical digestion is continued through the esophagus and in the stomach through its churning. Chemical digestion, meanwhile, also starts alongside mechanical digestion in the mouth through the release of enzymes in the saliva. Chemical digestion continues in the stomach and all throughout the small and large intestines. While food is in the mouth, swallowing propels the chewed food into the pharynx (throat) of the patient through the voluntary action of the muscles located in the tongue. The pharynx is the passageway for both food and air. It is about 12.5 centimeters long, and a small flap called the epiglottis, which closes over the pharynx, prevents the entry of food into the passageway toward the lungs.[4] Choking happens when food accidentally enters the trachea and blocks the airway.

From the pharynx, food is transported through a long, muscular tube called the esophagus. The esophagus connects the pharynx to the stomach and channels the food by way of peristalsis, which is the involuntary propulsion of the food inside the alimentary digestive canal through the repetitive motions of contraction and relaxation of the muscles lining the organ. Upon reaching the stomach, more of the mechanical and chemical digestion takes place. The stomach is the main "food tank" of the human body and is an integral portion of the digestive tract. It is a muscular, rounded, hollow organ located between the esophagus and the duodenum. The internal lining of the stomach is covered with inner foldings called *rugae*, or gastric folds, that account for the elastic property of the stomach, allowing it to carry greater volumes of food and also to help hold and move the food at the same time. Food is mechanically digested in the stomach through the mixing contractions of its walls.

Leaving the stomach, the churned food exits as a thick liquid called *chyme*, and enters the small intestine, where absorption takes place.[5] The small intestine is divided into three parts—duodenum, jejunum, and the ileum—and each makes its own unique contribution to the digestion of ingested food. The duodenum, which marks the end of the upper gastrointestinal tract, is around 25 centimeters long and five centimeters in diameter.[6] This is a C-shaped structure in which the digestive enzymes from the pancreas and the bile from the gallbladder are mixed together to break down major macronutrients of the food. Specifically, pancreatic juices have enzymes that break down proteins while the bile from the gallbladder begins the digestion of fats through a process called *emulsification*. The duodenum also performs a crucial role in maintaining the acidity of the stomach by secreting *bicarbonates* that neutralize its hydrochloric acid.

LOWER GASTROINTESTINAL TRACT

The second part of the small intestine, the jejunum, is where the lower gastrointestinal tract anatomically begins. This is the middle of the small intestine, where the major absorption of nutrients from food takes place. The jejunum has an extensive surface area due to its plicae circulares and *villi*. Plicae circulares, or circular folds, are large flaps projecting along the inside walls of the intestines. These folds delay the migration of the food and allow for better absorption of nutrients. On the other hand, villi are tiny projections from the inner linings of the celiac disease patient's entire small intestine. These structures are highly vascular, allowing the easy transport of digested nutrients from the food into the bloodstream of the celiac disease patient.[7]

The ileum is the last portion of the small intestine, and it connects it to the large intestine. This portion also has intestinal villi, where all soluble molecules are absorbed and carried into the bloodstream through capillaries located within the intestinal walls. In the large intestine, reabsorption of some minerals and especially water takes place. It is also in this large organ that unwanted parts of processed food are formed. The large intestine prepares the waste to be excreted from the body.

PHYSIOLOGICAL OVERVIEW
OF A HEALTHY DIGESTIVE SYSTEM

Key to Wellness

Healthy digestion is not a conspicuous process, and people are rarely concerned with their digestive system unless it starts malfunctioning. In fact, celiac disease sufferers oftentimes only become conscious of digestion when they start feeling the signs of unhealthy digestion such as discomfort, gastric pains, or excessive gastric gases.

Physiologically, digestion is performed by the body's system of organs on the ingested food, from which the nutrients are extracted before the residual waste is excreted from the body. This is not the only essential function of the digestive system. Equally important is its indirect role in defending the body from pathogens such as bacteria, virus, parasites, and fungi. As one will learn from the upcoming chapters, immune defense is important in the fight against celiac disease. [8]

The digestive system plays an important role in the entire body's well-being in general. A little problem with the digestive system at times may only affect the digestive system locally, but most of the time even a minute impairment of this system may start a chain of other diseases, such as celiac disease, and ultimately place the entire body at risk of a very serious ailment. Digestion is a vital process in that the most favorable performance of the organs depends on its proper execution. All the other systems of a celiac disease sufferer's body highly depend on the nutrients processed by the digestive system from the food consumed. For instance, the respiratory, circulatory, nervous, skeletal, endocrine, immune, lymphatic, reproductive, and urinary systems all require minerals and elements taken in by digestion that are used for its specific processes. The digestive system is an essential physiological "machine" that supplements the requirements of other systems, and the failure of this system to operate properly would definitely make it difficult for the organs to function at prime levels.

Managing Food Intake

Being careful with one's food intake is the best way to maintain and promote a healthy digestive system. However, this simple option is easily challenged by the number of processed foods available in the market. These foods are high in preservatives, rich in carcinogens, and packed with refined sugars, harmful fats, and other contents. This has been the most popular option for consumers nowadays due to the convenience these foods offer. Nevertheless, there are healthier alternatives, and though these foods require relatively more time to prepare, the benefits of choosing to eat healthy reward the celiac disease sufferer with ideal physiology.

Consequences of Taking Digestive Health for Granted

The digestive system (specifically, the small intestines) is where approximately 1,000 microorganisms responsible for aiding the immune system are localized.[9] "Good" bacteria have been seen to have a direct impact on the promotion of favorable metabolism of dietary components in the gastrointestinal tract.[10] These good bacteria aid in the metabolic processes by (1) assisting in the passive adhesion of substrates for proper absorption, (2) contributing to the number of enzymes used for digestion, and (3) helping in breaking down macromolecules such as lipids, lactose, carbohydrates, protein, and even ammonia.[11]

Without the aid of these microorganisms, immunity is greatly weakened, and this leaves the entire body highly susceptible and vulnerable to a wide range of diseases such as chronic inflammation, overfatigue, celiac disease, cancer, arthritis, poor skin and hair quality, allergies, premature aging, heart ailments, and other health issues.[12] These diseases are often in part due to faulty digestion (like that seen with celiac disease), which results in weakened (1) immune function, (2) nutrient breakdown processes, (3) absorption, and (4) metabolism, as well as accumulation of toxins in the body.[13] Optimum physiology of the immune system is highly dependent on the condition of the digestive system in that a decent intake of both vitamins and trace minerals and elements is required.[14] It is the immune system that protects the body from diseases, and a compromised immune system could result in serious infections and disease outbreaks. This problem can be a result of an improperly maintained digestive system.

Physiological Link between the Immune System and Digestion

The digestive system and the immune system are closely linked in such a way that a slight malfunction of one greatly affects the function of the other. Eighty percent of the immune system is located in the digestive tract, and this suggests that the immune system places good digestion at a higher priority than the body's overall immunity.[15] Therefore, a tiny effort to promote or maintain a healthy digestive system is a giant step toward boosting the immune system.

The presence of good bacteria in the intestinal tract is elemental to the efforts of the immune system in protecting the body from diseases. These good bacteria are termed the intestinal microflora. The intestinal microflora fight the harmful bacteria, termed bad bacteria, and keep it from multiplying in the intestinal tract. Also, the intestinal microflora double as a shield along the linings of the intestinal tract by creating a barrier on the intestinal wall so that these harmful bacteria cannot access the bloodstream and the other vital organs of the celiac disease patient's body.[16] To be able to grasp the importance of how closely the immune system depends on the health of the digestive system, professional caregivers will easily reach the conclusion that keeping a healthy digestive system is among the best steps to promoting overall wellness.

PHYSIOLOGY OF DIGESTION

The entire process of digestion is basically a systematic and intricate interplay of its main characters: the enzymes, the stomach acid, and the intestinal microflora. Each component plays a significant role in the digestion of food. Each prepares the ingested food for the next process, which the next component is subsequently able to perform better with the aid of the previous component. Malfunctioning or failure of a single component to deliver its optimum performance for food digestion leaves the other components compromised in executing their functions, and thus as a whole they disable the entire digestive mechanism. Having celiac disease does not make matters any better. Each component, therefore, contributes its role to the common goal of promoting a healthy and well-balanced body.[17]

Roles of Enzymes in Digestion

Digestive enzymes function in the initial digestion of food by breaking down protein, carbohydrates, and fats into smaller and smaller components. These enzymes enhance the degree of digestion primarily in the stomach. Enzymes make sure that most of the ingested food is broken down to a considerable degree so that less undigested food is subsequently transported into the intestines for nutrient absorption. Some of the most common digestive enzymes are the proteases, lipases, and carbohydrases. Proteases are responsible for the breakdown of protein, a common nutrient found in meats, nuts, cheese, and grains. Lipases break down fats that are found in oils, butter, meat, and dairy, to name a few. Carbohydrates break down starches, polysaccharides, sugars, and fiber, which can be introduced into the body through the consumption of fruits, vegetables, bread, and grains.[18]

There are two main physiological sources for enzymes: the food one eats, and the digestive enzymes that the body naturally produces.[19] Raw food is purportedly rich in the necessary enzymes for proper digestion. Plants, for instance, contain many enzymes that are naturally used by the human body for digestion. Cooking, processing, and other food-preparation techniques destroy these temperature- and pH-sensitive enzymes. The best way to preserve the enzyme content of the food is to serve and eat it raw. The consequence of inadequate enzymes to be able to fill the requirements for favorable enzymatic digestion requires more of the gastric acid of the stomach to digest more of the food. This is one way in which the celiac disease patient becomes healthier directly from a physiological standpoint.

Another consequence of insufficient digestive enzymes is reduced immunity, which can effect the prognosis of a celiac disease case. When enzymes used for digestion are not sufficient to execute proper digestion, the body automatically allocates other enzymes of the body to be able to meet the demands for the digestion. This reallocation of other enzymes lessens the body's immune enzymes intended for disease prevention and protection, weakening the body's defenses and making it more vulnerable to illness.[20]

These impairments can be minimized or avoided by increasing enzyme intake through eating food naturally rich in enzymes or by taking enzyme supplements. Increasing enzyme intake helps digestion by balancing the enzymes lost or reallocated and by relieving the digestive and immune system from the stress it was subjected to. These digestive enzyme supplements help to facilitate proper nutrient absorption into the blood and throughout the body.

Role of Stomach Acids in Digestion

A highly acidic stomach is indicative of a strong and healthy digestive tract.[21] As one ages, stomach acid tends to decrease, which results in more frequent indigestion.[22] Hydrochloric acid is the primary digestive acid of the stomach. This acid chiefly functions in ensuring that the food ingested by the body is free from harmful bacteria and cleanses it from pathogens before being transported into the gastrointestinal tract. Hydrochloric acid (HCl) also initiates protein digestion by triggering the release of the enzyme pepsin and regulates pH in the blood by promoting the production of alkaline bicarbonate.[23] Contrary to common belief, an increase of hydrochloric acid in the stomach does not cause acid reflux in the digestive tract. It is in fact the complete opposite that causes this condition.[24]

Hydrochloric acid is also highly important in the proper absorption of necessary minerals such as magnesium, chromium, copper, iron, manganese, magnesium, molybdenum, selenium, and zinc.[25] This indicates the importance of HCl in the use of various highly important minerals and nutrients. Strong stomach acid allows for the easy breakdown of food, provides a means for freeing the body from impurities or waste by-products, and eliminates harmful pathogens in the stomach such as bacteria, viruses, parasites, or fungi. When the celiac disease patient's body experiences a deficiency in stomach acidity, a number of diseases are bound to be expected, such as acid reflux, diarrhea, irritable bowel syndrome, constipation, eczema, hives, allergies, malabsorption, and gut infections.

Role of Intestinal Microbes in Digestion

The final step of digestion takes place in the intestines, where the crucial process of absorption is undergone. This is an important physiological concept to grasp since celiac disease primarily affects the abdominal organs. The natural microorganisms located in this long organ, sometimes referred to as the intestinal microflora, perform the terminal stage of converting the churned and liquefied food into absorbable nutrients or macromolecules. This process not only allows the nutrients to be ultimately transported into the celiac disease sufferer's bloodstream but also, most importantly during the course of the conversion, allows for the creation of by-products necessary for proper physiological function.[26]

There are two major types of beneficial bacteria in the intestinal tract. The first is the *lactobacillus acidophilus*, found primarily in the small intestine, and the second is the *bifidobacterium*, mostly located in the colon.[27] Both contribute to overall wellness and improved immunity differently. Lactobacillus acidophilus prevents the excessive multiplication of opportunistic pathogens such as *candida sp.*, *E. coli*, *H. pylori*, and *salmonella*.[28] It also aids in lactose digestion, nutrient absorption, the maintenance of the integrity of macromolecule absorption, lessening food poisoning occurrence, acidifying the intestinal tract, and preventing excretory infections.[29]

Bifidobacteria, on the other hand, contribute to a number of benefits, such as the inhibition of toxin-producing bacteria in the colon; the production of B-complex vitamins; the regulation of peristalsis and bowel movements; the manufacture of antibiotics, antifungals, and essential fatty acids; protecting against toxins and poisons; and the breaking down of bile acids, to name a few.[30]

These good bacteria are so important that the entire person's normal function would cease without them. Probiotics are naturally present at birth as microflora of the gut and are health boosters of the human body. They have been long studied to help promote proper growth of the beneficial microflora of the intestinal tract. These have been suggested and recommended for maintaining natural, beneficial bacteria populations in the intestinal tract and have been seen as a great avenue toward sustaining overall well-being by way of a healthy colon.[31]

PHYSIOLOGICAL DETAILS OF CELIAC DISEASE

Celiac disease is an autoimmune disease caused by the intake of the storage protein gluten. Autoimmune reactions occur when the immune system acts against substances locally present in the body, thereby attacking itself due to a false trigger that alerts its defenses against its own system.[32] Autoimmunity is a physiological process and only becomes harmful when the number of triggered reactive cells, particularly those receptive for autoantigens, is alarmingly high.[33] This typically exhibits diarrhea in patients suffering from the disease, but the manifestations have become varied, so that the only means to know for certain that celiac disease is present is through the biopsy of the small intestine.[34]

AN AUTOIMMUNE DISEASE

Not an Allergy

A common misconception associated with celiac disease is that it is an allergy to foods containing gluten. However, celiac disease is an autoimmune disease that is different from an allergy. The mechanism behind the autoimmune response of celiac patients to gluten is slightly dissimilar to the autoimmune response during an allergic reaction. Allergens, when brought into contact with a susceptible target, are typically responded to by an IgE-mediated response. Immunoglobin E (IgE) is an autoimmune antibody of mammals primarily functioning for immunity to pathogens such as parasites and involved in hypersensitivity reactions.[35] However, autoimmunity in celiac disease triggered by gluten involves the production of IgA and IgG by plasma cells of the immune system. This pathway of the immune response of celiac disease to gluten does not or seldom involves major participation of the IgE associated with an allergy.[36]

IgA and IgG are autoantibodies to *tissue transglutaminase (TTG)* produced by the plasma cells in response to the detection of antigens and are directed to attract inflammatory T-cells.[37] Celiac patients have IgA freely circulating in their bloodstream. These IgA antibodies attack the endomysium, which is the connective tissue in muscles, or the reticulin, which is composed of the fragile, extracellular fibrils.[38] Localizing this inflammatory response causes the flattening of villi and their eventual damaging, rendering them useless for effective nutrient absorption. Abnormal absorption of micronutrients and macromolecules leads to the diseases and disorders associated with celiac disease patients.

Microvilli of the Small Intestine

The physiological mechanisms that turn rogue and lead to the degenerative destruction of an individual positive with celiac disease are purportedly many, but most sources are conclusive that the site primarily targeted for damage is the intestinal villi. Celiac disease directly damages the mucous-secreting membranes lining the small intestine. Chronic inflammation can be observed in the mucosa, and this in turn causes cell death to the villi lining the small intestine. [39]

ANALYSIS

Celiac disease presents a serious case caused by genetic defect and induced by an environmental factor. From an anatomical standpoint, patients and caregivers should realize that the microvilli are damaged through autoimmune response to the macroprotein known as gluten. Physiologically, inflammation of the microvilli complicates the digestive system function and results in a number of other associated diseases, making it something of a life-changing disorder.

3

CAUSES OF CELIAC DISEASE

Ten thousand years ago, the protein gluten may not have been present in the human diet, and it was eight thousand years after the introduction of gluten before celiac disease officially surfaced.[1] Above all else, celiac disease is the condition in which the body's immune system mistakes substances or tissues typically present in the body for a foreign invader and fights against it. In a healthy person, the immune system will be able to differentiate between something usually found within the body and a foreign entity that can cause harm. When a person suffering from celiac disease ingests gluten, their immune system inappropriately creates antibodies, damaging or completely destroying villi.[2]

Gliadin is in fact a substance that can be found in wheat, barley, and rye that causes digestive problems for people with celiac disease. Other grains contain gluten as well, but they do not necessarily contain gliadin. That is why grains such as oats, flax, rice, wild rice, quinoa, flaxseeds, buckwheat, kasha, arrowroot, bean, lentil, maize corn, chickpea, millet, montina, almonds, sesame, sago soy, and amaranth, among others, are relatively safe for people with celiac disease to consume.[3]

Although celiac disease can affect people of all ages, genders, and ethnicities, it is most commonly contracted hereditarily.[4] First-degree relatives (parents, children, or siblings) of diagnosed patients have higher chances of inheriting this disease. The disease can remain unrecognized for years, and symptoms may surface at any age, some even starting from birth.[5]

LIFESTYLE IN CONNECTION TO CELIAC DISEASE

There are various lifestyle factors that affect the onset of symptoms, thus determining the extent of damage done by this disease. These lifestyle factors also pave the path to identifying the most effective methods for keeping the disease under control. For example, the later this disease is diagnosed in a person, the larger the effect might be in the small intestine. The greater the damage in the small intestine, the higher the chances of celiac disease starting a chain reaction of short-term or long-term complications that one may or may not notice.

Symptoms of celiac disease are as varied as the people they affect. People face different symptoms, depending on the lifestyle they lead. The main lifestyle factors affecting the onset of celiac disease include (1) how long a person has been consuming food containing gluten, and (2) how much gluten he or she is ingesting through food or other sources. [6]

Celiac disease can easily affect people who suffer from the following:

Type 1 diabetes

Neurological disorders such as epilepsy [7]

Hashimoto's disease [8]

Dermatitis herpetiformis [9]

Down syndrome

ADHD

Turner syndrome

Depression

Autoimmune thyroid disease

Migraine

Autoimmune liver disease

Irritability

Rheumatoid arthritis

Fatigue

Sjögren's syndrome

Anemia [10]

Addison's disease

Obesity [11]

Microscopic colitis [12]

Lactose intolerance [13]

Ulcerative colitis

The modern lifestyle and eating habits play a big role in the contraction of celiac disease. The fast and stressful nature of a busy life leads to a lot of clinical disorders these days, especially obesity, anxiety, depression, irritability, fatigue, migraine, and diabetes. Many prefer ready-to-eat meals and fast food for the sake of convenience. It is common knowledge that these foods are high in fat content and that this is also a factor that contributes to obesity. Along with obesity come various illnesses, but celiac disease is one such illness that has gone unnoticed for a long time.

One of the most overlooked factors is the exposure to hidden sources of gluten in daily life. These include medications, vitamin supplements, and cosmetic items such as lip balms.[14] The abovementioned nongluten-related health problems as well as food allergies or intolerances can also lead to the onset of celiac disease. Many medications that are prescribed for these conditions contain inactive ingredients known as fillers. These fillers act as lubricants and also absorb water, causing tablets to swell and then disintegrate, and also shape and give bulk to pills. Fillers, which are commonly made from starches extracted from corn, potatoes, rice, tapioca, or wheat, are also thought to be the primary source of possible gluten contamination in medications. Pharmaceutical companies are not required to specify the origins or the ingredients used to manufacture these fillers on the label, which is why this issue goes unnoticed and leads to the unintentional consumption of gluten. Medications with the following ingredients are safe for people with celiac disease: cellulose, dextrans, dextrose, glycerin, lactose, purified alcohol, stearates, and sucrose.[15]

A relatively large percentage of people diagnosed with celiac disease also display symptoms of and are diagnosed with lactose intolerance. Lactose intolerance can show up before or after being diagnosed with celiac disease. It can also develop after a patient starts following a gluten-free diet, and it may last either for a short period of time or permanently.[16] Lactase enzymes are necessary to break down lactose, also known as milk sugar and commonly found in dairy products. These enzymes are uniquely generated on the tips of the villi that line the intestinal tract. Once these villi are damaged, like those of a person suffering from celiac disease, the tips are the first to disappear and the last to heal and regenerate when the patient starts following a gluten-free diet. Depending on the extent of the damage in the intestine, there is no guarantee that the villi will fully regenerate. As such, it is understandable why a person with celiac disease is prone to lactose intolerance.[17] Ultimately, all the lifestyle factors mentioned above work both ways, since these illnesses lead to celiac disease, while celiac disease in turn also leads to illnesses.[18]

It was also found that a vitamin A derivative called retinoic acid, which is an element in some acne treatments, may also be responsible for causing celiac disease to a certain extent. Scientists quietly discourage vitamin A and retinoids for celiac disease patients because the vitamin A derivative seemingly fuels interleukin-15 (IL-15). Blocking of IL-15 would make retinoic acid harmless.[19]

CULTURAL FACTORS OF CELIAC DISEASE

Celiac disease most commonly affects people with Northern European ancestry. As such, it is prevalent among Caucasians in countries such as Australia, Ireland, Canada, Mexico, and Central and South America, and it is most widespread in Finland.[20] However, epidemiological studies conducted recently in North Africa, the Middle East, and Asia, where celiac disease was traditionally considered rare, revealed that the disease was underdiagnosed in these countries as well.[21] The world's population overall is underinformed about celiac disease. Too many general practitioners are unaware that such a disease exists.[22] This is because there is very little effort being taken to educate the public and to raise awareness about the true cause of this disease. There is also very little research being published in medical journals with regard to celiac disease.[23] Comparatively, countries such as Australia, Italy, and Ireland are six to eight times more informed about celiac disease than the United States. As such, almost 30–40 percent of patients are diagnosed with celiac disease in these countries, while less than 5 percent are diagnosed in America.[24]

What leads to this is the fact that in America, pharmaceutical companies are the major stakeholders in medical research, providing about 80 percent of the financing required for research and development of medicines as well as for postgraduate education. In other countries, these works of research and education are funded mostly by the government.[25]

Since there are no absolute medicinal methods to overcome celiac disease, pharmaceutical companies have very little or no chance at all to profit from encouraging research into causes of the disease. The culture of giving more priority to monetary gains and pharmaceutical interventions for illnesses instead of lifestyle counseling results in little or no motivation for people to take responsibility for their well-being.[26]

GENETIC FACTORS OF CELIAC DISEASE

Celiac disease is the most common genetically transferred disease, and first-degree relatives have the highest chance of inheriting it.[27] Statistics show that 3–6 percent of people in this category and about 2–4 percent of people with second-degree relatives (grandparent, aunt, uncle, or cousin) who have celiac disease or any of the diseases related to celiac disease may have it.[28] It is also frequently possible for patients with other genetic disorders such as Down syndrome and Turner syndrome to have celiac disease.[29]

Having a family member with another autoimmune disease increases the risk of another member having the genes responsible for celiac disease. In the case of twins, identical twins have a higher likelihood of sharing the genes for celiac disease as compared to fraternal twins.[30] Several diseases are brought about by the presence of an arrangement of genes that are either distinguished and strong or repetitive. However, the causative genes responsible for the occurrence of celiac disease are much more complicated. The major culprits, believed to play the most critical role in causing celiac disease, are class II human leukocyte antigens, also known as HLA-DQ2 and DQ8, where HLA refers to indicators found on white blood cells.[31] HLA-DQ2 is prevalent in Western Europe and Central Asia as well as Northern and Western Africa. The gene is present not only in patients with celiac disease but also in patients with other autoimmune diseases, such as Type 1 diabetes.[32] If one tests positive for HLA-DQ2, he or she could likely, though not certainly, fall prey to celiac disease.[33]

As genes are passed down through families, some celiac disease patients prefer to have their children genetically tested for the gene in order to avoid a later lab test to see whether genetics is in fact the cause of the disorder. One must, however, take note that this test will not confirm the presence of active celiac disease or silent celiac disease, for there still are many other causes for the disease to investigate.[34]

IMMUNOLOGICAL CONTRIBUTORS

As an autoimmune disorder, celiac disease is dependent not only upon genetic factors but also upon immunological contributors as well. In the presence of an accommodating genetic background, digesting gluten-rich products such as wheat, rye, and barley can expose the digestive tract to certain *immunoreactive epitopes*.[35] Exposure to these epitopes, coupled with the genetic contributors, can instigate certain maladaptive immune responses. Instead of completely digesting the food taken in, some products are presumed to remain undigested in the small intestine, thereby helping or aiding in the activation of the so-called T-cells that are present in the mucosa.[36] Derivatives of gluten, particularly those that have an affinity for binding to either DQ8 or DQ2, may cause the activation of the CD4+ T-cells that may, in turn, create a response that will target multiple endogenous autoantigens.[37]

Various reports show that there are a variety of different immune mediators that contribute to celiac disease. These immune mediators include plasma cells, macrophages, and even *natural killer cells*.[38] They also include CD8+ cytotoxic T-cells and CD4+ helper cells.[39] It must be noted, however, that celiac disease is still the subject of many different works of research and, thus, there has yet to be an agreement on the effect of antigen exposure on people afflicted with celiac disease. What can be gleaned from the wide array of works of research, conflicting as they sometimes tend to be, is that antibodies notably contribute to both the diagnosis of celiac disease and the monitoring of the response to celiac disease treatments.

Gluten: The Real Trigger for Celiac Disease

What makes celiac disease unique as an autoimmune disease is that gluten has been well defined as an official trigger. Gluten, which is a major culprit for celiac disease patients, is a storage protein that is found in barley, wheat, and rye. In wheat it is found as gliadin, in barley its similar storage protein is called hordein, and in rye it is secalin.[40] These storage proteins are collectively termed *prolamines*.[41] Variations of these proteins such as avenins of oats and zeins of rice are related to gliadins to a lesser extent.

For people afflicted with celiac disease, gliadin is changed into a toxic substance detected by the immune system as an antigen that activates its inflammatory response in the small intestine.[42] The inflammation, which is the body's automatic response to the "irritation," degrades the villi and diminishes the surface area available for nutrient absorption. The inflammation also destroys enzymes necessary for efficient digestion.[43] Gliadin is a glycoprotein that, when present in the enterocytes of celiac disease–afflicted patients, causes direct toxicity by promoting a lymphocyte-mediated cytotoxic response against *enterocytes*.[44] Gliadin is unaffected by the degradation property of digestive enzymes in an individual with celiac disease. Ordinarily, these harmful macromolecules are prevented from entering into the bloodstream through the nutrient-absorbing linings

of the intestines. Patients with celiac disease have an abnormally functioning intestine lining, where tight junctions that prevent the entry of
these toxins into the bloodstream are loose and thus allow for easy permeability to macromolecules. [45] This abnormality involves a complex interplay of enzymes and autoimmune processes that make gliadin highly
toxic to celiac disease patients.

ENVIRONMENTAL FACTORS OF CELIAC DISEASE

Although celiac disease is hereditary most of the time, it can sometimes
be triggered by environmental factors such as surgery, serious physical
injury, pregnancy, age at puberty onset, other autoimmune diseases,
childbirth, viral infections such as travelers' diarrhea, pneumonia and
rotavirus, severe emotional stress, the use of antibiotics or other medications that can cause alterations to the flora, or any other injury to the gut
that can initiate the celiac reaction in an already predisposed individual. [46]
   Celiac disease requires three factors to develop: a genetic predisposition, exposure to gluten through digestion, and a trigger to start this
atypical immune system response. [47] These environmental factors may
alter the functions of the small intestine of someone with these genes,
potentially increasing the immunologic response to gluten, hence aggravating the disease and leading to clinically apparent decompensation. [48]

Pregnancy

Pregnancy takes a toll on a woman's physical and emotional state, and
this could be bad news for women who are genetically vulnerable to
celiac disease, as active celiac disease could occur at the same time as the
pregnancy or slightly post-delivery. An apparently healthy pregnancy can
deteriorate and spawn various physical illnesses if the expectant mother is
prone to developing celiac disease. Other studies suggest that the method
of birth delivery may also play a part and that babies born by cesarean
delivery could be facing a higher risk of contracting celiac disease. A
retrospective multicenter German study conducted on 1,950 children revealed that, after 1,088 of them were checked by gastrointestinal (GI)
clinics while the remaining 862 served as controls, children with celiac
disease were 1.8 times more likely to have been delivered by the cesarean

method.[49] It is, however, curious that the method of birth did not seem to be responsible for Crohn's disease, ulcerative colitis, or other gastrointestinal conditions. In a recently published follow-up article, the researchers clarified why they thought cesarean deliveries potentially lead to celiac disease: during a cesarean section, the intestinal lining of the fetus that is normally protected and germ-free gets exposed to various bacteria.[50]

Food Contamination

Normally, oat grains do not belong in the wheat family that is classified as dangerous to a person with celiac disease. However, many people suffer the symptoms of celiac disease after eating oats. This has caused a great deal of confusion among doctors, patients, and nutritionists for many years. Over the years, as celiac disease started gaining more attention in the medical field, experts also looked into this issue with oats and learned that the oat, when in its most pure form, does not pose a threat to people suffering from celiac disease. It is often the cross-contamination of oats with other gluten-containing grains in processing facilities that causes the reaction in patients.[51] Contamination is a very real environmental factor that can trigger celiac disease.

Celiac Disease and Infections

Some infections trigger autoimmune diseases, as clearly discovered from the observation of animal study subjects. It is believed that viruses act by chemically modifying autoantigens, or by increasing immunogenicity of autoantigens secondary to local inflammation. Antigens are any substance that can stimulate the production of antibodies and combine specifically with them. Autoantigens are antigens of one's own cells or cell products. Infectious agents induce a variety of regulatory cells whose effects can extend to other specificities than those known to trigger nonregulatory cells' differentiation. This is known as *bystander suppression*. Infectious viruses may also interfere by using components that are not necessarily antigens but still link to specific cell receptors of the immune system.[52]

ANALYSIS

Different factors can trigger the onset of celiac disease, but it is mandatory that a person carry the specific genes in order to contract the disease. Previously thought to be prevalent only in people of Eastern European descent, recent studies have proved that others carry these genes as well.

Part II

Clinical Picture

4

PATHOLOGY OF CELIAC DISEASE

From the standpoint of pathology, celiac disease is a chronic immune-mediated disorder that can be observed, or occurs, in genetically predisposed people. This disease is often brought on by hypersensitivity toward wheat and, at the same time, related derivatives of rye and barley.[1] More specifically, it is a condition characterized by an increase in the responsiveness to prolamins, which includes the dietary wheat gliadin and such similar proteins as can be found in rye, barley, and, possibly, oats.[2] Pathologists sometimes also refer to this disease as celiac sprue, idiopathic sprue, gluten-sensitive enteropathy, idiopathic steatorrhoea, and nontropical sprue.[3]

IMPORTANCE

Looking into the pathology of celiac disease is important for pathologists and other medical practitioners for several reasons. For one, recent works of research reveal that celiac disease affects one in every 300 people, sometimes affecting as many as one in every 200 in Western countries.[4] Also, celiac disease, when untreated, is associated with various signs and symptoms. In severe cases, it can lead to neoplastic complications and even death.[5]

Considering that celiac disease is an autoimmune disease arising from an aberrant immune response of genetically susceptible people toward derivatives of gluten, diagnosing the disease early on could help in modifying the diet of susceptible individuals in order to prevent adverse reactions, especially since there is debate surrounding the safety of the consumption of oats for people affected with the disease. Unlike barley and rye, which are part of the Triticeae wheat tribe, oats are members of the Aveneae tribe of Gramineae.[6] As such, the prolamin in oats, more specifically avenin, is often more genetically disparate. On the one hand, this genetic disparity is thought to render the consumption of oats safer for patients with celiac disease, in contrast with the consumption of barley and rye.[7] On the other, it is proposed that the lower avenin to total grain protein percentage is not sufficient to render oats safe for consumption by people with this immune-mediated disorder. It is argued that the potential adulteration of oat products with gluten might be a sufficient condition for a small percentage of people with celiac disease to harbor a response to avenin.[8] For reasons of preventing adverse reactions toward gluten and understanding the condition better—along with possible cures, manifestations, symptoms, and other preventive measures—a categorical understanding of the pathology of celiac disease is highly necessary.

PATHOLOGICAL FORMS

Classic Celiac Disease

This form of celiac disease begins in childhood, and symptoms range from mild to severe gastrointestinal problems. The probability to develop serious risks is very narrow, as the biggest pain-inducing symptoms are bloating, gastrointestinal disturbance, cramps, reflux, and dyspepsia, also known as indigestion characterized by chronic or recurrent pain in the upper abdomen. The severity of pathology is directly related to the amount of intestine that is damaged.

Atypical Celiac Disease

This form of celiac disease is developed in adulthood, and symptoms are the exact opposite of those of classical celiac disease. This is because the majority if not all symptoms do not include the gastrointestinal tract, but bloating, cramps, and dyspepsia might be present. The malabsorption of certain nutrients, especially iron or calcium in the proximal upper portions of the small intestine, creates discomfort and nerve damage in the long term. This type of celiac disease increases the risks for other life-threatening conditions, including cancer and cirrhosis.

Silent Celiac Disease

This form of celiac disease is also developed in adulthood, and as the name suggests, it does not show any symptoms that would make it easily recognized. Therefore, severe, painful symptoms are not identifiable enough to pathologically distinguish celiac disease from another disorder. In a way, silent celiac disease is the most dangerous, as people could slowly develop life-threatening conditions, such as cancer in the small intestine.

Latent Celiac Disease

This category of celiac disease is developed in adulthood. Just as is the case with the silent version of celiac disease, the patient is relatively asymptomatic. Luckily, there is no extra risk of other diseases when it comes to latent celiac disease. People are diagnosed through pertinent genetic tests, but there is no pathological damage in the gastrointestinal tract as compared to other types of celiac disease. Even with latent celiac disease, each individual reacts differently and idiosyncratically to the lack of different nutrients (vitamins and minerals).

SYMPTOMS

Since the term *pathology* broadly means "the study of disease," this chapter will include symptoms and clinical presentations—all of which vary widely across individuals and are highly dependent on the age of a person.[9] The symptoms can be classified into two categories: (1) gastrointestinal symptoms and (2) extraintestinal symptoms.

Gastrointestinal Symptoms

While the manifestations of the symptoms could be rather dramatic and highly obvious in younger children, patients afflicted with the disease at a later age only exhibit very subtle symptoms, causing a considerable delay in the diagnosis of such. Gastrointestinal symptoms include a whole range of different conditions, including but not limited to abdominal pain, constipation, diarrhea, excessive gas, and even bloating. To alleviate these symptoms, what is often recommended is complete avoidance of food rich with or containing gluten. In order to identify these symptoms, a careful evaluation of an individual's diet history is advised.

Deficiencies of certain vitamins can also occur, primarily due to a malabsorption of fats. Among the vitamin deficiencies that a person with celiac disease can suffer from, vitamin D deficiencies are often deemed the most common. Deficiency of vitamin D can occur simultaneously with other longer-standing diseases, resulting in the onset of rickets, hypocalcaemia, tetany, or coagulopathy (which often happens secondary to a deficiency in vitamin K). In addition, anemia can also manifest, albeit secondary only to a deficiency in the amount or levels of iron and/or folate in the body. [10]

Among children and adolescents, the most common sign of celiac disease is a noticeably short stature. Children afflicted with celiac disease will often experience a decline in both height- and weight-growth velocity, thereby leading to a decrease in their growth percentiles. However, it is important to note that, for one, the setting of declining growth percentiles and data may not always be available, and, at the same time, such data may not always be comprehensive and reliable. As such, it is important to try other tests for pathology.

As for adults, the major symptom is diarrhea, with around half of the total cases showing such results. [11] Adults may already be symptomatic over a period of years prior to their diagnosis, or they may also have short stature (which, in fact, suggests the presence of long-standing celiac disease). Unfortunately, in a lot of cases, the regular onset of diarrhea is often misdiagnosed as plain irritable bowel syndrome, thus wrongly and unnecessarily leading to multiple clinical procedures and hospital admissions. Unknown to a lot of people, particularly to those already afflicted with celiac disease, the manifestations of symptoms such as this can often, and ultimately, be traced back to the usually undiagnosed affliction of celiac disease. [12]

As for patients who are identified through screening due to certain genetic risk factors, celiac disease can pathologically manifest itself as only mildly symptomatic, if not completely asymptomatic. Curiously, the number of individuals afflicted with celiac disease has grown rapidly over the years despite rapidly growing screening efforts. [13]

Extraintestinal Symptoms

Extraintestinal manifestations are such conditions that, while associated with the disease, are at least responsive, albeit only partially, to a gluten-free diet. It must be kept in mind that this distinction is (1) rather difficult to draw, and (2) not necessarily exact. Apart from this, certain pathology of the dental enamel can also be observed in celiac disease patients. These dental abnormalities include pitting or grooving, and they may be present in as few as 20 percent or as many as 70 percent of individuals afflicted with the disease. [14] Likewise, *aphtous stomatitis* (which is attributed to deficiencies in nutrition) can be observed in celiac disease patients. This symptom, however, can easily be treated or resolved with a gluten-free diet.

Certain pathologies of the liver may also be observed in celiac disease sufferers. They occur in about 40 percent of patients afflicted with celiac disease and can be resolved upon treatment. [15] Apart from these abnormalities, celiac disease is also often associated with some neurologic and psychiatric disorders that may be any of the following conditions: (1) anxiety, (2) irritability, (3) depression, (4) migraines, (5) cerebellar ataxia, and (6) peripheral neuropathy. In addition, patients suffering from celiac disease may also experience (1) hypotonia, (2) epilepsy, (3) headache, and (4) developmental delay. These conditions, in contrast to those previously enumerated, do *not* improve with the implementation of a gluten-free diet.

Clinical Symptoms of Celiac Disease

Celiac disease presents its manifestations in an uncharacteristically varied manner. In fact, its signs are widely different in each case and are highly dependent on the patient's age. [16] Most of the common manifestations of celiac disease, such as malnutrition, diarrhea, abdominal pain, and inability to cope and progress with digestion, are only a few of the signs that experts collectively refer to as the "celiac disease iceberg."[17]

Patients who live to an older age without knowing that they have this autoimmune disorder often have symptoms that are more elusive than those incurred by younger children who have had more obvious and devastating signs. For patients with such subtle signs, the diagnosis often comes late. The mutual symptoms include abdominal pain, diarrhea or constipation, bloating and excessive gas, vitamin and mineral deficiencies, and anemia.[18]

Infants and children with celiac disease typically exhibit these gastrointestinal expressions of the disease. Most of the severe cases in younger age groups are due to symptoms of malnutrition such as shortness in stature, dental problems, and development delay.[19] Nonspecific gastrointestinal problems are more commonly observed in adults with celiac disease than the extraintestinal manifestations. One of the most common extraintestinal signs for adults is fatigue and malaise, which may or may not be observed along with anemia. Anemia is very common for celiac patients and has long been considered one of the indicators of the disease. This kind of anemia for celiac patients may be due to folate, vitamin B12 deficiency, or chronic disease, but iron deficiency is the most likely cause. Iron deficiency anemia in celiac patients, coupled with the bleeding of the gastrointestinal tract, is one of the telltale signs of a patient suspected with celiac disease.[20]

What makes celiac disease more frightening is the reality that total treatment of the disease is yet to be discovered and only avoidance of the environmental trigger is the recognized cure. On top of this limitation to treatment is the necessity of immediate diagnosis; however, detection of celiac disease is not an easy feat because the clinical signs it manifests are tremendously varied. Signs that are common to other diseases, and understandably easily disregarded as less threatening, are the only indications of celiac disease. Invasive biopsy for the small intestine is the only sure means of detecting this disease.

Adult- versus Child-Specific Symptoms

Clinicians should note the classical adult symptoms (what the patient is complaining of) such as chronic diarrhea, weight loss, anemia, malnutrition, abdominal distension, lassitude (lack of energy), malaise, and edema (due to hypoalbuminemia). Every symptom should be described in detail. For example, pain should be described in terms of onset, duration, character, radiation of pain, and any other associated symptoms. Other adult symptoms, which have more than two times the prevalence compared to the general population, include oral aphthous ulcers, discolored teeth, and developmentally synchronous enamel loss.[21] However, gastrointestinal pathology alone cannot differentiate celiac disease from other illnesses such as irritable bowel syndrome. Improvement of symptoms after the introduction of a gluten-free diet has very low sensitivity for celiac disease. Around 60 percent of patients with diarrhea-predominant irritable bowel syndrome (IBS) show an improvement of symptoms after practicing a gluten-free diet.[22] Besides, ingestion of gluten that causes gastrointestinal symptoms is also not specific to celiac disease. This is why serology and biopsy are important when celiac disease is suspected in adults.[23]

Nonclassical symptoms may include abdominal pain, gastroesophageal reflux symptoms (such as heartburn), vomiting, constipation, and irritable bowel–like symptoms (distension, bloating, and *borborygmi*). Patients may even show nongastrointestinal symptoms (bone disease, skin disorders, and peripheral neuropathy) or few, or even none, of the above symptoms.[24] Other less common symptoms include dyspepsia, amenorrhea, and chronic fatigue syndrome.[25] Therefore, it is important for a clinician to review other body systems, such as the respiratory, cardiac, renal, and central nervous systems, that can be associated with celiac disease. Such diversity of symptoms can present a challenge to clinicians who might not be too familiar with the disease.[26]

Children may display similar pathology as adults in their complaints, such as vomiting, diarrhea, recurrent abdominal pain, irritable bowel–like symptoms, irritability, and unhappiness. Children can also show any atypical symptoms such as the ones described above in adults.[27]

PATHOLOGICAL ASSESSMENT

Initially, pathological assessment for the presence of celiac disease in an individual can be performed with the use of serologic markers that have very high sensitivity and specificity for diseases such as IgA antibodies to tissue transglutaminase (also known as TG).[28] With screening methods becoming more rapid nowadays, coupled with an increasing awareness with regard to celiac disease (its signs, symptoms, and causes), the number of individuals who are otherwise asymptomatic (or, if they have experienced manifestations of certain celiac disease symptoms, have what are often referred to as *subclinical symptoms*) have been diagnosed with the aforementioned disease.[29] Unfortunately, along with the advent of more advanced diagnosis techniques and procedures, the clinical manifestations of celiac disease have also been more varied and extensive. Such clinical manifestations are no longer isolated to the gastrointestinal tract. Also, celiac disease, in more recent works of research, has been associated with a number of other autoimmune disorders and conditions, such as Type 1 diabetes and autoimmune thyroid disease.

In terms of histopathology, there is a range of severity displayed with regard to the protean manifestations of celiac disease. Further adding to the complications of arriving at conclusive histopathological diagnosis of celiac disease is the array of entities that are known and recognized to produce consistent and parallel histopathological findings that include, but are not limited to, the following:[30]

inflammatory bowel disease
various autoimmune conditions
crypt hyperplasia
giardiasis
collagenous sprue
dermatitis herpetiformis
common variable immunodeficiency
blind loop syndrome
viral enteritis
bacterial overgrowth

Nevertheless, considering that the small bowel biopsy is regarded as essential to the diagnosis of celiac disease, it is thus important to know the major pathological characteristics of mucosa that are suggestive of celiac disease.

Mucosa Suggestive of Celiac Disease Pathology

In order to determine if the mucosa is pathological in an individual afflicted with celiac disease, certain features must be taken into consideration. Among these features are the following:[31]

> small bowel involvement that is characteristically proximal but de-
> creasing distally
>
> changes in terms of enterocytes—more particularly, loss of nuclear
> orientation (particularly basal nuclear), cuboidal morphology, and
> *cytoplasmic vacuoles* can be observed
>
> inflammation of the mucosa that involves (1) an increase in the num-
> ber of intraepithelial lymphocytes, and (2) an influx of immune
> cells existing in the lamina propria
>
> architectural changes in mucosa that include, but are not limited to,
> (1) a reduction in the number of goblet cells, (2) crypt hyperplasia,
> a thickening of what is termed a *basement membrane* that can be
> found just below the surface epithelium, and (3) villous atrophy

Histopathology of Celiac Disease

It is important to bear in mind that celiac disease, in terms of pathology at
least, appears to be related not to the degree of severity of the lesion in the
mucosa, but to the length of the affected bowel.[32] It is because of this
consideration that an observation of the compromise of the compensatory
ability inherent to the small bowel may, in some—if not most—cases, be
sufficient in unmasking compensated celiac disease. As there exist various ongoing works of research and reports on celiac disease and its pathology, among other things, it is no wonder that there are a lot of conflicting reports on the whereabouts of lesions along the small intestine
mucosa in cases of people with the aforementioned disease. A common
suggestion is that the villous lesions will rarely exist at the same time
with histologically normal mucosa.[33]

Another description of celiac disease is that relating to the presence of
a "patchy distribution." In an individual with celiac disease, a patchy
distribution of lesions is often exhibited, thereby demonstrating that there
is a need for experts to do multiple biopsy specimens. Traditionally, distal
lessening will depend on the degree of severity of intestinal pathology.[34]
This is because of the observation that lesions affect both the mucosa and

the submucosa. It is important to remember that, according to reports, celiac disease can also affect other mucosal sites, including the esophagus, stomach, and the large bowel.

It has also been previously discussed that the pathologist is confronted with a rather complex and heterogeneous population of granulocytes and lymphocytes in the mucosal biopsy specimens, primarily due to the very nature of the immunopathological basis of celiac disease. Despite the fact that the *lamina propria* can be properly considered the source of a brisk immunological response, and that grading such is as difficult as it is impractical, early work involving a murine model revealed that intraepithelial lymphocytes (IELs) can be a surrogate marker in terms of monitoring and assessing the immune activity in the lamina propria.[35] At present, a rate of 30 IELs for every 100 epithelial cells is considered "normal," although it has yet to be determined whether decreasing the upper limit for IELs will cause an adverse decrease in the specificity of the biopsy involving the small bowel in relation to the diagnosis of celiac disease. In the future, it is often argued, the figure stated above may still be further reduced, dependent upon the outcomes or the results of ongoing and future works of research.

Meanwhile, crypt hyperplasia refers to a condition (that initially precedes villous atrophy) in which the *crypts of Lieberkuhn* are elongated.[36] This elongation is often caused by any of these three factors: (1) the proliferation of stromal cells, (2) an influx of inflammatory cells, and (3) tissue remodeling.[37] Normally, there is a 3:1–5:1 ratio between villous height and crypt depth in adults. In children, the normal ratio would be around 2:1. A drastic departure from these figures is often indicative of the presence of celiac disease, in which case there is a perceived loss of villous height coupled with the stretching of intestinal crypts.

Another feature that aids in determining whether a person is afflicted with celiac disease is villous atrophy. Many clinicians consider the loss of villous height as pathognomonic for celiac disease. It is important to emphasize, however, that this finding has a nonspecific nature. Generally speaking, the height of the villous is three times the width of its base. There is no atrophy if the villi are of normal height. Villous blunting ranging from moderate to minor is indicative of mild atrophy, whereas the presence of truncated villous remnants is characteristic of marked atrophy. Finally, a third kind of atrophy, referred to as total atrophy, basically implies the complete—or total—absence of villi.

There are still a number of various histopathological observations that are often indicative of the presence of celiac disease. Among these are: (1) a loss in the columnar configuration of enterocytes, giving it instead a cuboidal shape, (2) a basophilic cytoplasm that may contain apical vacuoles at times, (3) a pyknotic nuclei that has lost its basal orientation, (4) changes in the intraepithelial tight junctions, and (5) differences in the mucous lining of the bowel lumen that can result from altered patterns of enzyme reactions that can, in turn, further promote the adhesion of bacteria to cells or to other surfaces.[38]

Differential Pathological Findings

Combining clinical and pathological findings leads to the confirmation of celiac disease in the majority of patients. Despite this, however, it must be taken into consideration how other conditions can, at times, mimic certain aspects of celiac disease without the association attributed to the conditions enumerated and discussed in the preceding paragraphs. Some of these differential findings and conditions are as follows:

- *Tropical sprue*: As in the case of the celiac disease, this disease is also characterized by a lack of *antiendomysial antibodies*. This condition also responds to therapy that makes use of folate and antibiotics.
- *Infectious (or viral) enteritis*: This disease is characterized by normal counts of IEL.
- *Common variable immunodeficiency*: This is characterized by the absence or the paucity of plasma cells. Infection of the giardia is also a common symptom of this condition, along with marked lymphoid nodular hyperplasia.
- *Autoimmune enteropathy*: This disease is characterized by either injury or total destruction of the crypts. In about half of the cases, antienterocyte antibodies have been diagnosed in patients afflicted with this disease. Its onset is roughly within the first six months after birth and, thus, it allows for early diagnosis.
- *Lymphoma development*: This condition is characterized by mass lesions, as demonstrated in imaging studies. Likewise, atypical lymphoid infiltrates can also be observed.

- *Intolerance of food protein*: In cases in which there is intolerance of food protein such as cow milk and eggs, there is an increase in the levels of eosinophils. Other manifestations of allergies can also be observed, ranging from asthma to atopy. As in the case of celiac disease, a response to elimination diets has been observed for this condition.[39]

PATHOLOGY SPECIMEN

In consideration of the distinctively heterogeneous distribution of lesions in celiac disease and the normal differences in terms of bowel histology, there are a number of biopsy specimens recommended by clinicians and pathologists for testing.[40] The specimens that should be routinely assessed by pathologists are the following:

architecture of the villi, including, but not limited to, the villous ratio
the lamina propria
enterocytes
the *brush border*
the primary structure of the inflammatory cell infiltrate that is present
    in the epithelium and the lamina propria—in particular, the pathol-
    ogist must conduct tests and examinations for intraepithelial lym-
    phocytosis
the muscularis mucosae
the lumen border, which must be checked for evidence of infection[41]

These are the starting points for pathologists in terms of assessing whether a patient is afflicted with celiac disease. The above enumeration, it must be emphasized, is not final, as ongoing works of research and studies have yet to fill in the gaps in the pathology of celiac disease. At present, however, the aforementioned specimens are given great importance.

RARE PATHOLOGY

Enamel Hypoplasia

Celiac disease affects the mineralization—growth and formation—of the permanent teeth.[42] The disease causes changes in the structure and color of the teeth, and may even interrupt their growth, especially when the disease appears while children's permanent teeth are still developing.[43] Interruption of dental growth may happen at the same time as gastrointestinal symptoms appear.[44]

Miscarriage

There are many factors that can cause spontaneous abortion or miscarriage, and this condition is not experienced exclusively among celiac patients. There is no definite reason as to how celiac disease can cause miscarriages. Nutritional deficiency could be one factor. Pregnancy complications are four times more likely to occur in women who have celiac disease than in those who do not.[45] There is also a significant connection in celiac disease to threatened abortion, gestational hypertension, placenta abruption, severe anemia, uterine hyperkinesia, and intrauterine growth restriction.[46]

Hyposplenism

When the spleen is unable to function normally, it may result in hyposplenism. Since the spleen is an important organ that helps the body fight against infections, having it damaged or impaired can put the body at risk of infection.[47] The connection between hyposplenism and celiac disease is not yet very clear.[48] It may be a result of nutrient deficiency that may cause atrophy or degeneration of body organs.

Lactose Intolerance

Celiac disease may trigger the nonproduction of lactase, which is essential in breaking down food that contains lactose. Because the small intestine is inflamed or damaged, it is hard for the body to produce lactase.

Hence, people would be unable to digest food that contains milk. Lactose intolerance can cause nausea, bloating, stomach pain, and diarrhea.[49]

ANALYSIS

The understanding of celiac disease pathology is continuously evolving. Various works of research and studies have allowed for a more in-depth and more accurate analysis and assessment of this disease. Whereas it used to be—or, at least, was perceived to be—rare, at present it is recognized that celiac disease is a rather common condition, with symptomatic manifestations ranging from asymptomatic to severely affected. The increase in the rate of celiac disease diagnosis can likewise be attributed to the apparent advancements in techniques and procedures that aid in the assessment of the condition.

It must be kept in mind, however, that procedural and research-based advances in terms of the pathology of celiac disease have given rise to some confusion in the same way that they have given rise to illumination. Comparison of the pathology of celiac disease with other conditions has led to the discovery of differential manifestations, showing that there is, to a certain extent, a similarity or parallelism in the manifestations and symptoms of celiac disease and other autoimmune diseases. As such, it prompts clinicians and pathologists to practice extra care in terms of diagnosis and treatment of celiac disease.

5

DIAGNOSIS OF CELIAC DISEASE

Overall, diagnosis of celiac disease requires a good patient history presenting with features of malabsorption and malnutrition, with focused clinical examination, followed by a battery of tests (blood tests, biopsy, and endoscopy) in investigations. Celiac disease to some extent can be associated with systemic diseases such as Type I diabetes mellitus, thyroid disease, and primary biliary sclerosis. [1] However, 60 percent of children and 40 percent of adults with celiac disease can be asymptomatic. [2] This chapter will discuss in detail the steps followed by a physician to confirm the diagnosis of celiac disease.

DATA ASSEMBLY AND SCREENING

Clinical Assessment

Clinical suspicion of celiac disease should arise if the patient presents with a family history of celiac disease in first-degree and second-degree relatives, medical history of Type I diabetes mellitus, thyroid dysfunction, autoimmune hepatitis, and osteoporosis. [3] The patient may also present with important symptoms of chronic diarrhea, weight loss, steatorrhea (presence of excess fat in feces), abdominal distension, and postprandial abdominal pain (abdominal pain after a meal). [4] The prevalence of celiac disease in the United States is about 1 in 141. [5] This means that a clinician could have a low threshold of suspicion for celiac disease when attempting a diagnosis. If celiac disease remains undiagnosed, it would increase the risk of life-threatening conditions such as malignancies (oropharyngeal cancer, non-Hodgkin's lymphoma, and small bowel adenoma), unexplained infertility, and osteoporosis.[6] Besides, a clinician should keep in mind other differential diagnoses that also cause similar clinical manifestations, such as tropical sprue (the flattening of villi and inflammation of the small intestine; found commonly in tropical regions) and *autoimmune enteropathy* (a rare disorder characterized by severe, prolonged diarrhea, and malabsorption due to immune-mediated damage of the intestinal mucosa). Diseases such as *Crohn's disease* (inflammatory bowel disease that can affect any part of the gastrointestinal tract) and intestinal tuberculosis should also be considered by a clinician.[7]

Investigative Procedures

Serological test and duodenal biopsy are the gold standard for the diagnosis of celiac disease. Celiac disease should be ruled out first before a clinician can consider other possibilities. A gluten-free diet would reduce the amount of autoantibodies to healthy levels. Therefore, ideally, the patient should not be on a gluten-free diet before serology testing so that false negative results do not occur. If the patient has a low probability of having celiac disease, a serological test for tissue transglutaminase antibody (TTGA, in the form of IgA antibody) should be done to measure the level of TTGA in the patient's serum. If TTGA rises above normal levels (positive), then the celiac disease patient should proceed with a duodenal biopsy. The total IgA in the serum should also be measured concurrently. This is because patients with IgA deficiency will give low values of TTGA, thus producing a negative serological result. Such patients should undergo a TTGA IgG antibody and deamidated gliadin peptide antibody (DGPA in the form of IgG antibody) serological test. If the IgG test is positive, then the patient should undergo a duodenal biopsy as the previous patient did. Celiac disease is unlikely in a low-risk patient if either the IgA or the IgG test is negative.[8]

If the patient has a high probability of having celiac disease, both a TTGA IgA and duodenal biopsy should be done as part of the entire diagnostic process. The patient is confirmed to have celiac disease if both tests are positive. If the TTGA IgA and duodenal biopsy are negative, then celiac disease is unlikely.[9]

If the patient's TTGA is positive but the duodenal biopsy histology is normal, he may still have disease, and he should be evaluated and monitored further depending upon his clinical circumstances. A follow-up can be arranged, and a biopsy can be repeated after one to two years. [10] MHC Class II HLA-DQ2 and -DQ8 molecular typing may be useful if such circumstances arise. If TTGA serology is negative but the duodenal biopsy is positive, or both serology and biopsy are negative but the patient is on a gluten-free diet, HLA-DQ2 and -DQ8 should be done to rule out celiac disease. If the result is negative, then celiac disease is very unlikely in the patient because the negative predictive value (NPV) of this molecular typing is more than 99 percent. [11] Then the clinician can consider other causes of the disease. Other diseases that show sensitivity to gluten usually do not have a strong hereditary basis, and they are not associated with malabsorption, intestinal malignancy, nutritional deficiencies, or autoimmune disorders such as celiac disease. If the molecular typing is positive, the patient should undergo a gluten challenge test (if he was on a gluten-free diet before this). For diagnostic purposes, sometimes doctors recommend that the patient take three grams of gluten daily for two weeks. If the patient is able to continue, then he can proceed until six weeks. Serology should be repeated at weeks two and six to access any changes of autoantibodies in the patient's serum. The gluten challenge test is the gold standard of diagnosis for patients who have normal serology and biopsy tests but are on a gluten-free diet. [12]

Availability of Resources

If a clinical setting has enough resources for diagnosing celiac disease, then the gold standard of diagnosis (serology and biopsy) should be used. Serology may be used as the only diagnostic tool for celiac disease if a trained expert is not available for duodenal biopsy tests. TTGA IgA is the most common test for the diagnosis, while the test for antiendomysial antibodies (EMA) requires a higher level of expertise. DGPA IgA and IgG may be used in children less than three years old (due to poor TTGA performance) and in patients with IgA deficiency. An intestinal biopsy can still be done if the disease is visible on an endoscopy, but clinical laboratories do not meet the actual standards. However, care should be taken while reading results given by nonexperts, because although the findings are characteristic of an intestinal atrophy, such an atrophy is not specific to celiac disease. The histological findings can then be combined with the improvement of symptoms when the patient was given a gluten-free diet. However, such practice is strongly discouraged because there are other diseases that also respond to a gluten-free diet, and it is only helpful in a minority of patients. [13]

In cases of clinical settings with low resources, the TTGA IgA diagnostic test can be done in a clinician's office by using self-antibody-based rapid assessments, carried out by pricking the tip of the finger for a blood sample. The test is quite simple and lasts only a few minutes. Endoscopic identification of mucosal atrophy of the duodenum only increases the suspicion of celiac disease but is not diagnostic of it. [14]

Patient Profile and Epidemiological Data

The patient profile should include the patient's name, age, gender, address, identity card number, ethnic group, occupation, and marital status. Generally, adults have their celiac disease diagnosed 10 years after their first symptoms appeared. [15] The ratio of diagnosed to undiagnosed cases of celiac disease in the United States is approximately 1:20. [16] Females have a higher risk of contracting celiac disease as compared to males, and the ratio is set to 2:1. [17] In 17 percent of pregnant mothers, such disease may manifest during pregnancy, or *puerperium*. [18] Celiac disease was traditionally associated with Caucasians, mainly located in Europe and North America. However, incidence of celiac disease is also reported in Amerindians and African Americans, as well as in people from the Middle East, India, Pakistan, and China. Such epidemiological data is diagnostically useful to get a general idea about celiac disease sufferers, starting from the patient profile itself. [19]

Other Aspects of the Patient's History

Other patient's histories are also important in the diagnosis of celiac disease. The estimated prevalence of each disease mentioned below will be shown in parentheses. Patients could present with the following medical histories:

Family history of celiac disease in first-degree (10 percent) and sec-
ond-degree (5 percent) relatives or personal medical history of
osteoporosis and osteomalacia of premature onset (2–4 percent)
Type I diabetes mellitus (2–15 percent, especially if there are any
digestive symptoms)
Thyroid dysfunction (2–7 percent)
Down and Turner syndromes (6 percent each)
Irritable bowel syndrome (3 percent)
Addison's disease and autoimmune hepatitis (3–6 percent)[20]

The patient may also have a history of neurological disorder, such as
tingling, numbness, loss of sensation in the limbs, and lack of voluntary
coordination of muscle movements.[21]

Screening for Celiac Disease

A physician may choose to advise the patient so that other relatives with
first-degree family members (who have been confirmed with celiac disease) undergo celiac disease confirmatory tests. Newly diagnosed patients with celiac disease should also inform family members of the risk
of contracting the disease. The testing of symptomless first-degree relatives is reasonable because studies indicate that patients often report improved health with a gluten-free diet and the resolution of previous unexplained symptoms. No new symptoms were reported after the initiation of
the gluten-free diet. Only a small proportion of patients reported increased health anxiety after the diagnosis. The overall satisfaction rate of
the diagnosis was high. Monozygotic (identical) twins presented the highest risk of having celiac disease if the other twin was confirmed as having
the disease.[22]

Screening patients with Type I diabetes mellitus (with gastrointestinal
symptoms) for celiac disease is reasonable because the incidence is relatively high (2–5 percent) and the gastrointestinal symptoms normally
resolve after a gluten-free diet.[23] The treatment of diabetic patients with
celiac disease for one year with a gluten-free diet is safe. Diabetic patients
with undiagnosed celiac disease carry a higher risk of developing diabetic
retinopathy and nephropathy as compared to asymptomatic diabetic patients, according to a large-scale study in Sweden. However, screening
for asymptomatic Type I diabetic patients is controversial. In addition to

that, parents with children who have Type I diabetes mellitus and children with parents of Type I diabetes should also be screened because of the increased risk of celiac disease. Besides, unexplained symptoms are also improved for Type I diabetic patients after a gluten-free diet.[24]

Differential Diagnosis

Other diseases that a clinician might also consider are the following:[25]

tropical sprue
enteropathy associated T-cell lymphoma
HIV enteropathy
chronic ischemia
autoimmune enteropathy
Zollinger-Ellison syndrome
combined immunodeficiency states
radiation damage
Crohn's disease
recent chemotherapy
graft versus host disease (GVHD)
giardiasis
eosinophilic gastroenteritis
refractory sprue
collagenous sprue

PHYSICAL EXAMINATION

A physical examination will help a physician confirm the symptoms given by the patient eliciting signs (what physicians can observe from the patient) of the disease. Celiac disease caregivers should be observant and should describe the general appearance of the patient, including the build, nutrition, gait, and position (sitting posture), as well as the measure of the body mass index (BMI). This is especially true if the patient is diabetic or hypertensive. The general appearance of the patient usually can be observed when the patient first enters the physician's office. Checking for vital signs (pulse rate, blood pressure, temperature, and respiratory rate) should become a routine practice for the clinician.[26]

Adults

During the general physical examination of the adult patient, clinicians should check for diagnostic signs of anemia such as koilonychia (spoon-shaped nails) and platonychia (flat nails), pallor in the nail bed, palms, face, palpebral conjunctiva (a transparent layer of the membrane covering the outer surface of the eye that also covers the inner side of the eyelids), and dorsum of the tongue. Checking for clubbing (the loss of angle between the nail bed and the adjacent skin) is only indicated when the patient is suspected of contracting chronic pulmonary or heart diseases. Fully white nails indicate chronic liver disease that can cause *hypoalbuminemia*, which in turn leads to edema in the patient. Checking for cyanosis in the tongue or nails is only indicated when the adult celiac disease sufferer has underlying pulmonary or cardiac problems. Clinicians can expect to find Heberden's nodules at the distal joints of the fingers if the patient shows up with osteoarthritis. Palmar erythema, also known as redness of the palms, is an indication of liver failure, thyrotoxicosis (excessive thyroid hormone secretion, which causes a variety of symptoms in the patient), and rheumatoid arthritis. Fine tremors of the fingers are an indication of Grave's disease (one of the causes of thyrotoxicosis). Flapping tremors of the hands are an indication of liver, renal, and respiratory failure. However, drugs such as alcohol, barbiturates, and phenytoin can also cause flapping tremors.[27]

Loss of the lateral one-third of the eyebrow indicates hypothyroidism. In older adults, puffiness in the eyelids almost always indicates generalized edema and nephritic syndrome, which is the thinning of the glomerular membrane in the kidneys that leads to protein and blood excretion in the urine. Thyrotoxicosis can cause exophthalmos, or bulging of the eyes. A physician should remember to check for yellowish discoloration in the sclera of the eyes and below the tongue for the presence of jaundice. Moreover, the practitioner can check in detail to see if there are any skin lesions or bruises on the skin and changes in the oral mucosa, especially glossitis, which is the smooth, reddened tongue occurring in 30 percent of patients with celiac disease.[28] Such changes would be prominent in cases of vitamin deficiencies because vitamin B2 is important for maintaining the integrity of the oral mucosa and skin while vitamin K is important for blood coagulation. A clinician should palpate for the enlargement of cervical (neck) and axillary (armpit) lymph nodes for any enlargements if malignancies are suspected. Examination for the dorsalis pedis (dorsum of the foot) and posterior tibial (back part of the tibial bone) arterial pulses in the lower limbs is also important. Low or absent arterial pulses are indicative of peripheral vascular disease or severe low blood pressure.[29]

A systemic examination mainly encompasses the respiratory system, cardiac system, abdominal area, and a neurological examination. Assessment of every system consists of four stages: inspection, palpation, percussion, and auscultation. In this case, abdominal examination is important, but careful observation of other systems is only indicated when irregularities are suspected in them. Inspection of the abdomen includes the observation of the abdomen if it is flat or distended, the fullness of flanks, the position of the umbilicus, and any swellings, scars, or sinuses on the abdomen. Palpation mainly involves the testing of abdominal tenderness and the enlargement of the liver and spleen. Listening for abnormal sounds while the surface of the abdomen is being tapped (percussion) is also used for finding tenderness points and the presence of any fluids in the abdomen. Auscultation with a stethoscope is used for finding any abnormalities in the bowel sounds. Neurological examinations such as tendon reflexes and vibration and touch sensations should be performed in cases when the patient complains of neurological symptoms. Nutritional deficiency, especially that of vitamin B6, is also an indicator for a neurological examination.[30]

Children

Anthropometry measurements reveal whether a youngster has the condition of "failure to thrive," which is basically low weight, low height, and irregular stature for the child's age. Most of the general and systemic examination procedures in adults are also applied here.[31]

NONIMAGING DIAGNOSTIC TESTS

Full Blood Count

Full blood count (FBC) is routinely done in patients who are admitted into the hospital and patients who are suspected of serious illnesses. It normally measures the following:

hemoglobin level in the blood
mean corpuscular volume (MCV)
total white blood cell count (TWBC)
mean corpuscular hemoglobin concentration (MCHC)
platelet count
count of each component of white blood cells
packed cell volume (PCV)

Blood indices measure the average size of a red blood cell (MCV), average amount of hemoglobin in each red blood cell (MCH), and average hemoglobin concentration in each red blood cell (MCHC). PCV measures the total volume of red blood cells in a given volume of blood.[32]

In celiac disease patients, a clinician can expect to find decreased hemoglobin levels in blood, with decreased values in all three components of blood indices and decreased PCV, which is a characteristic finding of microcytic anemia. This form of anemia may show increased MCV and MCH, but normal MCHC. TWBC and lymphocyte count may increase due to inflammatory reactions in the bowel or to autoimmune diseases.[33]

More on Serology

The serological test is useful in screening individuals who are at risk of celiac disease besides identifying individuals for duodenal biopsy.[34] In this case, only three antibodies are useful in the diagnosis of celiac disease—namely, TTGA, EMA, and DGPA. TTGA and EMA are autoantibodies (antibodies against human cells or proteins), while DGPA is against the gliadin component present in wheat and other cereals. TTGA and DGPA tests have high sensitivity toward celiac disease but have low positive predictive value (PPV).[35] In other words, it means that a positive test is not enough to confirm the diagnosis of a disease. Therefore, the

EMA test and biopsy are widely used to improve the accuracy of the diagnosis. However, only TTGA and DGPA are combined to produce reliable diagnostic results in low-risk patients because EMA requires expert observers. In addition to that, TTGA requires an enzyme-linked immunosorbent assay (ELISA) test, which requires only low expertise in the clinical setting. In high-risk patient populations, such a combination of serological tests does not yield any benefits to the diagnosis; therefore, either TTGA or DGPA is enough for diagnosis of this group of patients in combination with a biopsy.[36] Combined tests can improve the sensitivity, but with the expense, it is suggested that only patients with a positive serological test undergo intestinal biopsy so that the specificity of the overall diagnosis will increase.[37] Higher specificity should be able to prevent overdiagnosis and unnecessary treatment for the patient. However, diagnostic accuracy of the serological test also differs between laboratories. A large-scale international study found that when comparing the TTGA results among clinical and research laboratories, sensitivity varies from about 60 percent to just over 90 percent, and specificity ranges from 96 to 100 percent.[38] Serological tests in the clinical setting are usually less well performed than in the laboratory setting.[39]

If the suspicion is high toward celiac disease in the patient but the diagnostic serology is negative, then the patient can proceed with the intestinal biopsy. TTGA should be combined with DGPA IgA/IgG in children less than two years old because this group of children normally gives low values of TTGA irrespective of the presence of celiac disease. IgA deficiency normally occurs in 2–3 percent of patients with celiac disease and only 1 percent of those tested for celiac disease.[40] TTGA IgG and DGPA IgG testing is very helpful in this case. A negative serology test is produced in a few weeks if a gluten-free diet is introduced to a weakly positive patient. After 6–12 months of a gluten-free diet, 80 percent of the subjects will test negative for serology. By five years, 90 percent of the patients will show a negative serological test.[41]

EMA IgA binds to endomysium (connective tissue around the smooth muscles) and produces a characteristic staining pattern that can be seen with indirect immunofluorescent assays. EMA IgA binds to TTG that is presented on the endomysium, while TTGA binds to TTG that can be found in the intestinal epithelium. The antigens for TTGA were traditionally produced from liver extraction or the purification from human red blood cells, but recently, it has been produced by recombinant protein production.[42] A rapid form of TTGA test can also be performed in a clinician's office on a blood sample. In this test, TTGA is bonded to the TTG antigens released by lysed red blood cells instead of using antigens produced from the intestinal epithelium. The diagnostic accuracy of a rapid TTGA test is very similar to the conventional ones, but it should not replace the conventional TTGA test. DGPA IgA/IgG tests are similar to TTGA in the sense that they are using ELISA for the detection of antibodies and also have high sensitivity and specificity. With the combination of TTGA and DGPA, the sensitivity of detecting mild enteropathy (diagnostic grade greater than two) can be increased.[43] The antigliadin antibody (AGA) test, which was used previously, is no longer used now for the diagnosis of celiac disease because of low sensitivity and specificity. Its usage now is confined to biomarkers for patients with nonceliac gluten sensitivity.[44]

Gliadin Detection

Gluten sensitivity in celiac disease is due to the alteration of gliadin peptides by the enzyme *tissue transglutaminase (TTG)*, produced by almost all cell types, and in its inactive form it is kept intracellularly and is only released extracellularly upon mechanical or inflammatory stress.[45] Tissue transglutaminase catalyzes the permanent cross-linking of a protein with glutamine in another protein containing lysine, thereby resulting in a longer protein that is linked through a bridge called *glutamyl-lysine isopeptide* bond.[46] These altered gliadin peptides are then recognized by local intestinal T-cells as foreign and—by that diagnostic means—induce an immune response in the celiac disease sufferer. Although the specific mechanisms causing this T-cell mediation remain little understood, inflammation is closely linked to genetic and environmental factors.[47]

Duodenal Biopsy

Villous atrophy is characteristic but is not pathognomonic (confirmatory) of celiac disease. Celiac disease affects the proximal part of the intestine, especially the duodenum, and the intestinal lesion will decrease in severity as it goes from distal to the duodenum, with the exception of severe cases. Severity of the intestinal lesion diagnostically correlates with the severity of the symptoms. Such lesions are normally patchy inside the intestinal mucosa. A specific number of samplings is required for accurate diagnosis, and no lesions should be missed.[48] Some samples should be taken—four of the samples should be from the major duodenal papilla, which is the opening at the edge of the common bile duct and the pancreatic duct in the second part of the duodenum, while one or two samples should be taken at the duodenal bulb, the first part of the duodenum after the *gastric antrum*.[49]

For patients with a positive EMA test but with a normal duodenal biopsy, a second biopsy is warranted for testing. Since part of the duodenum that is above the papilla contains Brunner's gland, a gland that produces a mucus-rich alkaline secretion, which can stretch the mucosa of the duodenum, it will produce an appearance of villous atrophy because all the villi are being stretched flat. Acute inflammatory changes of the peptic duodenitis can also cause similar changes, such as villous atrophy.[50] In children and adults with positive diagnostic serologies, a duodenal bulb biopsy can increase the rate of diagnosis because 9–13 percent of the patients only have villous atrophy exclusively in the bulb.[51] A targeted biopsy at the nine or at twelve o'clock position of the duodenal bulb with the biopsies of the distal duodenum can increase the sensitivity to approximately 95 percent.[52]

Under a light microscopy examination of the duodenal specimen, the following diagnostic characteristics can be seen: atrophic villi, crypt hyperplasia, mononuclear cell infiltration of lamina propria, abnormalities of the epithelial cells, and *intraepithelial lymphocyte infiltration*. The staging of the histological characteristics of the duodenal mucosa is done by a modified *Marsh classification*, a common diagnostic scoring system for celiac disease.[53]

> Stage 0: This is the stage of preinfiltrative mucosa (normal mucosa without any infiltration). Such normal mucosa can be seen in up to 30 percent of patients with dermatitis herpetiformis and gluten ataxia.[54]
>
> Stage 1: Infiltrative mucosa where the number of intraepithelial lymphocytes (IELs) equals or exceeds 25 per 100 enterocytes, but the mucosa is normal. This is also called *infiltrative duodenosis*, and it is not specific to celiac disease because *Helicobacter pylori* infection, medications such as nonsteroidal anti-inflammatory drugs (NSAID), small bowel bacterial overgrowth, and systemic autoimmune disorders can also present with similar symptoms.[55]

IELs may still persist in more than 50 percent of the treated celiac disease patients.[56]

Stage 2: Crypt hyperplasia occurs when there is an increase in crypt depth but there is no reduction in crypt height in addition to increased IELs. Such changes can be induced by gluten ingestion and are seen in 20 percent of patients with untreated dermatitis herpetiformis and celiac disease.[57]

Stage 3: Villous atrophy with crypt hyperplasia and increased IELs is found in about 40 percent of dermatitis herpetiformis patients. Such changes are characteristic of celiac disease but are not pathognomonic because disorders such as severe giardiasis, chronic ischemia of the small intestine, and tropical sprue can also produce similar changes. This stage of disease can be subdivided into three more stages—namely, 3A (partial changes), 3B (subtotal changes), and 3C (total change, which means full-blown villous atrophy).[58]

Recently, there has been a new classification system named "simplified Corazza classification." Corazza Grade A is the same as Marsh Type 1, and Corazza Grade B1 is the same as Marsh Type 3A, while Corazza Grade B2 is the same as Marsh Type 3C.[59] In cases of lymphocytic infiltration only without any villous atrophy (stage 1), such a lesion is not specific for celiac disease and diagnostic factors should also be considered. However, if there is any histological response of the intestinal mucosa to a gluten-free diet with villous atrophy, then it is strongly suggestive of celiac disease. A biopsy has been traditionally carried out in three diagnostic stages: (1) biopsy on a gluten-containing diet, (2) biopsy on a gluten-free diet, and (3) biopsy on a gluten challenge test. Recent studies have indicated that a biopsy on a gluten-containing diet alone is enough to diagnostically confirm celiac disease in 95 percent of the cases in children.[60] The guidelines proposed by the European Society of Pediatric Gastroenterology, Hepatology and Nutrition (ESPGHAN) state that intestinal biopsies in children can be avoided as long as they meet the following criteria: characteristic symptoms of celiac disease with TTGA IgA levels more than 10 times the upper limit of the TTGA levels, and positive HLA-DQ2 testing. However, such a proposal needs further validation before being accepted as standard diagnostic criteria for children.[61]

Reliability of the histological diagnosis depends on a number of factors—namely, number of biopsies taken, quality of biopsy samples, handling of samples, patchiness of mucosal damage, different grades of lesion, and interpretation of lesions by experts. Therefore, an experienced expert is required to make an accurate diagnosis. A recent study showed that just over 65 percent of the 132,000 biopsies surveyed did not have enough samples.[62] This study also showed that the number of samples taken during a diagnostic biopsy is positively correlated with the number of newly diagnosed patients. In other words, an increase in the number of samples taken during a biopsy increases the chances of confirming celiac disease as the diagnosis.[63]

Molecular Typing

Celiac disease occurs almost exclusively in patients with MHC class II HLA-DQ2 and HLA-DQ8 molecules expressed from the genes. However, HLA genetic haplotypes alone only accounted for 30–40 percent of the genetic predisposition to celiac disease.[64] HLA-DQ8/DQ2 should not be used routinely in the initial diagnosis of celiac disease. Such molecular typing is only used in certain situations, such as a positive biopsy finding with seronegative results, patients on a gluten-free diet who show negative serology and histology, patients with suspected refractory celiac disease, patients with Down syndrome, or when serological and histological results do not match.[65]

A combination of the results for both HLA-DQ8 and -DQ2 is necessary because either one of the testing options only carries a positive predictive value of about 10 percent, which is somewhat unreliable.[66] DQ8 and DQ2 molecular typing carries a negative predictive value of 99 percent, which means that celiac disease is very unlikely if the result is negative.[67] The usefulness of HLA testing of family members of Type I diabetic patients is limited because around 70 percent carry the genes that could express DQ2 molecules anyway.[68]

Gluten Challenge Test

This test is designed for patients who tested negative for serology and biopsy but were on a gluten-free diet. Before a gluten challenge test is taken, celiac disease should be ruled out by HLA-DQ2 and HLA-DQ8 molecular typing. Such molecular testing is not affected by the consumption of a gluten-free diet. Only when the molecular typing is positive should the patient undergo gluten challenge tests. This is because positive molecular typing does not confirm the presence of celiac disease; only negative molecular typing is able to exclude it.[69] A gluten challenge test is now less frequently used because serology and biopsy have a high positive predictive value to exclude low-risk patients from celiac disease and high-risk patients who give consistent serology and biopsy results.[70] Former results of the gluten challenge test should be considered to exclude the probability of having celiac disease in patients who are adhering to a gluten-free diet. Patients are exempted from gluten challenge tests if they express severe symptoms following gluten ingestion. Patients who refuse to undergo a formal gluten challenge test with unconfirmed celiac disease should be managed similarly to a patient with celiac disease confirmed. However, such measures will increase unnecessary expenditure in monitoring and treatment because the patient may or may not have celiac disease.[71]

If the duration of a gluten-free diet is less than one month, the serologic and biopsy results usually do not normalize immediately. On such occasions, the serology and biopsy results are often positive. However, there is still a possibility that the serology and biopsy results can revert in no time under a gluten-free diet. Thus, a negative serology and biopsy result does not rule out celiac disease in patients with a gluten-free diet.[72] Although traditionally 10 grams of gluten per day for six to eight weeks was the usual dosage for gluten challenge tests, such a dosage is not justifiable in recent studies because a high gluten dosage does not improve the diagnostic efficacy of celiac disease.[73]

Liver Function Tests

Parameters for liver function tests include prothrombin time (PT), activated partial thromboplastin time (aPTT), albumin levels, bilirubin levels (direct and indirect), and liver enzyme levels. PT measures the extrinsic pathway of coagulation, while aPTT measures the intrinsic and common pathways of coagulation that involve different clotting factors in each pathway.[74] Liver function tests to some extent can act as a screening test for celiac disease. When no other etiology is found for the elevation of serum liver enzymes, such as alanine aminotransferase (ALT) and aspartate aminotransferase (AST) levels, then the patient should be tested for a diagnosis of celiac disease.[75]

Other Nonimaging Tests

Biochemical tests may reveal a reduced concentration of calcium, magnesium, and total protein, albumin, or vitamin D.[76] Blood magnesium, calcium, protein, and albumin levels are measured when the patient is suspected of losing such nutrients when they experience prolonged vomiting, diarrhea, hypertension, and uncontrolled diabetes mellitus (magnesium is important for the regulation of blood pressure and blood sugar levels). For an adult, the normal blood level of magnesium is around 1.5–2 mg/dL.[77] Calcium level tests are indicated in bone diseases, chronic kidney disease, intestinal malabsorption, and disorders of thyroid and parathyroid glands. Normal levels of calcium should be 8.5–10.2 mg/dL.[78] Moreover, intestinal permeability tests using D-xylose are neither sensitive nor specific enough to warrant a diagnosis of celiac disease. Stool studies and salivary tests for TTGA do not have enough backup evidence for an accurate diagnosis; therefore, they are not recommended for the diagnosis of celiac disease.[79]

IMAGING TESTS FOR CELIAC DISEASE

Endoscopy

Upper gastrointestinal endoscopy or endoscopy through the mouth allows histological sampling of the mucosa, which is less invasive and less time consuming than a peroral biopsy, or biopsy through the mouth. Observation of typical lesions in the duodenum can provide an indication for biopsy, but it is not sensitive enough for fully diagnosing celiac disease. Some of the characteristic findings in endoscopy include scalloped, flattened mucosal folds, with fissures, or a mosaic pattern, which disappears or becomes small after maximum insufflation (blowing air into the intestinal lumen). Such findings will prompt a duodenal biopsy to confirm the endoscopy observations.[80] Upper endoscopy with duodenal biopsy is important for the clinical diagnosis of persons with suspected celiac disease.[81]

Capsule endoscopy, when a capsule the size of a pill that contains a tiny camera takes photos inside the gastrointestinal tract, should not be used in patients except in cases when the serological result is positive but the patient does not wish to undergo upper endoscopy and a biopsy. Capsule endoscopy is useful because it is not invasive to the celiac disease sufferer as compared to an upper endoscopy. Capsule endoscopy has better overall sensitivity (95 percent) in the detection of the gross changes of the villous atrophy in the intestinal mucosa as compared to upper endoscopy (55 percent).[82] However, the sensitivity is less for lesions with Marsh stages 1 and 2 celiac disease. Capsule endoscopy is also useful in detecting complications of refractory celiac disease, such as extensive mucosal damage, stenosis, ulceration, and lymphoma. Erosions or ulcerations are normally found in patients who are using NSAID. Such findings of complicated celiac disease may prompt further enteroscopy of the small intestine, especially for the patients suspected of lymphoma, adenocarcinoma, and ulcerative jejunitis.[83]

Bone Density Measurements

Bone density measurements are useful in celiac disease patients who are suspected of osteoporosis and bone fracture.[84] Such a procedure is painless, with minimal exposure to radiation. Normally, dual-energy X-ray absorptiometry is used for measuring bone densities. Such testing is indicated in (1) females over 65, (2) males over 70, (3) individuals with hyperparathyroidism and vertebral abnormalities who have undergone long-term steroid therapy, and (4) celiac disease sufferers who have a previous fracture following bone trauma. The normal bone density value is 1500 kg/m^3.[85] One major limitation of this test is that the increase in bone mineral density does not correlate well with the increase in bone resistance to fracture because bone strength also depends upon other factors, such as connectivity and arrangement of the bone mass, elasticity, and stress/strain response of the bone to trauma.[86]

Other imaging tests, such as computed tomography enterography, magnetic resonance imaging enterography, and enteroclysis, which is a fluoroscopic X-ray for the small intestine, may be useful for complicated celiac disease. Radiological signs of malabsorption such as dilation, flocculation (when barium comes out from a suspension to form flakes), and segmentation of barium (barium suspension divided into compartments by invagination of intestinal walls) in barium swallow tests are not specific to celiac disease and therefore remain unused in the diagnosis.[87]

LIFESTYLE AFTER DIAGNOSIS

The right attitude is very important for adapting to life after being diagnosed with celiac disease. Patients diagnosed with celiac disease are encouraged to view their diagnosis as an opportunity to explore, discover, and create a healthy, new lifestyle.[88] The damage done to the intestine lining results in malabsorption of nutrients needed by the body, since the villi play an important role in absorbing nutrients from food. This can lead to other health conditions such as malnutrition, nutritional deficiencies, rickets, kidney stones, osteomalacia, anemia, osteoporosis, infertility, and low blood glucose levels.[89]

Though celiac disease can cause various side effects depending on various factors, changing certain parts of a patient's lifestyle after diagnosis can help them recover and adapt well to their condition. At the same time, each person's system rebounds and heals at different rates.[90] It is widely known that the only permanent remedy for patients suffering from celiac disease is to maintain a gluten-free diet throughout their lifetime. Only by maintaining a strict gluten-free diet can one's body manage to completely heal and naturally regenerate the villi. Often, after being diagnosed with the disease, the doctor will put the patient in touch with a dietician who can explain in detail how to identify and live a gluten-free lifestyle.

There are various associations and aid groups dedicated to helping people suffering from celiac disease cope with their condition and maintain a healthy lifestyle after diagnosis. It is often helpful for newly diagnosed patients to contact and join these help groups. Interacting with others who are facing the same situation can help newly diagnosed patients learn more about celiac disease, as well as how they can keep their condition under control while still living their lives to the fullest. Support groups also play an important role in promoting ideal mental health following diagnosis. Another option for gaining confidence and getting to know coping strategies from others who have experienced celiac disease firsthand is opening oneself to forums, blogs, and social media outlets.

The ideal way for a celiac disease patient to ensure that well-informed care is within hand's reach is by requesting a "care conference" with his or her doctor, dietician, family members, pharmacist, registered nurse, and a member of a support group for celiac disease. Organizing this meetup after diagnosis is a good way to get to know valuable information about the disease and achieve a more positive outcome after starting a gluten-free diet. This meeting can be arranged on a one-to-one basis as well, as these professionals represent the different important disciplines and will share important information that will affect the rest of a patient's life. The doctor, who will be aware of a patient's total medical condition and prescribed medication, may share a specific follow-up plan, while the dietician can provide recommendations for the mandatory dietary changes as well as educational opportunities. Professional caregivers such as registered nurses can coordinate all disciplines and even act as patient advocates, while family members will be able to have a better understanding of the challenges, genetic predisposition, common symptoms, and the necessity of maintaining a strict, lifelong gluten-free diet once the patient has been officially diagnosed. Just as importantly, the pharmacist can evaluate the medications prescribed for the possibility of hidden gluten, while the support group members can share the challenges they personally faced and foster a sense of community and help fight the feeling of isolation. Ultimately, this care collaboration is the most effective way for all disciplines to understand and develop a personalized approach that will work best for a particular patient.[91]

Celiac disease sufferers will have to get regular health screenings to make sure their condition is kept under control and that it is not affecting them in any other way or leading to other health problems such as osteoporosis or a thyroid or calcium deficiency.[92] Recently diagnosed patients should encourage their immediate family members to take the necessary tests required to detect any chances of celiac disease in their bodies. The issue of the age at which gluten should be introduced to a child's diet has been greatly studied, discussed, and debated. Current studies show that the best time for introducing gluten to children who are predisposed to celiac disease is between four and six months after birth.[93] Studies also show that breastfeeding children can possibly reduce their lifelong risk and offer protection from inheriting the disease.[94] This is one way new mothers with celiac disease can protect their children from contracting the disease from them.

ANALYSIS

Diagnosing individuals with celiac disease is constantly improving. Looking into the dynamics among reliable antibodies, on the one hand, and self-antigens (TG) and modified environmental antigens such as *de-amidated gliadin peptide (DGP)*, on the other, has made the diagnosis for celiac disease both easier and more reliable.

6

NEW ADVANCES IN CLINICAL RESEARCH

The complexity of celiac disease lies not only in the wide variety of symptoms it exhibits, which may coincide with other diseases, but also in its association with multiple conditions that involve several known and unknown signalling pathways. That is why clinical research on the subject of celiac disease must be adaptive to changes. The vulnerability of celiac disease to wrongful assumptions and diagnosis, as well as misinterpretations, has prompted extensive research over the years to discover its detrimental effects, which, along with the rapid advancement of science, is necessary for a better understanding of its prevention, diagnosis, and long-term therapy.

CLINICAL TRIALS

Before proceeding with the discussion on the current drugs in development, it would be best to understand the clinical development process itself—the different phases in clinical development as well as the purposes of each phase. The clinical development process, even for experimental celiac disease drugs, starts in the creation and testing of compounds in a laboratory. A safety test is then done by running experiments on animals. After such, approval from the U.S. Food and Drug Administration should be obtained for further testing in humans. If obtained, clinical trials on humans will be conducted to test safety and efficacy. There are three different clinical trial phases. These may be done in clinical research centers, doctors' offices, or hospitals. If the medicine shows positive results throughout all the phases, the drug may then be marketed once approved by the FDA.

Each clinical trial phase is designed to provide an answer to specific concerns. After a preclinical trial that lasts about five years, a Phase 1 trial begins. In a Phase 1 clinical trial, the new drug or treatment is tested in a small group (20–80) of human respondents to evaluate if it is safe, to determine a typical range of dosage, and to know if there are side effects. Phase 1 clinical trials usually last for two years. It should be noted that Phase 1 trials are not designed to check effectiveness, so positive results do not imply that the drug will work. A Phase 2 clinical trial is performed in a larger group of people (100–300) to evaluate the effectiveness of the drug or treatment and to further test its safety. Phase 2 clinical trials are further subdivided into two stages, Phase 2a and Phase 2b, which are completed in about three years. In Phase 3, the drug or treatment is administered to a much larger group of people (1,000–3,000) to (1) confirm effectiveness, (2) further monitor the possible side effects, (3) compare the drug to a treatment already in use, and (4) gather information that supports the safe use of the drug or treatment in the study. This would take about three to five years. Pivotal 1 and Pivotal 2 are the subphases in Phase 3 clinical trials. Postmarketing studies may be done to draw further information, including the risks, benefits, and optimal use of the drug or treatment.

Patients who wish to participate in these trials should be aware of the potential risks, as well as the benefits, that they could get in doing such. When a drug is tested on a patient, the condition may get better or worse. There is no guarantee, as this is just a test. In *double-blind experiments* specifically, a patient may get a placebo drug. Patients should also understand that the drug or treatment they receive during the trial stage could lead to side effects. On the brighter side, participating in clinical trials is a good chance for a patient to work closely with a medical team that can evaluate the respondents' conditions. To top it all, this would be a great opportunity to contribute to the community. If the treatment is proven successful, it would be favorable not only to the respondents but also to the greater public.

ADVANCES IN CELIAC DISEASE PREVENTION RESEARCH

Although genetics is now known to play a role in the development of celiac disease, prevention of this disease is still possible.[1] While pharmacological alternatives to a strict gluten-free diet (GFD) are still a long way from being officially incorporated in celiac disease patient therapy, some measures, which may be applied even as early as infancy and which may delay, if not prevent, the onset of celiac disease, have already been explored.

Recent clinical studies have shown that breastfeeding significantly lowers the risk of developing celiac disease in children and infants, depending on the duration.[2] In the majority of the cases studied, infants breastfed for longer than two months had a considerably reduced risk of celiac disease than those breastfed for a shorter period of time. Evidence has also emerged regarding the protection that breastfeeding confers to infants while they are gradually and simultaneously introduced to gluten-containing food, although how long this protection against celiac disease lasts and what underlying mechanisms are involved is still uncertain.[3] On the other hand, the time of gluten introduction also has an impact on celiac disease development, with a window of the first gluten exposure between four and six months of age being the most advantageous period for lowering the risk of celiac disease.[4] The amount of gluten consumed during these first critical months, especially after weaning, is crucial as well, as gliadin, a component of gluten, was recently found to trigger a pathway that ultimately leads to increased intestinal permeability to certain antigens, and continuous exposure to large amounts of gluten at an early age can potentially make it worse.[5] Based on these findings, it is therefore safe to say that breastfeeding, along with the introduction of moderate amounts of gluten during the favorable "window period," is the recommended method of prevention, as it reduces the risk of developing celiac disease, especially for those who are genetically predisposed to have the disease early or later on in life.

Aside from breastfeeding and the right timing of gluten exposure in infants, the use of probiotics and regular vaccinations have also been proposed in the prevention of celiac disease. Large amounts as well as the abnormal composition of intestinal microbiota have been researched in patients with celiac disease, and although a concrete link between these two has yet to be established, regulating the intestinal microflora and how it induces inflammatory responses in the gastrointestinal tract and affects its permeability may be beneficial in combating the onset of celiac disease.[6] Since there is a correlation between the disease and EBV (Epstein-Barr virus) infection—one of the most common viral infections in humans, which has been found to activate the production of a key player in celiac disease development—vaccination might also be able to contribute to the prevention of celiac disease, but further studies are still needed to prove this.[7]

ADVANCES IN CELIAC DISEASE DIAGNOSTICS RESEARCH

Diagnosis of celiac disease has come a long way from what was initially a simple combination of serological examination and histological confirmation via duodenal biopsy, which, until now, still remains the gold standard in celiac disease diagnosis. Over the years, extensive research has shown that celiac disease is embodied by a wide variety of "generic" symptoms, such as anemia, weight loss, fatigue, steatorrhea, and immunoglobulin A deficiency (IgA), among others, all of which may or may not be entirely present in suspected patients and may or may not be caused by it.[8] This broad spectrum of clinical manifestations, along with complex associations with other conditions (e.g., osteoporosis, dermatitis herpetiformis, and malignant lymphoma), has prompted researchers to find better, more efficient methods of diagnosis that will not only lead to more conclusive results but also eliminate the possibility of false-positive correlations in the process.

Serological Testing

Initially, serological testing for celiac disease relied primarily on the presence and/or absence of antireticulin antibodies (ARA) and antigliadin antibodies (AGA) in patient serum. However, issues regarding the low specificity and sensitivity of these markers (particularly AGA, which has been reported to give highly false-positive results in patients whose intestinal problems are not caused by celiac disease) led researchers to the discovery and use of endomysial antibodies (EMA) and antitissue transglutaminase (ATA) antibodies usable for the diagnosis of celiac disease.[9]

Quantification of the antibodies for EMA and TTG or tissue transglutaminase in patient serum allows for a more specific method of verifying immunological response to gluten because TTG—which is normally present in the intestine—is attacked by ATAs during gluten-triggered immune response, while EMA is specifically produced by the body when it considers gluten as an antigen. Tests involving ATAs and EMAs have been found to increase in specificity and sensitivity considerably, providing a better diagnostic alternative and less uncertainties, especially when used in combination. [10]

EMA is detected via indirect immunofluorescence, a method that employs two different types of antibodies, one of which is specific to EMA (primary), while the other is targeted to the primary antibody (secondary) and labeled with a fluorescent dye. This dye emits a colored signal or fluorescence when exposed to a certain wavelength of light, and because any number of secondary antibodies can attach to the primary, this signal can be amplified, allowing for greater sensitivity. [11] The EMA assay, however, is qualitative rather than quantitative, and despite being more accurate than AGA-based tests, it corresponds more correctly to the degree of villous atrophy or erosion of the small intestine lining—which could vary between patients—introducing another undesirable possibility, this time for a false-positive result. [12] Hence there arose the necessity of developing a more appropriate method with parallel sensitivity and specificity to EMA tests, an assay now known as the tissue transglutaminase (TTG) test.

Due to advanced clinical- and evidence-based research, the TTG test is now one of the most commonly used diagnostic tests for celiac disease and employs ELISA, which shares a similarity with immunofluorescence in that it also makes use of two antibodies, a primary and a secondary, but differs in that the secondary antibody is chemically bound to an enzyme, which will enable the determination of a positive result by producing a colored reaction once it reacts with its appropriate substrate. Quantification is then made possible using a machine known as an ELISA reader, which translates the results into numerical data in a matter of minutes. Compared to other tests like those of AGAs and EMAs, TTG testing is more reliable, quantitative, and sensitive, as well as specific. However, since immunoglobulin (IgA) deficiency has also been observed in some patients with celiac disease, AGA, EMA, and TTG tests now also include

IgG-based tests in order to eliminate the possibility of false-negative results, which may arise in IgA-deficient patients. [13]

Interest in using the gliadin peptide as a marker in serological testing was rekindled only after the discovery that deamination of gliadin, an event facilitated by the enzyme TTG, enhances its binding to human leukocyte antigen HLA-DQ2. [14] Clinical researchers have found that this deamination process, meaning the removal of an amino group from an amino acid compound, converts glutamine residues within the gliadin peptide into glutamic acid, an event that eventually triggers a drastically amplified T-cell-mediated immune response. [15] Since these exaggerated immune responses that ultimately lead to damages in the small bowel have been established as typical, observable symptoms of celiac disease in positive patients, deamidated gliadin peptide (DGP) tests are now included in the repertoire of serological assays needed in order to confirm the presence of celiac disease. Indeed, compared to nondeamidated gliadin peptides used in early AGA tests, DGP performs much better as a serological marker, having been able to accurately correlate AGA positivity to celiac disease as opposed to the normal gliadin marker, which reportedly has a high rate of giving false-positive results. [16]

HLA-DQ Haplotyping

Despite the many advances in serological testing, which now provides a clearer picture of whether a person is really positive for celiac disease as compared to before, a more in-depth, DNA-based test was developed that does not rely on serum antibody levels in order to support, invalidate, or confirm uncertain diagnostic test results. This test, now widely used in celiac disease diagnosis, is the human leukocyte antigen (HLA) haplotyping. This genetic test screens for HLA genes (alleles) belonging to the HLA-D region of the chromosome, specifically HLA-DQ2 and HLA-DQ8, which are known to play a role in celiac disease progression via antigen presentation. [17] DNA for HLA typing is extracted from patient blood samples then subjected to a procedure called a polymerase chain (PCR) reaction in order to produce a large quantity of DNA copies. Because the prevalence of DQ2 is higher than DQ8, a positive result for either or both is possible, though it does not immediately mean a positive diagnosis for celiac disease, as DQ2 is found to be present even in people who lack celiac disease. [18] On the other hand, while a positive result might help corroborate serological and histological data pointing toward celiac disease, a negative result (for both) can completely eliminate the possibility. Hence, instead of being a stand-alone research method for celiac disease, HLA haplotyping is more a tool to aid in the diagnosis of persons with increased risk of developing celiac disease due to genetic associations (family), as well as to help clarify uncertain results from serological and/or histological tests.

ADVANCES IN LONG-TERM THERAPY RESEARCH

For many years since the discovery of celiac disease, the only long-term therapeutic option presented to patients has been a strict gluten-free diet (GFD). Recent research particularly in the fields of biochemistry and genetics have opened doors to patients for a wider therapeutic variety, but most of these alternatives are yet to provide a novel therapy that, in and by itself, completely eliminates the necessity to exclude gluten-containing food sources. Although a diet free of gluten has proven itself quite efficient in alleviating the symptoms of celiac disease in most cases, it is not without disadvantages. Aside from being relatively costly and isolating for patients mentally as well as socially, GFD also requires the use of supplements to provide nutritional needs that cannot be met by avoidance of gluten-containing foods, and there are some cases in which adhering to a strict GFD does not deliver the desired results.[19] Hence the need to find the means to address this problem has commanded great importance in recent years.

Gluten Modification and Detoxification

Initially, oats have been proposed as a substitute to wheat, barley, and rye products, but contamination with flour during production and the intolerance of some celiac disease patients to oats have led researchers to steer their focus toward gluten, the main culprit of celiac disease, and eventually to identify the toxic sequences present in the two main components of gluten: gliadins and glutenins.[20] Advances in genetics and, particularly, genetic manipulation techniques have since put these discoveries to good use and enabled the production of wheat variants with significantly reduced toxicity by either deleting or altering part of the gene that encodes for the immune-response-stimulating portion of gluten.[21] Similarly, enzymatic treatment and bacterial fermentation of flour utilizing lactic-acid-producing bacteria can alter the toxicity of gluten.[22] The use of TTG from a microorganism to introduce modifications in the immunodominant part of gliadin, a research process known as *transamidation*, has been reported to effectively reduce T-cell-mediated immune response and subdue gliadin activity in intestinal T-cell lines, respectively.[23]

Like genetic modifications, gluten detoxification offers another means of avoiding GFD by lowering the immunogenicity (the ability to trigger an immune response) of gliadin peptides, and this is usually achieved through oral therapy. Prolyl-endopeptidases (PEPs), which are enzymes found in bacteria, were found to be capable of digesting gluten into small fragments that lack T-cell stimulatory properties, making these enzymes potentially useful as components for oral supplements to be taken by celiac disease patients desiring gluten.[24] SC-PEP has since undergone modifications over the years in order to augment its activity and resistance to degradation by gastrointestinal enzymes. Moreover, SC-PEP has been tested together with EP-B2, an endoprotease enzyme that cleaves peptide bonds from germinated barley seeds for possible combination therapy.[25] Clinical researchers are also looking into another type of enzyme known as AN-PEP, which is produced by the fungus *Aspergillus niger* and which can help degrade gluten inside the body more rapidly.[26] This endorses the possibility of safe ingestion of gluten by celiac disease patients without inducing harmful inflammatory responses. The potential of *polymeric binder molecules* is also currently being explored, as these binders have the ability to bind gliadin in simulation studies, ultimately preventing the formation of immunogenic peptides and subsequently inflammation in the gastrointestinal tract.[27]

Although these recent developments show attractive benefits, the presence and involvement of gluten in these proposed treatments still threatens to cause unwanted effects despite lower toxicity and thus, potential substitutes to gluten have also been investigated. *Triticum monococcum*, for instance, an ancient wheat strain that possesses low immunogenic properties, has shown potential as a candidate for use in cereals that can be safely ingested by patients.[28] Psyllium, a plant used to produce mucilage commercially and another possible gluten alternative, has also been recently reported to produce promising results after dough made from it was used to bake bread and was tested in celiac disease sufferers.[29] All of these possible alternatives, however, are still undergoing preclinical or clinical trials in order to determine their safety for human consumption.

Regulation of Tissue Permeability

It has long been established by clinical research that permeability of the gastrointestinal tract is involved in celiac disease progression and that in celiac disease patients, this permeability, which is controlled by tight junctions, is compromised to a deleterious degree. Indeed, these junctions, which are responsible for controlling the extent to which ingested macromolecules may pass through the epithelial barriers of the gastrointestinal tract, are rendered weak and unregulated, resulting in antigens such as partially digested gluten and its components being free to travel across and induce responses such as severe inflammation. Therefore, modulation of these tight junctions, and, consequently, GI tract permeability, is of utmost importance and presents a logical target for new celiac disease research.

Zonulin inhibitors present a prospective solution to the problem of GI hyperpermeability in celiac disease patients. By inhibiting zonulin, a protein that increases intestinal permeability produced in large quantities by celiac disease patients due to the binding of gliadin to a signaling protein receptor CXCR3, absorption of these immunogenic gliadin peptides can be prevented. Larazotide acetate, a synthetic peptide also known as AT-1001, has been generated as a zonulin antagonist and reportedly invoked ideal responses in advanced clinical trials.[30] AT-1001 is a derivative of the Zonula occludens toxin (ZOT) produced by the bacteria *Vibrio cholera*, which binds to ZOT receptors to inhibit tight junction impairment.[31]

Scientists observed that when the intestine is exposed to gluten, zonulin is released in unusual amounts.[32] This is now known as pre-haptoglobin 2. It seemingly causes the tight junctions to open and thus increases permeability in the intestine, which is also known as leaky gut. Larazotide acetate, or AT-1001, is a peptide molecule engineered to induce the body to close the intestinal cell junctions in order to reduce or even eliminate leaky gut problems. Leaky gut is what causes inflammation among celiac disease patients. It should be taken at or shortly before gluten exposure to keep gluten effects in moderation.

AT-1001 once showed potential in treating celiac disease. Alba Therapeutics had a $25 million deal with another corporation for AT-1001 rights outside the United States and Japan. When trial results did not meet expectations, the latter company terminated the deal. This was a major development setback for AT-1001. However, in early 2011, a global bio-pharmaceutical company agreed with Alba for an option to acquire its total AT-1001 assets.[33] Indeed, the clinical trials done for larazotide acetate are a landmark in celiac disease research. It was the first clinical trial to be published detailing results of medical prevention of gluten-related toxicity. This drug is not expected to be a total remedy but, at best, it could protect a celiac disease sufferer from minimal amounts of gluten intake.

Inhibition of Antigens

Inhibition of the antigen process presents another possible treatment route for celiac disease. *Tissue transglutaminase* 2 (TTG2) in the individual with celiac disease mediates and enhances antigen presentation by enabling a process called deamidation, which causes specific gluten amino acid residues to be converted into glutamate. Glutamate, in turn, increases the affinity of T-cells to bind immunogenic gluten peptides due to HLAs, molecules present on the surface of antigen-presenting cells. This cascade of reactions leads to exaggerated immune response characteristics of symptomatic celiac disease in patients, but it opens up another therapeutic approach for celiac disease via inhibition of TTG2.[34] As a result, TTG2 inhibitors such as cystamine and imidazolium derivatives (L682777 and R-283), as well as dihydroisoxazole compounds, have been developed and subjected to animal studies with varying successes, necessitating further studies in order to assess and improve this mode of treatment for celiac disease.[35]

HLAs, especially of the DQ2 and DQ8 subtypes that are genetically linked to celiac disease development, are also good targets of antigen-presentation blockers. Because of the role HLAs play in celiac disease—that is, in presenting gliadin peptides to T-cells—HLA-DQ2- and HLA-DQ8-specific inhibitors have also been developed, respectively. In particular, HLA-DQ2 inhibitors are synthesized by altering a specific part of it that is said to trigger inflammatory response, rendering it insusceptible to T-cells, all the while retaining its affinity to DQ2.[36] New research suggests that the use of a positional scanning nonapeptide library in the generation of HLA blockers was reported to yield optimum results.[37] This strategy is derived from positional scanning synthetic combinatorial libraries (PS-SCL), a biometric analysis commonly used in T-cell-related cancer research that allows for the generation of new chemical libraries (an index of various chemicals and their corresponding structures) from already existing ones.[38] By using a nonapeptide library in a positional scanning format, HLA blockers with desirably high affinity to HLA-DQ2 have been synthesized.

Inflammation and Immune Suppression

Inflammation in the gastrointestinal tract due to gluten-induced immune activation is one of the most common symptoms of celiac disease. This, however, can easily be alleviated by consistent adherence to GFD, except in patients with *refractory celiac disease (RCD)*. RCD type 1 is defined by the appearance of histologically normal lymphocytes (one type of white blood cells), whereas RCD type 2 is defined by the presence of abnormal intraepithelial lymphocytes (IELs), followed by the possible development of a cancer called enteropathy-associated T-cell lymphoma (EATL). However, persistent inflammation, among other symptoms, is common in both RCD types.[39] The use of corticosteroids such as budesonide in RCD patients has been found to be effective, although not consistently.[40] Immunosuppressive therapy, including the use of interferon-gamma (INF-γ) and tumor necrosis factor-alpha (TNF-α) inhibitors, seems beneficial to RCD type 1 patients, while RCD type 2 patients may respond more to drugs such as cladribine, a medication used to treat hairy cell leukemia (HCL) and multiple sclerosis (MS), and stem cell treatment.[41] Both INF-γ and TNF-α are pro-inflammatory factors that activate the expression of metalloproteinases (MMPs), enzymes that trigger villous atrophy, another symptom of celiac disease. Therefore, inhibiting these factors may alleviate the onset of celiac disease.[42]

New research also suggests a better way of blocking interleukin-15 (IL-15), which plays a major role in the development of RCD and its associated conditions by enhancing the binding of epithelial MICA, a stress-induced antigen, resulting in a reversal of intestinal damage in animal models.[43] This suggests a possible solution to the extreme gastrointestinal injury sustained by patients suffering more severe types of celiac disease. A University of Chicago research study conducted in mice that went through genetic alterations to exhibit celiac disease showed that blocking interleukin-15 or IL-15, an inflammatory protein, may help treat celiac disease symptoms and prevent celiac disease development in people who are possibly at risk.[44] The study on mice showed a reversal of disease symptoms, enabling the mice to eat gluten again. According to the researchers, IL-15 may drive intolerance to gluten. It is essential to find pathways to block it to develop potential celiac disease therapies.

Alvine Pharmaceuticals is a private company that develops biological products targeting autoimmune or inflammatory diseases. By far, it has made the most progress among the drug companies in the clinical research race to develop a new treatment for celiac disease. Proteins are made up of amino acids. The sequence of amino acids, which are contained in the middle of protein segments or peptides, determines the characteristics of each protein. Glutamine and proline are amino acid sequences in gluten molecules responsible for triggering celiac response. In order to eliminate gluten effects, the peptides should be broken up. This would require an enzyme. ALV003 is a mixture of two proteases, potent digestive enzymes that can help break down gluten proteins before obtaining reaction from the immune system. For optimal results, ALV003 must rapidly and effectively degrade gluten proteins at locations that will stop or destroy any peptides that could cause an immune response.[45]

Two separate Phase 1 studies were completed: pharmacokinetic—how the body reacts to the drug—and pharmacodynamic—how the drug affects the body.[46] These studies involved both celiac disease patients and nonceliacs as controls. In the data presented at the Digestive Diseases Week Conference in 2009, ALV003 was found to be pharmacokinetically stable and exhibited pharmacodynamic effects in the human stomach.[47] A Phase 2a study included a daily administration of ALV003 for six weeks to celiac disease patients.[48] This was in conjunction with a gluten-free diet. To the delight of scientists around the world, the study demonstrated that ALV003 could lessen the density of mucosal injury in the small intestine.

Test results of the drug P(HEMA-CO-SS) (now called BL-7010) on mice showed a reduction of the immune system response to gluten.[49] The drug binds to gluten protein, which lessens gluten's toxicity. It then ushers the gluten through the digestive system and out from the body with the stool. Although it has not been tested on humans, laboratory experiments performed with biopsy specimens from people with celiac disease proved that BL-7010 may help to pacify the reaction of the immune system to gluten. As with the other drugs currently in development, BL-7010 is expected to protect celiac disease sufferers from mild to moderate cross-contamination of gluten in food. It still will not allow large amounts of gluten intake.

Clinical trials have been completed in people with celiac disease observing a gluten-free diet and purposefully infected with *necator Americanus*, a species of parasitic hookworm that thrives in the small intestines of hosts, including humans. [50] Study results showed that hookworm infection led not only to parasite-specific immunity but also to the modification of the respondent's immune response to gluten. [51] The use of *necator Americanus* is in experimentation at Princess Adelaide University in Australia. It aims to provide better tolerance and reduced symptoms in gluten challenges. [52]

Traficet-EN is engineered to inhibit C-C chemokine receptor type 9, a protein encoded in humans by the CCR9 gene, for gut T-cell homing. [53] Phase 2 clinical trials were initiated by ChemoCentryx to study the potential of this treatment for celiac disease patients. The study evaluated its effect on respondents in terms of mucosal morphology and inflammation in the small intestine, comparing it to that of the placebo. Further trials will be launched to gain an indication for Traficet-EN in the treatment of people with celiac disease. [54]

Clinical Research Advances for Refractory Celiac Disease

People with Type II RCD usually observe that their symptoms are being resolved through steroids and azathioprine, but they do not experience intestinal healing. Worse, it seemingly does not give them protection against NHL. Cladribine, a powerful intravenous drug for chemotherapy particularly administered to patients with leukemia, has been tested in Type II RCD patients. A clinical trial performed in the Netherlands showed a positive effect of Cladribine in calming refractory celiac disease, causing symptoms to be resolved and the intestine to begin to heal in almost 60 percent of respondents. Despite this, it is still doubted that the drug will prevent EATL or *enteropathy-associated T-cell lymphoma*, which is a rare but deadly type of lymphoma.

Type II RCD patients suffer a disproportionate degree of affliction. Cladribine has been the first choice of drug treatment for Type II RCD. About 50 percent of the patients experienced intestinal healing and symptomatic relief. Additionally, there was an 83 percent overall three-year and five-year survival observed in respondents who responded to the treatment. No significant increase in lymphoma rates was noted. The researchers concluded this treatment to be promising, with excellent clinical and histological responses and a less frequent EATL transition. [55]

For Type II RCD patients who respond negatively to all the treatments, autologous hematopoietic stem cell transplant (auto-SCT) is being considered. A celiac disease center has tested this procedure, in which stem cells are harvested from the bone marrow, grown in a laboratory, and transplanted back through a process of high-dose chemotherapy. If not done properly, the risk of this procedure could even lead to death. A trial result shows that eleven of thirteen Type II RCD patients who have undergone auto-SCT experienced significant improvement within a year. A patient was reported dead due to complications, one developed EATL after four years, while the majority exhibited favorable clinical improvement. The authors concluded that auto-SCT is feasible and promising. [56]

Vaccination

Following the success of a study on a mouse model immunized with an immunodominant DQ2-specific gluten, a gluten vaccine called Nexvax2 has been designed and has gone through clinical trials. [57] This vaccine contains a mixture of highly recognized gluten peptides and, following the same principle behind the vaccination for common viral infections, it aims to induce immune tolerance to gluten in people with celiac disease. Nexvax2 is developed using ImmusanT, a peptide-based vaccine. Approximately 90 percent of celiac disease sufferers have the HLA-DQ2 gene. These patients are the candidates for Nexvax2. Vaccines are commonly known as a way to protect the body against infectious disease, in which materials based on a bacteria or virus is introduced to the tissues and organs. This would provoke an immune reaction to that specific material. If the person is later exposed to that infectious agent, the body has the ability to attack it. The Nexvax2 vaccine does not work in the same way. The treatment approach is called *immunotherapy*, in which the idea is not to provoke a strong gluten response, but rather to repeatedly introduce small amounts of this so-called foreign substance so that the immune system would be tricked into considering gluten as not foreign at all. Simply said, it is designed to reduce the intestine's reaction to gluten.

This vaccine works through the concept of immune-system tolerance to a foreign antigen or entity. When the immune system has already learned to react badly or develop sensitivity to a foreign antigen through continuous exposure, especially if there are no danger signals, it may tolerate or suppress its response to that specific foreign antigen. The goal in developing Nexvax2 is to identify protein sequences or peptides that trigger celiac response. At best, it is expected to suppress such peptide response even to other sequences in the gluten molecule triggering a response to celiac disease. The Nexvax2 vaccine targets the gluten-specific T-cells and reprograms them to act as allies. They stop T-cells or immune cells from being activated by, and responding defensively to, gluten. The goal is not only immune response prevention but also the restoration of gluten tolerance and intestinal health. [58]

This therapeutic treatment has already undergone a proof-of-concept preclinical development and Phase 1 clinical trial in Australia, New Zealand, and the United States to ensure safety and potential effects at larger doses. Patients could therefore have a normal diet without causing injury to the intestinal wall. The lining of the intestine could also be repaired over time and will remain healthy. Booster shots would be recommended for periodic treatment reinforcement, and, in addition, Nexvax2 is designed to help improve the quality of life of people suffering HLA-DQ2-related celiac disease. All in all, vaccination has been proven to be safe and well tolerated by volunteer patients, but further clinical trials are still needed in order to determine its efficacy. [59]

ANALYSIS

The development of celiac disease involves numerous factors, including genetic and environmental ones. The complicated interplay among these elements during celiac disease progression has urged clinical researchers to continue to delve deeper into its mysteries, arming people with enough knowledge at present to prevent, manage, and alleviate its symptoms, if not cure it completely.

Part III

Other Manifestations

7

MENTAL OUTCOMES OF CELIAC DISEASE

A person's mental health can be affected by a diagnosis of any disease, including celiac.[1] Mental disorders may arise if the person is unable to cope with a distress (i.e., pain) or disease (i.e., celiac disease). There have been reports of psychiatric symptoms and disorders linked to celiac disease. The most commonly occurring are anxiety disorders and depressive and mood disorders.[2]

GENERAL MENTAL OUTCOMES

Many works of research show that celiac disease can develop through psychological problems and that it influences general mental health.[3] A person's thinking (cognition), emotions, and behaviors may be affected by celiac disease. Although there has been limited research conducted to find out more about the relationship connecting mental health and the restrictiveness of the gluten-free diet, the research conducted until the present does show some link between mental functioning and celiac disease. A celiac disease patient's thought processes are directly affected when a person has a problem with cognitive functions. Examples include attention and concentration difficulties, brain fog (mental confusion, difficulty thinking clearly), memory lapses, and forgetfulness. Nutritional deficiencies and behavioral issues related to celiac disease, both pre- and postdiagnosis, may have an impact on cognitive function, which stymies mental health. It can also result in irritability, fatigue, lack of energy, eating issues, impatience, anxiety, and ADHD-related problems. Emotionally acknowledging that they are not normal while not knowing the exact reason as to why they are feeling such a way can cause severe emotional and mental stress in already diagnosed patients as well as undiagnosed patients with a genetic predisposition for celiac disease, which can even worsen or aggravate the situation.[4]

Celiac Disease and Mental Stress

The development of autoimmune diseases, including celiac disease, implicates physical and psychological stresses. Various studies conducted on animals and humans give evidence of the effects that sundry stressors have on immune function. Moreover, a high proportion of patients reported uncommon emotional stress before disease onset, as found in many retrospective studies. Research has shown that stress is a contributing factor, and it may also be a disease aggravator. Unfortunately, this is a vicious cycle because not only does the disease cause considerable stress in patients, but the stress can also trigger the disease.[5]

Celiac Disease and Cognition

Cognition is the ability of the brain to process, retain, and manage information. This includes the ability to reason, judge, perceive, comprehend, be attentive, and keep a memory. These abilities are imperative in a celiac disease sufferer's daily life. A disruption or impairment in these functions can cause the person to have memory lapses, attention and concentration difficulties, and mental confusion.[6] Researchers have suggested that nutrient deficiencies related to celiac disease can lessen cognitive functioning, particularly in newly diagnosed patients.[7] Furthermore, there are studies showing that the immune response triggered by the disease can lead to inflammation that can impede the flow of blood going to the brain, resulting to *hypoperfusion*. A decreased cerebral oxygen level is detrimental to mental health, for it causes decreased brain activity. This will lead to headaches, memory lapses, difficulties in concentrating, and inattentiveness.[8]

Celiac Disease and Behavior

There are studies that show that sometimes, individuals with celiac disease have reported issues that influence their behavior and interpersonal relationships.[9] The most common are hyperactivity or hypoactivity, ataxia, and problems with eating and weight.

Hyperactivity

When the celiac disease patient gains an excessive increase in muscular functions and activities, he or she is said to be hyperactive.[10] Clinical studies prove that patients with celiac disease are hyperactive because they have attention and concentration difficulties.[11] A person suffering from celiac disease can become restless and talk excessively while interrupting others often. These can have an impact on behavior, thus causing strains in relationships.

Eating and Weight Problems

There are numerous ways in which these issues are manifested in patients with celiac disease. Some celiac sufferers find it difficult to abide by a prescribed diet. Gluten-free diets often have more calories and fats.[12] Thus, the patients fear gaining weight. Others become overly cautious with their food. This may lead to a decrease in food intake for fear of ingesting something that will aggravate their condition.[13] Individuals with these symptoms are prompted to lessen their social interactions. These issues create a negative impact on the person's social and emotional well-being.

IN-DEPTH DISCUSSION OF SEVERE MENTAL OUTCOMES

Schizophrenia is a severe disorder characterized by partial or total loss of contact with reality, intellectual breakdown, and bizarre emotional reactions or none whatsoever. Celiac disease sufferers who also have schizophrenia can experience symptoms such as flattened affect, delusions, hallucinations, and dissociation from self and from the real world. Even though there are still differences of opinion on whether schizophrenia is purely psychological or neurological, or a combination of both, what is becoming very clear is that schizophrenia has a connection with wheat, rye, barley, gluten intolerance, and, therefore, celiac disease, at least in people who already have a predisposition, be it genetic or environmental, for schizophrenia or related personality disorders such as schizoid and schizotypal personality disorders. The link between schizophrenia and celiac disease was originally uncovered during a study that was trying to discover the connection in gluten intolerance, schizophrenia, and celiac disease.[14]

According to researchers, gluten may be an environmental factor for developing schizophrenia when the patient is already genetically predisposed to celiac disease.[15] When genetic and environmental risk factors come together, the chances of developing schizophrenia, diabetes, or any other disease are dramatically increased. A study has shown that more than 30 percent of people with schizophrenia had high levels of antibodies against gluten.[16] Researchers claim that, should this theory prove correct, a change in the patients' diet could improve their quality of life by reducing or controlling the symptoms of diabetes, schizophrenia, and its related disorders.[17] Not only would changing to a gluten-free diet be beneficial for patients who are already suffering from schizophrenia or diabetes, but an early diagnosis of both schizophrenia's risk genes or risk environmental factors (such as gluten) and celiac disease could also set in motion an early conversion to a gluten-free diet, which would effectively stop schizophrenia from developing later in life.[18]

Anxiety Disorders

When anxiety no longer functions as a signal for needed response to stimuli, it instead becomes chronic and permeates a major role in a celiac disease patient's life, leading to maladaptive behavior and emotional disability. Of all mental disorders in the United States, anxiety disorders have the highest prevalence. One out of four adults is affected, and it is more prevalent in women than men.[19]

Anxiety, which is more or less a vague feeling of apprehension or dread, is the body's natural response to external or internal stimuli. Experiencing anxiety is inevitable in life, but it can serve as a positive motivation to the person to resolve a crisis.[20] Normally, when a person experiences anxiety, the body responds by activating the autonomic nervous system, which generates the involuntary activities involved in self-preservation. It stimulates the adrenal medulla to secrete adrenalin, causing the body to shunt blood from the gastrointestinal and reproductive systems and increasing the release of cortisol (stress hormone) to free glucose to fuel the heart, muscles, and central nervous system.[21] In celiac disease, the surface epithelium of the small bowel is damaged. Due to the decreased blood flow to the gastrointestinal system during the presence of a stressor, the reparation of the small bowel is delayed, resulting in the leakage of undigested food particles and toxins in the bloodstream and eliciting the immune system to respond.[22] When these toxins are left unresolved, they will reach the brain, leading to inflammation. Inflammation in the hippocampus region of the brain, which is responsible for mood, will interfere in the production of certain neurotransmitters such as serotonin and gamma-aminobutyric acid.[23] These neurotransmitters are responsible for regulating anxiety. Symptoms of anxiety include the following: [24]

agitation: the person feels tense, confused, or irritable
restlessness: inability to relax, with a mild feeling of discomfort
irritability: sensitivity to stimuli
lack of sleep: may cause irritability and agitation
anger: severely anxious patients express anger as a result of decreased thought processes

Anxiety may be beneficial or harmful for an individual with celiac disease. It depends on the degree and duration as well as the ability of the person to cope with the stimuli. There are four levels for anxiety: mild, moderate, severe, and panic.

- Mild anxiety is when the person senses that there is something amiss and needs special attention.[25] This in fact helps the celiac disease patient to focus and be attentive to learn, think, act, feel, and come up with a solution for the problem. Mild anxiety motivates people to engage in activities directed toward the resolution of the problem.[26]
- Moderate anxiety is felt when there is an alarming feeling that something is definitely wrong.[27] Despite still being able to learn and process information to solve the problem, assistance is needed.

In this case, the patient is having difficulty staying attentive and becomes nervous and agitated easily.[28]

- Severe anxiety is demonstrated by the inability to focus and solve basic problems.[29] Reasoning abilities decrease, and the person becomes restless, irritable, and angry.[30] The sympathetic nervous system is activated, thereby increasing the vital signs and muscle tone.
- Panic occurs when the celiac disease patient's area of focus significantly decreases compared to severe anxiety. He or she is unable to cope, and cognitive processes focus more on the defensive.[31]

Causes of Anxiety Disorders

The pathophysiology of anxiety disorders is not too clear. It is believed that gamma-aminobutyric acid or GABA and serotonin, both neurotransmitters, have a major role in regulating anxiety.[32] GABA is an inhibitory neurotransmitter that functions as the body's natural anti-anxiety agent. It reduces cell excitability, resulting in a decrease in the rate of neuronal firing.[33] In anxiety disorders, GABA seems to be dysfunctional, impeding the management of anxiety. Serotonin is essential in regulating anxiety. Any interruption in the synthesis of this neurotransmitter can affect mood. Norepinephrine, an excitatory neurotransmitter, is responsible for physiological shifts such as cardiovascular changes during high stress. Research has identified that dysregulation in norepinephrine in the parts of the brain associated in regulating anxiety can be either overactive or underactive.[34]

Diagnosis of Anxiety Disorders

Undiagnosed celiac disease patients often report feelings of anxiety, nervousness, short temper, or irritability, which are associated with their physiologic symptoms. These are brought about by malabsorption resulting from nutrient deficiencies.[35] The damage in the small intestines disrupts the absorption of essential nutrients, such as vitamin B complex, iron, calcium, and vitamin K, needed in the proper functioning of some organs. Without these nutrients, the celiac disease sufferer is unable to produce tryptophan and monoamine precursors required in the synthesis of key neurotransmitters such as serotonin and gamma-aminobutyric acid, upsetting the biochemical balance and thereby triggering anxiety-related symptoms.[36]

In addition, the damaged small intestines cause the undigested food particles and toxins to escape to the bloodstream through the small openings in the small bowel.[37] These by-products circulate throughout the body, triggering an autoimmune response.[38] Antibodies are produced to attack these foreign bodies, but these can also attack normal cells or tissues. As a result, inflammation occurs. If this reaches the brain, its functions are compromised. Neuronal signals will be disrupted, and release of neurotransmitters and hormones will be unregulated, leading to emotional imbalance in the person with celiac disease. It is difficult to determine if the individual is, in fact, suffering from an anxiety disorder in relation to present disease condition, life events, or both, because anxiety can be experienced at any point. Works of research pertaining to the association of existing celiac disease and the possibility of anxiety disorders before the individual is diagnosed are very unclear. There is a study negating the link between anxiety and celiac disease, but another suggests that symptoms are present even before an official diagnosis.[39]

Diagnosed individuals are found to be at a higher risk of acquiring anxiety disorders. A longitudinal study has learned that anxiety is more prevalent in women with celiac disease in comparison with women who do not have the disease.[40] Furthermore, experts discovered that children with celiac disease are more prone to anxiety than their healthy counterparts.[41] Anxiety in celiac disease is usually related to the challenges they will encounter during the disease management. Those who worry over the outcomes of the treatment may develop generalized anxiety disorder or panic disorder, while those who fret about cross-contamination may develop obsessive-compulsive behavior through a preoccupation with cleaning surfaces—behavior that, if left unmanaged, may turn into an official clinical disorder.

Treatment

Combining medication and therapy is the most effective form of treatment for anxiety disorders in celiac disease patients. Drugs used to treat these disorders are benzodiazepines for all types of anxiety disorders; tricyclic antidepressants such as clomipramine for obsessive-compulsive disorder; a beta blocker such as clonidine for panic disorder; and selective serotonin reuptake inhibitor (SSRI) antidepressants such as fluoxetine for panic disorder, obsessive-compulsive disorder, and generalized anxiety disorder.[42] Cognitive-behavioral therapies used for the management of these disorders are the following: [43]

Positive reframing: The therapist instructs the patient to turn negative thoughts into positive ones during panic episodes. These positive thoughts can be listed to be used in case of panic attacks.

Decatastrophizing: The person is encouraged to use thought stopping as well as distraction techniques to keep him from focusing on pessimistic thoughts.

Assertiveness training: Fostering self-assurance is the goal of this therapy. It helps the celiac disease sufferer to take control over life events and create interpersonal negotiations by being able to communicate concerns to other people.

Dementia

Dementia is the general loss of mental function, such as memory, to the point that it becomes a clear mental disability to the sufferer, affecting almost every sense of the celiac disease patient's life. If a person were to hear the term *dementia*, the first two things that would come to mind are most likely lunacy or psychosis (which is entirely false), or Alzheimer's disease, the most common form of dementia. Though less known, dementia can be caused by several other factors, such as vitamin deficiency, a common consequence of celiac disease.[44] Research from the Mayo Clinic's neurologists has shown a possible connection between celiac disease and dementia.[45] They did this through the examination of 13 patients' medical histories, all of which showed severe mental decline in a two-year period since the gastrointestinal symptoms of celiac disease manifested. In five of the cases, gastrointestinal and mental symptoms appeared simultaneously.[46] Two of the patients followed a gluten-free diet, which helped with celiac symptoms and even reversed dementia, and mental function was fully restored in one of the patients.[47] Besides vitamin deficiency, another common factor in celiac disease and dementia is copper deficiency and/or toxicity. In fact, the relationship of autoimmune diseases and environmental factors, such as the ones that could provoke copper toxicity, is becoming more apparent. The discovery of this connection can lead to the development of new therapies for improving intestinal permeability and mucosal regulatory T-cells, as well as the neutralization of inflammatory cytokines.[48]

Mood Disorders

Occasionally, everyone (including celiac disease patients) has their low periods in which they feel sad and mentally exhausted. Sadness in mood may be a response to misfortunes such as an existing disease. When these become excessive and start interfering with an individual's life, mood disorders, also called affective disorders, develop.[49] Mental health experts have found that the mood disorders common in patients with celiac disease are major depressive disorder and dysthymia, although there are studies indicating that bipolar disorder is included as well.[50]

Simply put, celiac disease has been linked to depression.[51] A disturbance in mood, thoughts, and body that involves feelings of sadness, disappointment, hopelessness, loneliness, doubt, and guilt in varying degrees is known as depression.[52] It interferes with the celiac disease sufferer's cognition, affect, behavior, and physical health. Although the celiac disease patient may not suffer from depression, the condition is persistent when he or she does.[53] When an individual encounters a provocation, whether external or internal, he or she may choose how to respond by either denying or accepting its existence. During this period of depression, activities of daily living (ADLs) are compromised, which may lead to the suppression of some of the functions of the body such as the production of certain biochemical substances necessary for regulating mood. Patients with celiac disease, particularly the newly diagnosed, have nutrient deficiencies due to malabsorption in the small bowel.[54] This all results in the inability of the body to produce tryptophan and monoamine precursors essential in synthesizing key neurotransmitters such as serotonin and norepinephrine.[55] These neurotransmitters function by energizing the body to mobilize during stress.[56] Inadequate serotonin and norepinephrine are found to promote depression.[57] Symptoms of depression include the following:

moodiness: a condition in which the person becomes temperamental
   and sullen
anergia: lack of energy
loss of appetite: this may be attributed to anergia

sleep disturbances: this may cause moodiness

Causes of Mood Disorders

There are a handful of theories regarding the cause of mood disorders, but the most recent studies focus on biochemical imbalance as the cause.[58] Psychosocial and interpersonal stimuli seem to trigger changes in the physiologic and chemical aspects of the brain, resulting in an alteration in the balance of neurotransmitters.[59] The neurotransmitters believed to be involved in mood disorders are serotonin and norepinephrine.[60] Serotonin plays a major role in regulating behavior. Deficits in this particular neurotransmitter have been found in individuals experiencing depression. Similarly, norepinephrine may also be deficient in depression.[61]

Diagnosis of Mood Disorders

Depression symptoms (part of the group of symptoms seen in mood disorders) are often reported both before and after the diagnosis of individuals with celiac disease. Prior to diagnosis, many individuals report feelings of depression. This may be due to the untreated symptoms of celiac disease, such as gastrointestinal distress, taking their toll on the person's physiological and psychosocial well-being. Similar to anxiety disorders, nutrient deficiencies contribute to the development of mood disorders such as depression. It has been observed that malabsorption of key vitamins such as B12 and folic acid results in depression by decreasing the precursors needed in the production of serotonin and norepinephrine.[62]

Moreover, patients exposed to continuous stressors have a consistent signal for the brain to release the stress hormone cortisol, which stops digestion by further aggravating the damage in the small bowel. Autoimmune response is triggered, and inflammation occurs.[63] Undigested food particles and toxins escape through the openings in the celiac disease sufferer's small bowel and into the bloodstream. These particles will further invoke a response from the immune system, which will release cytokines, which are pro-inflammatory peptide or protein molecules known to cross the blood/brain barrier, thereby gaining direct access to the brain.[64] Cytokines may inadvertently cause inflammation in the brain, resulting in the decreased regeneration rate of brain cells. Slow regeneration of brain cells affects its functioning; thus, depression develops.[65]

Diagnosed celiac disease patients have difficulty coming to terms with living with an additional chronic condition. Treatment for celiac disease throughout the person's entire life can be a source of frustration and isolation when most social events and interactions involve eating. Also, restrictions in diet can cause grief and loss. If these symptoms intensify and become persistent, they can interfere with the patient's life and cause a severe mood disorder, particularly major depressive disorder and dysthymia.

Types of Mood Disorders

The following are the types of mood disorders related to celiac disease:

- According to official psychiatry guidelines, major depressive disorder is diagnosed when sad mood or lack of interest in daily life activities last for around two or more weeks with at least four other symptoms of depression.[66] These symptoms can be anhedonia or having no pleasure or joy in life, changes in eating habits, weight gain, self-esteem issues, energy deficiencies, difficulties in concentrating and decision making, and altered goals.[67]
- Dysthymic disorder is found in a celiac disease patient when there is a depressed mood for most days for a minimum of two years, with some symptoms that are less in severity and do not meet the criteria for major depressive disorder.[68] Two of the following symptoms are included in this mental disorder: decrease in energy and self-esteem, disturbances in sleeping and eating habits, feelings of hopelessness and irritability, fatigue, and difficulty concentrating.[69]
- A celiac disease sufferer can have bipolar disorder when his or her mood switches between extremes of mania and depression.[70] Mania is described as an abnormally and constantly elevated or irritable mood lasting for about a week or more.[71] During an episode of mania, at least three of the following symptoms must be manifested: distractibility; racing, unconnected thoughts or ideas; pressured speech, sense of grandeur or exaggerated self-esteem; decreased need for sleep; and psychomotor agitation. Hallucinations and delusions may also be experienced during a manic episode.[72]

Past works of research have observed that depressive disorders are features of celiac disease. It has been found that symptoms of depressive disorders are present upon diagnosis of celiac patients.[73] At present, researchers are still studying the relationship of celiac disease and mood disorders. A recent survey involving over 175 women with celiac disease yielded a result of 37 percent of these women having depression.[74]

Treatment

Drugs used to treat major depressive disorder in celiac disease sufferers are called antidepressants. These include atypical antidepressants, selective serotonin reuptake inhibitors, cyclic antidepressants, and monoamine oxidase inhibitors. The medication of choice is chosen based on the client's symptoms and age. Physical health needs and history of past drug intake are also taken into account.[75]

- Selective serotonin reuptake inhibitors (SSRIs) inhibit serotonin reuptake and have few sedating, cardiovascular, and anticholinergic side effects. For most patients, SSRIs are effective for their relatively safe usage and low side effects, which make people more apt in complying with the treatment regimen, especially for older adults.[76]
- Cyclic antidepressants, particularly tricylics, are the oldest known medication used for depression. They alleviate symptoms of depression such as hopelessness, anhedonia, and helplessness. Cyclic antidepressants are also indicated for panic disorder, obsessive-compulsive disorder, and eating disorder. There are two categories for these antidepressants—namely, tricylics and heterocyclics. Both medications need 10–14 days (a lag period) prior to achieving the desired serum level for altering symptoms and six weeks before reaching full effect. Being the oldest, they cost less and have generic forms available.[77]
- If the person does not respond adequately or they have side effects from SSRIs, atypical depressants are usually used. They include the following medications: venlafaxine (Effexor) to block serotonin, norepinephrine, and dopamine (weakly) reuptake; bupropion (Wellbutrin) prevents norepinephrine and dopamine (weakly) reuptake; duloxetine (Cymbalta) selectively inhibits serotonin and norepinephrine; nefazodone (Serzone) blocks the reuptake of serotonin and norepinephrine with few side effects; and mirtazapine (Remer-

on) inhibits serotonin and norepinephrine as well and it has fewer sexual side effects, although it has a higher incidence rate of sedation, weight gain, and anticholinergic reactions.[78]

- Monoamine oxidase inhibitors (MAOIs): Of all antidepressants, monoamine oxidase inhibitors are infrequently used due to their adverse effects, which are fatal, such as hypertensive crisis. The crisis is a life-threatening condition in which the person can have symptoms leading to cerebral hemorrhage resulting in death. In addition, interactions with a variety of prescription and over-the-counter drugs are also observed. A celiac disease patient who is undergoing an antidepressant therapy must allot five to six weeks of washout period prior to shifting to MAOIs.[79]

- Electroconvulsive therapy (ECT): This type of therapy is only used for select groups who do not respond to any antidepressants or those who suffer from adverse effects of therapeutic doses. ECT is done by applying electrodes to the head and delivering an electrical impulse to the patient's brain, causing a "healthy" form of seizure. The resultant shock is believed to stimulate the brain to correct the biochemical imbalance of depression. Usually, a person undergoes ECT for 6–15 treatments, which are scheduled three times a week. Improvement can be seen after a minimum of 6 treatments and maximum benefit after 12–15 treatments.[80]

  Preparing a celiac disease patient for ECT is similar to preparing for an outpatient minor surgery: the patient is placed on nil per os (NPO) after midnight, removing nail polish, voiding prior to the procedure, and starting an intravenous line for medication administration. The medications given are the following: a short-acting anaesthetic so the patient will not be awake during the process, and a muscle relaxant or paralytic (succinylcholine) to achieve muscle relaxation for safety reasons. Oxygen is also provided. After the procedure, the patient is mildly confused or disoriented. Short-term memory loss may also happen. The health care professional also assesses whether the gag reflex has returned before introducing anything by mouth. ECT is also indicated for individuals who had a relapse. After ECT, the patient is prescribed an antidepressant therapy to prevent relapse.

- Psychotherapy: The most effective treatment for affective disorders, specifically depressive disorders, is combining both medications and psychotherapy.[81] Interpersonal therapy can help a celiac disease patient to deal with difficulties in interpersonal relationships. Behavior therapy aims to decrease the negative interactions of the patient and encourages positive ones, while cognitive therapy turns the person's distorted thinking into positive, realistic thoughts.

NEURODEVELOPMENTAL DISORDERS

Attention Deficit Hyperactivity Disorder

Clinical reports prove that ADHD is associated with celiac disease.[82] Untreated celiac disease in children and adolescents tends to manifest a very disruptive behavior, and they seem to have difficulty concentrating. In celiac disease, toxins from the villi lesions can escape into the bloodstream.[83] When these toxins reach the brain, inflammation occurs, and *cerebral perfusion* is compromised.[84] Decreased blood flow to the brain will decrease the oxygen levels, resulting in an impairment in its functions, such as concentration difficulties in ADHD patients.[85]

Inattentiveness, impulsiveness, and overreactiveness are characteristics of attention deficit hyperactivity disorder (ADHD). This mental health disorder is common in children. An estimated 3–5 percent of all school-aged children are affected by this mental health disorder.[86] Usually, attention deficit hyperactivity disorder is diagnosed once the child starts attending school because this is the time when the symptoms significantly affect behavior and performance.[87] Some parents report that symptoms start to manifest earlier, although it is difficult to distinguish between normal active behavior and excessive hyperactive behavior.[88] It had been formerly believed that diagnosed children outgrew this disorder, but recent studies confirm that it can persist into adulthood. Approximately 30–50 percent of these children manifest symptoms well into adulthood.[89]

Causes of ADHD

Even with extensive research, the specific cause of ADHD still remains unknown.[90] Environmental toxins and damage to the brain altering its structures and functions combined with any brain abnormalities present during childhood may precipitate ADHD.[91] Studying the brain images of people diagnosed with ADHD, researchers have suggested that metabolism in the frontal lobes has decreased.[92] The frontal lobes are necessary in controlling impulse, attention, and organization.[93] Other studies show that there is a decreased cerebral perfusion in the frontal cortex in children with ADHD and atrophy in the said structure in young adults with a history of ADHD.[94]

Diagnosis

Very active or difficult-to-handle children are often misdiagnosed with ADHD. To avoid misdiagnosis, a pediatric neurologist or child psychiatrist must be the one to assess and evaluate the child for ADHD. To diagnose a child, in at least six months he or she must have manifested at least six persistent symptoms of inattention and/or hyperactivity-impulsivity.[95] Symptoms of inattentive behaviors, whether speaking of a celiac disease patient or not, are as follows: missing details, making careless mistakes, being forgetful of daily activities, difficulty focusing or paying attention, being easily distracted, avoiding mentally taxing tasks, difficulty organizing, and not following through on assignments or chores.[96] Meanwhile, symptoms of hyperactive-impulsive behaviors are as follows: intrusive, fidgety, impatient, leaving his or her seat often, always interrupting, excessively running or climbing, often blurting out answers, always playing loudly, and seems to be always driven or on the go.[97] These symptoms must be evident at seven years of age and occur in two or more different settings, such as at school or at home.[98] Diagnosis of ADHD in mature celiac disease sufferers involves a careful examination of the person's past and current difficulties.[99] An expert will assess and review the patient's recollection of behavior during childhood. Evaluation of academics and work, as well as interpersonal relationships with family and friends, is also done. [100]

Treatment

Similar to other mental health disorders that may be found in celiac disease patients, the most effective way for treating ADHD is a combination of pharmacotherapy and psychotherapy.[101] Medications given to ADHD patients are directed at decreasing symptoms of hyperactivity and impulsiveness. They also improve attentiveness, enabling the individual to participate in interpersonal events.[102] Methylphenidate, amphetamine, and dextroamphetamin are the most common medications given.[103] Methylphenidate helps the child by improving attention and reducing hyperactive-impulsive behaviors. Stimulants are also used, such as dextroamphetamine and pemoline. Some of these medications—namely, methylphenidate, amphetamine compounds, and dextroamphetamine—are available in sustained-release form to be taken once a day, eliminating the need for another dose.[104] When stimulants are ineffective or the side effects become intolerable, antidepressants are the second treatment of choice. Atomoxetine is an antidepressant that inhibits the reuptake of norepinephrine selectively.[105] However, this drug can cause liver damage, so celiac disease sufferers who are taking this must undergo liver function tests.

Studies have shown that removing gluten from the diet can decrease the symptoms of ADHD. In one study, ten participants with celiac disease reported a remarkable improvement in behavior after six months of a gluten-free diet.[106] Another study yielded a similar result.[107] After six months of dietary intervention by taking out gluten, there was a significant improvement in the participants' behavior and functioning, such as persistent attention, better concentration, completion of tasks, and less distractibility to other stimuli.

Autism

Autistic disorder, also called childhood autism, is a pervasive developmental disorder that is characterized by significant abnormal development in social communication and interaction.[108] The child has a limited capacity to become involved in activities.[109] Autism affects 1 in 1,000 U.S. children from 1 to 15 years of age.[110] In general, boys are more prone to this disorder than girls.[111]

Causes

The definitive cause of autism remains unknown, but a genetic link has been confirmed to be a precipitating factor. Those children diagnosed with autism have a relative with the same disorder or traits. Some suggest that measles, mumps, and rubella (MMR) vaccines may contribute to late-onset autism. However, no sufficient evidence has been put forth to prove this claim.[112] Studies have yet to determine any direct link between autism and celiac disease, but researchers believe that the inability to digest gluten in these patients will eventually result in autism.[113] This is due to the opiates found in both gluten and casein, a protein found abundantly in dairy products.[114] Intestinal malabsorption will lead to the indigestion of these proteins, which can pass through the lesions in the small intestines and into the bloodstream.[115]

Diagnosis

To diagnose a child with autism, regardless of whether celiac disease is present, specialized physicians and psychiatrists are needed for proper assessment and evaluation. Usually, autism is identified as early as 18 months and no later than three years old.[116] An estimated 80 percent of autism cases are early onset, and the 20 percent occurs when the child reaches two to three years old because this is the time when the regression of development is manifested.[117] Children with autism tend to display minimal eye contact with others. They also have few facial expressions, limited gestures, and impaired verbal communication. They do not have spontaneous enjoyment and experience the inability to engage in playtime. Stereotyped motor behaviors are also observed, such as head banging and hand flapping. They have fixations with parts of objects.[118]

In some cases, autism improves when children learn to communicate by acquiring and using language. This is especially helpful if the child also suffers from celiac disease. When behavior in adolescents begins to deteriorate, hormonal changes and difficulty meeting social demands are said to be the cause. In adults, autism is only viewed as an odd behavior or may be diagnosed as other mental health disorders.[119]

Treatment

Reducing behavioral symptoms and encouraging development by learning are the goals of treatment for autistic children with celiac disease. Special education and language therapy are used because of their more favorable results.[120] For pharmacologic treatments, antipsychotics such as haloperidol and risperidone may be used to treat specific symptoms such as aggressiveness and temper tantrums.[121] When disease is present, a gluten- and casein-free diet is implemented to improve behavior. It has been observed that removing gluten and casein in the child's diet can yield a remarkable improvement in interpersonal communication and relationships.[122]

EATING DISORDERS

Anorexia Nervosa

Anorexia nervosa, an eating disorder, is characterized by a remarkable disturbance in perceiving body size, with an extreme fear of gaining weight.[123] This usually begins at adolescence, particularly 13–18 years of age.[124] Reports suggest that there may be a minimal link between celiac disease and anorexia nervosa.[125]

Causes

Causes of anorexia may be traced to a combination of factors, biological and genetic.[126] Any changes in the balance of serotonin, dopamine, and norepinephrine may contribute to the development of anorexia. Those individuals who have relatives diagnosed with eating disorders are at least five times more prone to acquire an eating disorder.[127] Other factors to be considered are rooted in relationships. Disturbance in early life relationships may render the child vulnerable to eating disorders. A distorted body image may come about if there is a misperception with internal needs. Some people seem to have decreased anxiety when they control their bodily functions such as eating. When children are raised in strict environments where perfection is highly valued or they have yet to separate successfully from parents' wishes or desires, they might think that the only area in which they can exert control and make decisions is their bodies.[128] This is also considered a form of rebellion.[129]

Furthermore, the promotion of an ideal body image of thinness and peer pressure play a role in eating disorders.[130] While researchers have yet to determine a very strong, direct link between eating disorders and celiac disease, a study has reported that the development of eating disorders in patients with celiac disease may be due to the preoccupation with food.[131] Adolescents diagnosed with celiac disease have a higher risk of developing eating disorders.[132] The reason may be due to the difficulty in complying with the gluten-free diet because of the unwanted weight gain.[133] Signs and symptoms of anorexia are as follows:[134]

preoccupation with food and weight
excessive weight loss
body image distortion

amenorrhea
withdrawal from activities
unawareness that the above behavior is unusual

Diagnosis

Due to the nature of celiac disease, exacerbation of eating disorders may occur.[135] Physicians or psychiatrists specializing in eating disorders assess and evaluate these individuals by checking their history of family relationships, binging or purging, and anxiety control.[136] Height and weight are also taken to see if the body mass index is appropriate for the person's age.[137] A series of blood tests may be done to check for any underlying complications.[138]

Treatment

Anorexic patients are very difficult to treat because they are often resistant and deny any problems.[139] Those with major life-threatening complications are sometimes admitted at a hospital to correct dehydration, electrolyte and metabolic imbalances, severe weight loss, and cardiovascular complications.[140] Outpatient treatment is indicated to those who are more willing to gain weight. Furthermore, cognitive behavior therapy is used to prevent relapse.[141] For medical management, weight restoration and correcting its complications are the focus of treatment. Nutritionally balanced meals and snacks are prepared, and caloric intake is gradually increased. If severely malnourished, total parental nutrition or tube feedings is recommended.[142] Access to the bathroom is also supervised to prevent purging.[143]

Medications used for anorexia are amitriptyline and cyproheptadine, an antihistamine, to promote weight gain. For the antipsychotic behaviors, olanzapine is prescribed. Fluoxetine is used to prevent relapse, but close monitoring is necessary due to its side effect of weight loss.[144]

Bulimia Nervosa

Individuals with recurring episodes of binge eating, then purging behaviors after, may be suffering from bulimia nervosa.[145] This usually begins during late adolescence, typically in ages 18–19 years.[146]

Causes

Anorexia and bulimia have the same generalized causes, but the exact cause is still unknown.[147] While celiac disease may exacerbate or precipitate bulimia, bulimics find it difficult to comply with a gluten-free diet because of weight gain, thereby worsening both disorders.[148]

Nonetheless, bulimia and celiac disease are still being studied rigorously for a correlation. As with anorexia, preoccupation with food and weight gain may add up to the development of bulimia.[149] Although the death rate for bulimia is estimated at less than 3 percent, the recurrence of binge eating and purging episodes is at 30 percent.[150]

These individuals are aware that their behavior is beyond the norm and try to hide it from others. They even secretly store food in various locations throughout the house, and they often manifest compensatory behaviors such as misusing laxatives, enemas, or diuretics.[151] Self-induced vomiting or excessive exercising may be used by bulimics to lose weight. Some may experience depressive or anxiety symptoms. Other symptoms are as follows: calorie consumption restriction between binges, use of substances involving alcohol, dental enamel loss and an increase in dental caries, irregularities in the menstrual cycle, laxative dependency, esophegeal tears, fluid and electrolyte imbalances, metabolic alkalosis, and slightly elevated serum amylase levels.[152]

Diagnosis

To diagnose bulimia, there must be at least two episodes of bulimic behavior a week for three months.[153] A dental examination is indicated to show if there are any cavities or gum infections that are a result of self-induced vomiting.[154] A physician will ask a series of questions, and body mass index is measured.[155] Blood tests may be done to assess for complications.

Treatment

Cognitive-behavioral therapy is the most effective treatment for bulimic patients who also suffer from celiac disease.[156] Strategies are used to change the patient's thinking and actions regarding food to instead focus on interrupting the psychological cycle of bulimia. Combined with self-esteem enhancement and assertiveness training, cognitive-behavioral therapy yields positive results.[157] Antidepressants are prescribed to reduce binge eating and preoccupation with body image.[158] They also help improve mood. However, these results are only short term, with some patients relapsing within two years.[159]

AVOIDANCE OF NEGATIVE MENTAL OUTCOMES

When an individual is diagnosed with celiac disease and a mental health disorder, acceptance can be difficult. Sometimes, it might aggravate the condition if he or she refuses to cooperate with the treatment plan. Proper health teaching and counseling, along with reasonable goals that are attainable and realistic, are necessary to help the celiac disease patient recover. Moreover, compliance with the medications and therapies is a must because it can assist the person to overcome the factors and situations that worsen mental health disorders. The therapies are designed to facilitate a sense of control that these persons lack and to properly learn how to use coping mechanisms in managing the disorder. The goal of these treatments is to yield a positive outcome by enhancing the person's self-esteem.

Lifestyle changes are also essential to achieve enhanced self-esteem. These changes are geared toward the alleviation of depressive and anxiety symptoms. Eating a well-balanced, healthy, and gluten-free diet, rich in nutrients such as vitamin B complex, is essential for maintaining mental health and achieving good nutritional status.[160] This can improve sleep, mood, and reduce gastrointestinal symptoms. Scientists have documented that those who adhere to these lifestyle changes have reported a significant improvement in mental health and a decrease in stress.[161] Participating in an exercise regimen has also been found to help improve self-esteem. During exercise, the body releases endorphins that trigger positive feelings, and pain perception is reduced. It has likewise been shown that regular exercise helps lessen stress by decreasing anxiety and depression. Self-confidence and self-esteem are also improved.[162]

ANALYSIS

After taking all the above into consideration, it appears that additional ways of achieving good mental health as a celiac disease sufferer include:

(1) keeping a journal or diary to express feelings rather than internalizing them, (2) seeking help by joining support groups who can help increase the ability to cope and reduce the feeling of loneliness, and (3) learning ways to cope with and manage stress. Above all else, self-care is important to help manage stress and improve self-esteem in a person with celiac disease.[163]

In managing patients with celiac disease and mental health disorders, it is imperative that they are not isolated. Caregivers can encourage them to participate in social events and establish interpersonal relationships to improve their mental and physical health.[164] Many links between celiac disease and mental health disorders remain undetermined, but further works of research can potentially prove that celiac disease indeed causes a disturbance in mental health.

8

PHYSICAL DISORDERS ASSOCIATED WITH CELIAC DISEASE

The focus now is on the nonpsychological disorders that are commonly associated with celiac disease. The causes, pathology, and diagnosis of celiac disease itself have already been discussed and are therefore beyond the scope of this chapter. Celiac disease has been associated with an increased risk of certain other disorders, illnesses, and medical conditions, and treating it early and consistently can help prevent or alleviate some of these secondary issues. Talking to a medical professional to zero in on a plan is a good way to start, but knowing the risks is essential to cultivating better overall health.

BONE AND JOINT DISORDERS

Osteoporosis

One study has shown that 47 percent of women and 50 percent of men who suffer from celiac disease also has osteoporosis.[1] In women, a strong link between the age at menopause and bone mineral density (BMD) at the lumbar spine and femoral neck was also found. Osteoporosis is a disease in which bone density lowers, making bones more fragile and more likely to fracture. Osteoporosis can lead to severe pain and even disability, when bones become so fragile that it is virtually impossible to achieve simple tasks such as standing up without fracturing them in the process.[2] Osteoporosis can result as a complication of celiac disease. Due to the fact that it blunts the intestinal villi in the small intestine's jejunum, celiac disease interferes with nutrient absorption, including calcium, though many others are also malabsorbed.

Calcium is critical in the making and maintenance of healthy bones. Because of the interference with nutrient absorption, people who suffer from celiac disease can suffer from osteoporosis even when their intake of calcium seems right, if celiac disease is left unchecked or undiagnosed. Once celiac disease is recognized and diagnosed, the patient will most likely start a gluten-free diet. This can restore nutrient absorption in just a few months, though older patients may take up to two years for the intestinal villi's functions to be fully restored and bone density to be improved.[3]

In addition to a gluten-free diet, traditional bone care steps are also recommended. These steps include weightlifting, walking, climbing, dancing, not smoking, avoiding the excessive use of alcohol, and consuming proper amounts of calcium and vitamin D, maybe even using osteoporosis treatment medications, such as bisphosphonates, estrogen antagonists, calcitonin, and parathyroid hormone.[4] In extreme cases of celiac disease, following a gluten-free diet does not help due to the fact that the intestine is too damaged and repair is impossible. For such cases, nutrition supplements must be taken through an IV.[5] Strenuous exercise is also not recommended for these particular cases.

People who have been on a gluten-free diet throughout their life have normal bone mineral density (BMD), effectively preventing osteoporosis from taking place.[6] One study has shown that osteoporosis in celiac disease may not only be related to malabsorption of calcium but also be part of an autoimmune process, having found antibodies that attacked osteoprotegerin, a protein that controls the speed at which bone tissue is removed and replaced, and obtaining positive results when neutralizing harmful antibodies.[7]

Osteomalacia

Osteomalacia is described as the softening of bones by an insufficient amount of phosphorous, calcium, or vitamin D in the bones. This is usually caused by a resistance to the effects of vitamin D or a malabsorption of calcium from the intestine. It is easy to understand why osteomalacia is related to celiac disease. As is the case with the more common osteoporosis, a deficiency in the function of the intestine causes bones to be at a high risk of fracture due to weakness in their structure. Through gluten-free dieting and proper consumption of vitamin D and calcium, the celiac disease patient's bone and muscle functions are greatly improved, and abnormalities in the bone often become less evident. Unfortunately, it must be noted that osteomalacia has some everlasting effects that no amount of treatment can mollify.[8]

Arthritis

A physical manifestation of celiac disease is arthritis, particularly one that involves not only the peripheral skeletal but also the axial skeletal. Arthritis has been reported to be present in up to 25 percent of all the celiac disease–afflicted patients who participated in a study and were observed as test subjects.[9] This figure, however, changes depending on the techniques for ascertainment used as well as the populations of patients afflicted with celiac disease that were screened for arthritis. In order to dispel confusion, and so as to distinguish arthritis as experienced by celiac disease patients from other types of arthritis, it is necessary to point out that this particular arthritis is acute and nonerosive. This type of arthritis, generally speaking, resolves with the implementation or institution of a diet free of gluten and its derivatives. The two most common arthritides are osteoarthritis and rheumatoid arthritis, both of which can appear in comorbidity with celiac disease. Osteoarthritis can exist in comorbidity with celiac disease simply because one of celiac disease's most common symptoms is a lack of nutrients caused by the obstruction of the small intestine's villi. Joints need nutrients to repair themselves, and a lack of nutrients would negatively affect that endeavor.[10]

Rheumatoid arthritis is an autoimmune disease in which the immune system attacks the body's joints, causing inflammation and pain. It is different from mere joint pain in that it is not simply a telltale warning sign of an autoimmune disorder but an autoimmune disease in and of itself.[11] It is also distinguishable from joint pain in that it can damage several organs, including the heart, if left undiagnosed and untreated.[12] There is no definitive cure for rheumatoid arthritis. However, symptoms can be temporally alleviated through medication.[13] Unfortunately, this same medication often leads to secondary effects, such as asthma, chronic rhinitis, and skin rashes. Worse yet, it can also lead to complications in the gastrointestinal tract, such as ulcers, bleeding, and irritation on the gastrointestinal surface.[14]

It is important to note that even though it might be tempting to avoid any form of physical activity due to inflammation and pain, it is precisely physical exercise, along with appropriate rest, that stops the joints from becoming stiff, thereby increasing pain and diminishing the body's mobility.[15] Simply put, there is a link between celiac disease and arthritis. Arthritis can appear as a complication of celiac disease if left untreated. It can also appear before gluten enteropathy.[16]

It has been observed in patients who have both celiac disease and rheumatoid arthritis that joint inflammation and pain occurs within hours of consuming wheat-containing food.[17] Following a gluten-free diet as well as using medication for arthritis and regular exercise can eventually lead to a full remission from celiac disease as well as arthritis symptoms.[18] Simple allergic arthritis can also exist in comorbidity with celiac disease. Allergic arthritis is a form of food allergy that causes inflammation and pain in the joints when eating new kinds of food, or a familiar food in excess.[19] Given that wheat is one of the most common triggers for allergic arthritis, it is simple to understand why comorbidity between it and celiac disease can develop.

Growth Problems

A body's growth depends on several factors: genetics, exercise or lack thereof, and nutrient intake, just to name a few. When that last factor, nutrient intake, does not reach the adequate requirements, problems with the body's growth begin to appear. The person, usually a child or teenager, visually seems to be stuck in a much younger person's body. This is especially pervasive, since approximately 1 percent of children suffer from celiac disease, making it one of the most widespread childhood diseases.[20]

In certain cases, growth issues may be the only symptom of celiac disease, making the diagnosis particularly difficult.[21] With that in mind, it is fairly easy to understand the connection between celiac disease and growth problems. Celiac disease obstructs the intestinal villi, whose purpose is to absorb nutrients. This causes a below average nutrient intake, and eventually nutrient deficiency, leading to several problems, including growth issues. An Italian research study was developed to show the relation between celiac disease and growth-hormone deficiency and their comorbidity in children. Some 210 of the children in this study had common growth hormone deficiency, and 12 more had celiac disease.[22]

Out of those 12 children, nine showed remarkably positive results in their growth issues when subjected to a gluten-free diet for one year. However, the three remaining children did not respond to it.[23] After screening those three, researchers found that two of them had an isolated growth-hormone deficiency, while the other child had multiple growth-hormone problems.[24] Due to these results, growth-hormone therapy was initiated on the three nonresponsive children. Growth rate was eventually achieved through the growth-hormone therapy along with the gluten-free diet.[25] Researchers concluded that patients who fail to thrive under a strict gluten-free diet should be screened for growth-hormone deficiency and, if the results show such deficiency exists, include growth-hormone therapy as a complement of the gluten-free diet in order to ensure the patient's proper growth.[26]

CIRCULATORY ISSUES ASSOCIATED WITH CELIAC DISEASE

The circulatory system is divided in the lymphatic and the cardiovascular system. Lymph flows through the lymphatic system, which is later distributed to all parts of the body, as opposed to blood, which never really leaves the circulatory system. The cardiovascular system comprises numerous veins and arteries that transport clean blood to and from the heart. Through the lymphatic system flows a clear liquid called lymph, and it contains salts, electrolytes, nutrients, and, of course, water.

It is also the waste disposal system of the body, carrying diverse waste and depositing it on the skin, liver, bladder, lungs, colon, and kidneys, which then ensure that waste is properly disposed of, eliminating it from the body. The circulatory system, including both the cardiovascular and lymph mechanisms, has a strong connection to celiac disease.[27] The lymph system's center is the abdomen. Lymph is the fluid that transports chyle—a combination of lymph and fat absorbed by the intestinal villi and then in turn absorbed by lacteals, a special kind of lymphatic capillary—and then delivers it throughout the body. Those very same intestinal villi are obstructed by celiac disease through inflammation. The same thing applies for the cardiovascular system. With the exception of fat, all other digestive products—carbohydrates, amino acids, and proteins, for example—are infused directly into the bloodstream.

Therefore, when celiac disease is active, neither nutrients nor waste can be properly absorbed into the lymphatic system and, as a result, into the rest of the body. Nutrients are lost and waste stacks inside the colon, congesting it and further obstructing the intestinal villi. In fact, celiac disease has several effects on both the cardiovascular and the lymphatic system that will be explored.

Mesenteric Lymph Node Cavitation Syndrome

Characterized by cystic change in mesenteric lymph nodes and signs of hyposplenism, this syndrome is a rare complication of celiac disease. Even though it is often the consequence of a failure to control celiac disease, it can also exist from the beginning of diagnosis and treatment of the disease.[28] Due to its rareness and the obscurity of the term even among the medical community, this physical disorder is very poorly understood.[29] More often than not, the cause of *mesenteric lymph node cavitation syndrome (MLNCS)* is not defined. It causes central necrosis of the mesenteric lymph nodes. It may present due to a poor response to a gluten-free diet. It can also lead to further complications, such as sepsis and lymphoma, often resulting in death.[30] An important element of this syndrome is hyposplenism, described as a reduction in normal spleen function. This syndrome causes structural changes in the spleen, which cause it to malfunction.

Because the spleen ceases to work, or works at a slower pace than it originally did, the celiac disease patient is at higher risk of infections, such as bacterial sepsis, which can result in death.[31] The risk of sepsis, and, by extension, death, seems to be higher if celiac disease is detected in adulthood rather than in childhood.[32] The risks are also greater for solid tumors and several thrombotic, vascular, and autoimmune disorders in adult celiac disease.[33] It is possible that the cavitation changes caused by this syndrome lead to excess antigen exposure through damaged mucosa, provoking lymphoid cell depletion in the spleen and lymph nodes.[34]

This same cavitation change can cause necrosis in the mesenteric nodes triggered by intravascular blockage and immune complement activation.[35] Spleen function can be restored, but not before the small intestine's issues and changes caused by MLNCS have been resolved.[36] Even though mortality is high (up to 50 percent), improvement and even normalization of mesenteric lymph nodes have also been reported when a strict gluten-free diet is followed and celiac disease does not resist it.[37]

Lymphoma

Lymphoma is a type of blood cancer caused by the abnormal reproduction or life span of B and T lymphocytes, the white cells that defend the organism from diseases and infections, eventually forming a solid tumor from the aforementioned white cells. There exists the true physical relationship linking celiac disease and lymphoma. Specifically, there is a connection between enteropathy-associated T-cell lymphoma, the most common gastrointestinal lymphoma, and the results of the intestinal biopsy performed on celiac disease patients to observe its mucosal healing.[38]

Those patients whose intestinal villi remain atrophied are at a higher risk of acquiring lymphoma as a result. Likewise, a follow-up biopsy may stratify patients with celiac disease by risk for lymphoma.[39] Patients whose biopsies shown mucosal healing are at lower risk than those whose intestinal villi remained totally or subtotally atrophied.[40] Partial atrophy, however, does not bear a connection with lymphoma. The only known method for obtaining mucosal healing in celiac disease is through following a strict gluten-free diet.

As time passes and celiac disease is kept under control, the risk of death and lymphoma is also lowered. However, it remains relatively high in comparison to people without celiac disease. Because of the importance of mucosal healing, it is recommended that a follow-up biopsy be performed on patients with celiac disease to confirm healing and to prevent lymphoma and other complications derived from persistent intestinal villi atrophy.

Thromboembolism

Thrombosis is the formation of a blood clot inside a vein or artery, causing it to block the flow of blood through that particular passage. Even though blood clots are usually created after a traumatic injury to the blood vessel, it can be formed for other reasons, such as a complete stop of blood flow, causing the blood to accumulate and form blood clots. Embolism is when the said blood clot separates itself from its point of origin, traveling through the system and therefore leaving the point of origin free for blood traffic, but with the potential to obstruct yet again at some other point in the circulatory system.

The blood clot is then referred to as an embolus, and once free from its point of origin it is even capable of moving on to an artery when its point of origin was a vein, or vice versa, if the appropriate conditions are met. It must be mentioned that although only blood clots will be discussed in this chapter, both veins and arteries can be blocked by several different things, such as fat or a gas bubble. That said, it is important for caregivers to remember that venous and arterial thromboembolism has been found in comorbidity with celiac disease, and it may be the initial symptom. [41] The fact that it is often found in patients with celiac disease may point to the disease increasing the tendency of the blood to coagulate, and create clots as a consequence. [42] Increased amounts of thrombin-activatable fibrinolysis have been reported in patients with celiac disease, which has been identified as a risk factor for thromboembolism. [43]

Coagulopathy

Coagulopathy is, in a way, the exact opposite to thrombosis. Rather than an excess of clotting of the blood, or its clotting when it is not needed, coagulopathy is the loss or impairment of the blood's ability to clog. In other words, when a blood vessel is opened because of a trauma, the blood will not clog at the wound to avoid (1) bleeding out or (2) the entrance of pathogens into the blood system. This leaves the body defenseless to each of these threats, causing excessive or constant bleeding at random or after a trauma is inflicted upon the body.

In celiac disease, coagulopathy may occur as a result of a combination of vitamin K as well as several fat-soluble vitamin deficiencies. [44] These deficiencies are caused by the obstruction of intestinal villi in the small intestine's jejunum. It is important to note that, while thrombosis may be very common among celiac disease patients, coagulopathy is not, but it still exists in comorbidity with celiac disease. [45] Due to the fact that coagulopathy in celiac disease is caused by a lack of nutrients—which is consistent with the malabsorption of nutrients in the intestinal villi—following a strict gluten-free diet must be complemented with the intake of vitamins D and K and calcium supplements in order for the manifestations of both celiac disease and coagulopathy to be treated.[46]

Anemia

Iron-deficiency anemia is a form of anemia that can be caused by insufficient absorption of iron. It can be related to celiac disease, since celiac disease causes malabsorption of nutrients. A case exists of a 14-year-old male student who was found to have a low hemoglobin level during a routine medical examination. He had no cardiovascular or gastrointestinal symptoms. While determining the cause of his anemia, a biopsy of his duodenum revealed villous atrophy. Further serologic testing revealed a high level of the antibody anti-immunoglobulin A (IgA) tissue transglutaminase, a possible indicator of celiac disease. After being on a gluten-free diet for one year, his hemoglobin level returned to normal.[47]

Anemia is characterized by the deficiency of hemoglobin in the blood. Since hemoglobin transports oxygen, a lack of hemoglobin basically *equals* a lack of oxygen. Because cells require oxygen to survive, an insufficient amount of oxygen could very well prove fatal to the body. The lack of hemoglobin in a celiac disease patient can be attributed to a wide range of reasons, from physical blood loss and hemorrhage to lack of nutrients in the blood, which is where celiac disease comes into play. Anemia is both the most common blood disease and the most common blood disease caused by celiac disease. Furthermore, celiac disease–related anemia is often due to a lack of micronutrients such as iron, folic acid, and vitamin B12, caused by a deficiency in the absorption of nutrients by the small intestine's villi.[48]

Anemia may be the first symptom to appear, indicating that celiac disease is present.[49] It may also be the only symptom to indicate the existence of celiac disease, specifically in children.[50] Iron-deficiency anemia is very common among celiac disease patients; up to 46 percent of celiac disease sufferers have comorbid iron-deficiency anemia, out of which the majority are adults rather than youngsters.[51] Even though the most common reason for existence of iron-deficiency anemia is malabsorption of iron by the intestinal villi, it may also exist as a result of internal bleeding in the intestinal tract, or a combination of both.[52]

It is important to note that while internal bleeding in the intestinal tract may be a cause for iron-deficiency anemia in celiac disease, it is not as common as simple iron malabsorption, which is a direct consequence of celiac disease.[53] Occult gastrointestinal bleeding seems to be responsive to a gluten-free diet.[54] Doctors should consider celiac disease as a possible cause for an otherwise unexplained iron deficiency anemia, especially when it comes to menstruating women.[55] In the case of iron deficiency anemia and celiac disease, a combination of a strict gluten-free diet and iron supplementation is the best and safest treatment. Iron supplementation must continue to be taken until the amount of hemoglobin in the blood is normalized and iron stores have been restored, which could take up to a year for hemoglobin and up to two years for iron.[56]

A lack of folic acid can also result in macrocytic or *megaloblastic anemia*. Folic acid is a type of vitamin B (B9 to be precise), and it is a crucial element for the metabolism and metabolic regulation of amino acid and nucleic acid.[57] Folic acid is also a requirement for proper hematopoiesis and development of the nervous system in the celiac disease patient.[58] Folic acid is absorbed in the small intestine's jejunum, so malabsorption of vitamin B9 is often caused by infections and diseases of the small intestine.[59]

Comorbidity between celiac disease, folic acid, and iron deficiencies can show atypical findings in the blood smear.[60] Severe folic acid deficiency may result in a decreased number of leukocytes and platelets, or cause severe pancytopenia.[61] Studies have shown that folic acid deficiency anemia is common among patients with celiac disease, particularly those who have recently been diagnosed with it or who have failed to follow the required treatment.[62] It has also been found that children with celiac disease often have a vitamin B9 deficiency; yet it rarely becomes anemia.[63] A combination of vitamin B9 supplementation and a strict gluten-free diet is recommended for the treatment of patients who suffer from both celiac disease and folic acid deficiency.[64] Vitamin B12 deficiency anemia can also coexist with celiac disease.

Even though vitamin B12 is mostly absorbed in the distal ileum of the small intestine, some of it is also absorbed passively throughout the said organ.[65] As a result of this, vitamin B12 deficiency is common among celiac disease patients and often leads to anemia.[66] Even though a dysfunction in the small intestine could be the reason behind vitamin B12 anemia in celiac disease, this is probably not the case, since the amount of vitamin B12 absorbed in the small intestine is not enough to cause a significant imbalance in the amount of vitamin B12 in the body. Therefore, other alternatives have been proposed as the possible reasons behind the existence of vitamin B12 anemia in celiac disease patients, such as decreased gastric acid, autoimmune gastritis, bacterial overgrowth, or decreased efficiency in the mixing with transfer factors in the intestine.[67]

Vitamin B12 deficiency anemia should be considered as a possible comorbid disease for all patients who have celiac disease and who also suffer from other hematological or neurological diseases.[68] Patients who suffer from celiac disease in combination with vitamin B12 deficiency should adhere to a gluten-free diet as well as parenteral, intramuscular vitamin B12, since no study has found oral vitamin B12 to be as effective as parenteral when the patient also has celiac disease. Celiac disease sufferers who have vitamin B9 and B12 deficiency anemia as well as celiac disease may not present the usual macrocytosis present in comorbidity between vitamin B9 and celiac disease alone, and examining the blood smears may present a dimorphic picture showing the effects of both deficiencies at the same time.[69]

RELATED SKIN MANIFESTATIONS OF CELIAC DISEASE

Dermatitis Herpetiformis

The most common dermatological manifestation of celiac disease is dermatitis herpetiformis. This skin disease is characterized by a prolonged and painful and severely itchy rash with small blisters. It affects approximately 10 percent of the patients with celiac disease, and it is more common in people of Northern European descent than in African Americans and Asian Americans.[70] When misdiagnosed, it can be more painful and stressful, as it can be mistreated by inappropriate remedies or even hidden or disguised.[71]

In older studies, the relationship of celiac disease and dermatitis herpetiformis was determined through intestinal biopsies and physical and histological examinations. Their individual occurrences were then recorded and matched. The results showed that only 9 out of 47 Caucasian patients (19 percent) with dermatitis herpetiformis have no detectable mucosal abnormality.[72] This means that roughly 80 percent of dermatitis herpetiformis have biopsy evidences of celiac diseases. Presently, the relationship of these two diseases is more understood as mechanisms, and research on their prevalences became a focus of a number of studies. For instance, it was discovered that both celiac disease and dermatitis herpetiformis are autoimmune diseases and are facilitated by IgA autoantibodies triggered by the ingestion of the intake of grains with gluten content. The only difference is the major autoantigen for celiac disease is tissue transglutaminase, while for dermatitis herpetiformis the major autoantigen is epidermal transglutaminase.[73] It was also previously emphasized that people with one autoimmune disease are more likely to have one or more additional autoimmune diseases.

Because of the well-established association of celiac disease and dermatitis herpetiformis, patients with the latter disease were recommended to follow a consistent gluten-free diet originally designed for patients of the former disease. Topical and oral medications—for example, dapsone and sulfapyridine—were also strongly suggested for faster skin healing. This is because the diet may take months to years to manifest in the skin because IgA deposits in the dermal-epidermal connection of the skin take such a long time to react, unlike in the gastrointestinal tract.[74]

Alopecia Areata

Alopecia areata is another autoimmune disease in which there are patchy areas of total hair loss in the scalp, or even on other hair-bearing parts of the body. It was found in 1–2 percent of patients with celiac disease.[75] Also, it was found that a gluten-free diet helps patients with alopecia areata regrow their hair completely.[76] Though not yet proven biochemically, this result could indicate the possible contributing role of gluten in the mechanism of the development of this disease, which would make it more closely associated with celiac disease than just the prevalence of one celiac disease incident in every 85 patients with alopecia areata.[77]

Chronic Urticaria

Chronic urticaria is a skin rash distinguished by the presence of a long-term (up to six weeks or more), reddish, raised urticaria, commonly known as hives or bumps. Oftentimes, the reason for the occurrence of this disease is unknown or idiopathic. Also, the major mechanism that could be the cause of this skin disorder is an autoimmune reaction. This is once again similar to the mechanism of celiac disease. Because of this, some case studies and reports have been documented in order to analyze the association of the mentioned diseases. There are various studies proving the association of chronic urticarial and celiac disease. This was determined through the improvement of the skin condition as well as malabsorption through the gluten-free diet.[78]

In contrast to the isolated case studies mentioned above, there is one study that proved otherwise. This study, involving 80 patients with idiopathic chronic urticaria and 264 healthy controls, compared the prevalence of celiac disease in both groups of an adult population. They found that 1 out of 80 patients with idiopathic chronic urticaria, and 1 out of the 264 controls, had celiac disease detected through serology and biopsy. The results indicated a statistically insignificant prevalence of celiac disease for each group. This means that people with idiopathic chronic urticaria are not at a greater risk of having celiac disease than the general population.[79] Although there may be contrasting results, the coexistence of chronic urticaria and celiac disease could not be neglected and may be attributed to an increase in the mucosal permeability due to celiac disease, which might be the cause of the urticarial lesions.[80]

Psoriasis

Psoriasis is an autoimmune disease of the skin in which there are reddish, raised, and scaly patches that are usually covered by a silvery white accumulation of dead skin cells. It is reportedly connected with a number of systemic comorbidities.[81] Studies have shown the relationship of celiac disease and psoriasis. One large-scale study involved 12,502 patients with psoriasis and 24,285 healthy controls. Results show that the prevalence of celiac disease was higher in patients with psoriasis than in healthy controls. This proves that, statistically, psoriasis is indeed associated with celiac disease.[82]

Other clinical research involving a smaller number of subjects also investigated the association of celiac disease and psoriasis.[83] This time, the antibodies associated with the mentioned diseases were the basis for the association. The antibodies gliadin IgA, gliadin IgG, and tissue transglutaminase IgA are associated with celiac disease, while HLA-Cw6 is an allele associated with psoriasis. Fifty-six patients with psoriasis and 60 healthy controls were tested for their antibody levels and allele typing. Results show that the celiac-associated antibodies were statistically greater in the serum of the patients with psoriasis than in the healthy controls, but no correlation was found between any one of the antibodies and the HLA-Cw6 allele. This means that patients with psoriasis could also have celiac disease.[84] An additional proof that psoriasis is associated with celiac disease is the fact that recent case reports show an improvement of psoriatic skin lesions when a gluten-free diet is followed. Psoriasis in those with celiac disease was observed to be more severe.[85]

Eczema

Similar to psoriasis, eczema is another disorder of the skin associated with celiac disease. Eczema is characterized by red patches of skin, usually with lumps or blisters. It is also distinguished by very intense itchiness and inflammation. The cause of eczema is not yet established, but the physical skin conditions point to a genetic predisposition as well as environmental factors. Previous research shows that eczema is somehow associated with celiac disease because it occurs three times more in patients with celiac disease than in healthy control subjects. Many eczema cases have been documented to be alleviated through a gluten-free diet, making it one of the recently accepted approaches to healing.[86]

Acne

Acne is a very common human skin disease, and its formation is affected by various genetic, hormonal, psychological, and microbiological factors. For this reason, it would be hard to test for the association of acne with celiac disease. Since patients of celiac disease undergo some hormonal imbalance, which is one of the factors contributing to acne formation, celiac disease has some indirect effect on the formation of acne in the skin.[87]

Dry Skin

Having dry skin is a very common complaint of patients with celiac disease. Though this is not really a disorder, it could also be one of the indirect skin manifestations of celiac disease. This is because patients with celiac disease cannot absorb vitamin E into their intestines, resulting in lower skin quality. Celiac disease patients avoid grains that are rich in this vitamin. Therefore, consuming enough of the vitamin is not always that easy.[88]

NEUROLOGICAL DISORDERS

Neuropathy

Up to 50 percent of patients with celiac disease may present with peripheral neuropathy.[89] Peripheral neuropathy is damage to the peripheral nervous system's nerves. Symptoms include numbness, pain, tremors, tingling, and itching on limbs or even on the face. It is important to objectively prove that the patient has neuropathy, since these symptoms are also found in other diseases. Interestingly, these symptoms for neuropathy were sometimes displayed before the gastrointestinal symptoms for celiac disease appeared. One 2003 study showed that 5 percent of the patients who suffered from peripheral neuropathy also had celiac disease.[90] The studies into the effectiveness of a gluten-free diet to counteract celiac neuropathy have yet to show conclusive results. Some claim the diet has helped ease the symptoms of neuropathy, while others have observed no difference or have even reported worsened symptoms.[91]

Ataxia

In celiac disease, ataxia is often related to neuropathy.[92] Ataxia is defined as the lack of voluntary muscle movements, which implies dysfunctions in the nervous system, particularly in those parts responsible for coordination and movement, such as the cerebellum. In the case of ataxia caused by celiac disease, that is precisely the case. As the name implies, this form of ataxia is caused by the ingestion of gluten in those who are sensitive to it, such as celiac disease sufferers. As opposed to some cases of gluten neuropathy, a gluten-free diet has shown positive results. It can diminish symptoms and prevent further progression of this neurological impairment.[93] Furthermore, antigliadin antibodies have been found in ataxia patients.[94] Since it has been claimed that such antibodies are neurotoxic to the cerebellum, this was to be expected. Vitamin E supplementation has also been useful for some patients, but others have had normal

vitamin E levels while still suffering from ataxia. Therefore, a 100 percent clear connection with nutrient deficiency and the triggering of ataxia
has not been possible to establish.[95]

Epilepsy

A Swedish analysis has shown that patients with celiac disease have an
increased risk of developing epilepsy later on. This was discovered
through a comparison of the databases of patients who suffered from
celiac disease against those who did not, from 1969 to 2008.[96] The analysis also showed that people with celiac disease had greater susceptibility
to epileptic seizures no matter their age, leading to the conclusion that all
celiac disease patients were at a moderately higher risk of epilepsy.[97] It
has been established that in order for epilepsy to occur, the patient must
have an extreme intolerance toward gluten, to the point that the patient's
nervous system would be so affected by it that epileptic seizures occur
when consuming gluten or even items whose protein structure resembles
that of gluten, referred to as cross-reactive food.[98]

Studies have shown that an early diagnosis of celiac disease for epilepsy sufferers can slow down the evolution of epilepsy and help the
patient's cognitive status.[99] Likewise, starting a gluten-free diet leads to
progressive control over epileptic seizures, allowing for the use of less
antiepileptic drugs or even eliminating the need for their use entirely.[100]
In contrast, a late diagnosis of celiac disease or failing to follow a gluten-
free diet can lead to severe complications for both celiac disease and
epilepsy, as well as sabotage the overall treatment process.[101]

RELATED BACTERIAL AND VIRAL MANIFESTATIONS

Bacteria

In addition to the gastrointestinal and extraintestinal manifestations, dis-
arrangement in the natural levels of microbial biota can also be associated
with celiac disease. For instance, infants with celiac disease had been
characterized to have significantly higher numbers of both gram-negative
and gram-positive bacteria.[102] This result was supported by another study
in which the diversity of fecal microbiota was found to be significantly

higher in children with celiac disease than in the control group.[103] In support of the claim stated above, a similar study also ascertained that the number of gram-negative bacteria and the total bacteria were significantly higher in children patients with active celiac disease than in symptom-free patients and healthy controls.[104] The scientists also determined that the ratio of lactobacillus bifidobacterium (beneficial bacteria) to bacteroides *E. coli* (potentially pro-inflammatory bacteria) was significantly reduced in youngsters suffering from celiac disease.

Viruses

Viruses are small, infectious particles that invade cells of other living organisms in order to replicate themselves. They are comprised of either DNA or RNA strands that contain their genetic information and a protein coat for their protection. Once they invade their host cell, they incorporate their genetic material into the genetic material of the host cell, thereby disrupting the host cell's normal functions, and they cause or activate certain diseases of the host itself. In the case of celiac disease, it was discovered that celiac patients had an excess of adeno-type virus antibodies in their bloodstream. This means that some specific types of viruses are also associated with celiac disease. For instance, the adenovirus type 12, usually isolated from the intestinal tract, shares some similar protein sequences (12 amino acid residue) as those of the A-gliadin, an alphagliadin component known to be the trigger for celiac disease. This could indicate that if the immune system detects this virus and produces an antibody against it, the next time it encounters a similar particle (this time it may be the same virus again or the gliadin already) it will have already produced an antibody, and hence it may show some manifestation of celiac disease.[105] Another virus that can be associated with celiac disease is Epstein-Barr virus. This is because through the polymerase chain reaction (PCR) method, a significant 72 percent of patients with complicated celiac disease were positive for the said virus, while only 15.3 percent of patients with noncomplicated celiac disease were positive.[106]

OTHER INTERNAL ASSOCIATIONS
WITH CELIAC DISEASE

Oral and Dental Manifestations

The digestive tract starts in the oral cavity, so, in a sense, the degree of celiac disease may also start there. One of the common oral manifestations of celiac disease is enamel defect. This is because while celiac disease develops at any age, abnormalities in the structure of children's dental enamel may occur if it develops in children as their permanent teeth are forming.[107] Moreover, there are four classifications of systemic dental enamel defects in patients with celiac disease.[108] Grade 1 enamel defects are characterized by single or multiple cream, yellow, or brown opacities/discoloration of the enamel. Grade 2 enamel defects include slight structural defects such as rough enamel surface, horizontal grooves, and shallow pits, in addition to the patchy symmetric opacity/discoloration. Grade 3 enamel defects are distinguished by the evident structural defects that include deep horizontal grooves, large vertical pits, and linear discoloration. Lastly, Grade 4 enamel defects are differentiated through severe structural defects, in which the shape of the tooth may be totally changed.[109]

Studies show that these enamel defects are more common in patients with celiac disease than in the control group. To be specific, 69 percent of the adult patients with celiac disease also had enamel defect, in contrast to the control group, with only 19 percent.[110] In addition, enamel defects found in celiac patients were more "specific," meaning the enamel defects were symmetrically and chronologically ordered, as compared to the control group, in which the defects were mostly "unspecific."

Dental enamel is one out of four major tissues that make up the tooth in humans as well as some animals. It is the white, visible part of the tooth, serving as a protective layer for the rest of the tooth, but one that can easily decay or be destroyed in a patient with celiac disease. Oddly enough, some people find out about their celiac disease due to a visit to the dentist as opposed to a visit to the gastroenterologist. This is due to the fact that defects on the dental enamel, such as brown, white, or yellow spots, ridges, or abnormal formations of the teeth, can be a telltale sign of celiac disease. They can make the dentist, or any other doctor, suspect it, and they therefore refer the patient to the appropriate doctor (a gastroenterologist) for diagnosis and treatment. Of course, this does not mean that all dental enamel defects are a direct effect of celiac disease, but rather that dental enamel defects are common among celiac disease sufferers, especially children.[111]

The reason dental enamel defects are more common among children with celiac disease is for the same reason that dental defects are common among children in general: dental care is not always top priority. It is usually later in life that visits to the dentist are made, and if the dentist is unaware of the existence of celiac disease, the signs will simply not become a cause for alarm. One reason why dental enamel defects may not be immediately identified as a celiac disease symptom is because it is similar to other defects that are caused by excessive fluoride or a maternal or childhood illness.[112]

It is also important to note that dental enamel defects may be the only observable sign of celiac disease.[113] If both celiac disease and dental enamel defects are diagnosed early, before the teeth are fully formed, the child has a chance of having normal teeth later in life, as long as the child adheres to a strict gluten-free diet. Dental enamel defects are not reversible or treatable in adults—not even through a strict gluten-free diet.[114]

Thyroid Diseases

The thyroid is a gland located in the neck. It produces hormones that control the rate of metabolism of body cells, oxygen consumption, and nutrient absorption. Hypothyroidism, or the reduction in the amount of thyroid hormones; hyperthyroidism, or the increase above the normal levels of thyroid hormones; and thyroiditis, or the infection and inflammation of the thyroid gland, are among the common disorders occurring in the thyroid.[115] These diseases, along with other autoimmune diseases, have formerly been suggested to be associated with celiac disease.[116] For instance, recent studies show that adults with celiac disease are four times more at risk of hypothyroidism and nearly three times more at risk of hyperthyroidism than healthy individuals. In children with celiac disease, results were higher, at six times more for hypothyroidism and almost five times more for hyperthyroidism.[117] Additionally, 4 percent of adults with autoimmune thyroid disease also have celiac disease, while almost 8 percent of children with autoimmune thyroid disease also have celiac disease.[118]

Grave's disease is the overproduction of thyroid hormones by the immune system. It is also the most common cause of hyperthyroidism. On the other hand, Hashimoto's thyroiditis is the negative reaction of the immune system against the thyroid gland itself, and it is the most common cause of hypothyroidism. These two diseases are included in the autoimmune thyroid diseases strongly associated with celiac disease. The reason why celiac disease is strongly associated with autoimmune thyroid diseases is because they both involve an autoimmune process, in which the body attacks itself: the small intestine and the thyroid for the celiac disease and the autoimmune thyroid disease, respectively. A person who has a preexisting autoimmune disease is inclined to develop another autoimmune disease. The increased possibility, despite treatment, may be due to overlapping genetic predispositions. Lastly, symptoms of celiac disease and autoimmunity are nonspecific and often overlap with each other. This includes weight loss; diarrhea and/or constipation; fatigue; depression; joint, bone, or muscle pain; and infertility.[119] That in turn can affect thyroid health.

Liver Disorders

Hepatobiliary disorders pertain to the disorders or diseases affecting the liver. The main function of the liver is to (1) process the oxygen-rich blood from the aorta and also the nutrient-rich blood from the intestines, (2) regulate the different chemical levels in it, and (3) convert them into more usable forms or to less harmful ones—whichever is applicable. It also produces the bile that helps carry away toxic substances. The liver also has many other vital functions, such as the production of certain proteins, cholesterols, and immune factors; the regulation of blood clotting; the removal of bacteria from the blood; and the processing of hemoglobin. Having these various essential functions, disorders that occur in it immensely affect and are manifested in other body systems, and vice versa. Celiac disease of the gastrointestinal tract is no exception. Some of the liver disorders that have been documented to be associated with celiac disease include the abnormal elevation of liver enzyme levels, nonspecific hepatitis, nonalcoholic fatty liver, and autoimmune and cholestatic liver disease.[120]

Regarding the unexplained elevated liver enzyme levels, the result of one study showed that 5 out of the 55 patients with cyptogenic elevation of liver enzyme levels suffered from celiac disease.[121] Another study also found some association, though slightly lower: 19 (6 percent) out of 327 patients of chronic liver disorder had celiac disease.[122] Still another study showed a similar result: 13 out of 140 (9 percent) were found to be positive for celiac disease.[123]

To counter these findings, studies were also done to determine the prevalence of abnormal liver enzyme levels in celiac disease patients. Researchers showed that 30 had increased liver enzyme levels (out of the 75 patients with celiac disease).[124] Another study reported that 60 percent of children with celiac disease also had increased liver enzyme levels.[125] Subsequent surveys showed parallel results, in which 62 of 132 patients (47 percent) and 67 of 158 (42 percent) had been documented to have abnormally elevated liver enzyme levels.[126] To date, the reason or mechanism of how and why there are increased liver enzyme levels has not been proven. Theories and preliminary studies, though, were conducted. One study found that liver damage, manifested through increased liver enzyme levels, could be the result of an abnormality in the increase in intestinal permeability of celiac disease patients. This is because intestinal permeability was significantly greater in patients with elevated liver enzyme levels than in those with a normal liver enzyme level.[127]

Another liver disorder that had been documented to have an association with celiac disease is *primary biliary cirrhosis*. A large-scale epidemiological study found that 3 percent of patients with celiac disease had primary biliary cirrhosis, and 6 percent of patients with primary biliary cirrhosis had celiac disease.[128] Other investigations showed increased prevalence of primary biliary cirrhosis in patients with celiac disease.[129] Though additional evaluations proved otherwise, the association of celiac disease and primary biliary cirrhosis appears to be solid.[130]

One more cholestatic liver disease that has some proof of association with celiac disease is *primary sclerosing cholangitis*. One published study reported that approximately 3 percent of patients with primary sclerosing cholangitis were found to have celiac disease.[131] The second one found that 1 in approximately 60 patients with primary sclerosing cholangitis had celiac disease.[132]

Autoimmune and nonspecific hepatitis is another liver disease that has some association with celiac disease. Results of one study showed that 4 percent of 157 patients with Type 1 autoimmune hepatitis, plus 24 patients with Type 2 autoimmune hepatitis, were diagnosed to have celiac disease. This result is eight times greater than the occurrence of autoimmune hepatitis in the general population. [133] To add to this, there are other clinical reports suggesting the association of celiac disease to autoimmune hepatitis. [134]

Other liver diseases that had some cases reported to be coexistent with celiac disease include other autoimmune liver diseases, fatty liver, and end-stage liver disease. Because patients involved in these case studies are small in number, it would be too rash to generalize. Moreover, associations were not too strong as compared to the other liver diseases previously discussed. In addition, because the mechanisms and cases are not yet well established, associations could just be coincidental instead of being a true manifestation of each other. [135]

Urinary Tract and Kidneys

Celiac disease may cause a urinary tract infection if left undiagnosed or untreated, especially among children. Urinary tract infection was found to be significantly more common among children with celiac disease than the control group. [136] Out of the different urinary infections that were found in children with celiac disease, the one caused by *E. coli* was found to be the most prominent, being in more than 80 percent of the tested children. [137] *E. coli* infection usually vanishes on its own, so no exceptional treatment is really needed. [138]

Kidney stones in the urine, called urolithiasis, but commonly referred to as the former, are associated, albeit rarely, with celiac disease, both in adults and in children. [139] The reasons behind this connection are yet to be uncovered. As with most other celiac disease–related disorders, following a gluten-free diet can be helpful in treating celiac disease and also in avoiding the formation of new kidney stones. [140]

A 45-year-old Caucasian man was diagnosed with proteinuria, possibly an early symptom of kidney disease, during a routine physical examination in February 2005. Despite being treated for the anomaly, his condition worsened. It was then that malabsorption was considered as a possible diagnosis. After serological testing for celiac disease turned out positive, he started a gluten-free diet by January 2006. Within three to six months, his condition improved. [141]

Pancreatic Disorder

The pancreas is an internal organ that secretes enzymes and hormones. The enzymes help break down carbohydrates, fats, and proteins while the hormones regulate the level of glucose in the blood. Exocrine pancreatic insufficiency (EPI) is one of the major diseases of the pancreas, in which the pancreas does not produce sufficient digestive enzymes to enable adequate digestion and nutrient absorption in the body.[142] Celiac disease is associated with EPI, and the first study that described and reported this association was more than 50 years ago.[143] A number of studies have already validated this finding.[144]

The level of an *elastase* called Fel-1 can be evaluated to determine the exocrine pancreatic function. Fel-1 levels are significantly lower in adult patients with celiac disease and chronic diarrhea than in the control group. Also, the prevalence of low Fel-1 was 11 percent for the patients with new celiac disease, 6 percent for the celiac disease patients on a gluten-free diet without gastrointestinal symptoms, 30 percent for the celiac disease patients on a gluten-free diet with chronic diarrhea, and 4 percent for the patients with chronic diarrhea but without celiac disease. These results suggest that EPI is the cause of the persisting symptom of celiac disease (chronic diarrhea), accounting for about one in three adult patients examined.[145]

More recent research confirms that Fel-1 can indeed be used to identify exocrine pancreatic insufficiency in adult patients with celiac disease. Celiac disease symptoms were lessened due to the supplementation of pancreatic enzymes. In detail, almost 20 patients presented a significant increase in Fel-1 levels over time as they took supplementation, and only 1 out of 19 did not show any symptomatic benefit, while 8 out of 19 already stopped supplementation because their celiac disease–related symptoms had already improved. This suggests that long-term supplementation is unnecessary, and the dosage may be lowered or even discontinued as symptoms are reduced.[146]

Inflammatory Bowel Diseases

Inflammatory bowel diseases are long-term disorders in which there is inflammation of the gastrointestinal tract. These include ulcerative colitis and Crohn's disease. Ulcerative colitis is a disease that causes ulcers and irritation in the inner lining of the large intestine, the colon, and the rectum. Meanwhile, Crohn's disease affects any part of the digestive tract.[147]

These diseases have previously been reported to be associated with celiac disease. In one study, out of 455 patients who had celiac disease, 10 also had inflammatory bowel disease (five had ulcerative colitis while the other five had Crohn's disease) based on their biopsy results. This means that inflammatory bowel disease was more common within their group of patients with celiac disease than in the general population, because recorded data show that the worldwide occurrence of ulcerative colitis is only up to 25 out of 100,000 individuals, while that of Crohn's disease is only up to 16 out of 100,000 individuals.[148]

Research that included a control group composed of healthy people also reported the prevalence of association between the two diseases. The experts have concluded that the prevalence of inflammatory bowel disease was ten times higher in patients with celiac disease than in the controls, while the prevalence of celiac disease was comparable in those with inflammatory bowel disease and the healthy group.[149] In addition, science has found that patients with inflammatory bowel disease have a lower risk of having celiac disease than the general population. Moreover, the prevalence of celiac disease was two times greater in patients with ulcerative colitis than in those with Crohn's disease.[150]

Irritable Bowel Syndrome

Irritable bowel syndrome (IBS, not to be confused with inflammatory bowel disease, which includes ulcerative colitis and Crohn's disease) is a common gastrointestinal disorder without any known organic cause. It is characterized by any of the following: crampy abdominal pain, gassiness, bloating, and changes in bowel habits (constipation, diarrhea, or both).[151] It is commonly confused with celiac disease, for it shares similar symptoms. However, they are differentiated based on where and how they affect the gastrointestinal tract. Celiac disease causes damage to the small intestines, while irritable bowel syndrome mainly involves the large intestines and does not really cause damage to them—hence it is just called a syndrome and not a disease. Recently, studies have been conducted to evaluate the association of these two conditions with similar symptoms.[152]

One study concluded that irritable bowel syndrome was significantly associated with celiac disease when compared with matched controls. In this regard, it was suggested that patients with irritable bowel syndrome should be consistently evaluated for the presence of celiac disease. Also, duodenal biopsy is suggested for a more accurate confirmation of the presence of celiac disease than testing for *endomysial antibodies*. Therefore, regular testing for celiac disease in patients with irritable bowel syndrome already is recommended. [153]

In light of these findings, 12 of the 105 patients with irritable bowel syndrome that were studied had celiac disease, while none of the 105 healthy controls had it. [154] Another survey involving a larger number of subjects (4,204 individuals in all) concluded that the prevalence of celiac disease detected through biopsy in patients meeting diagnostic criteria for irritable bowel disorder was four times greater than those in healthy individuals. [155] On this note, another study determined that celiac disease serological testing in patients with suspected irritable bowel syndrome is cost-effective. [156]

Intestinal Cancer

At times, when the genetic material of the cells of living organisms develop some errors or mutation due to exposure to radiation and/or carcinogenic substances, the cells fail to repair or correct themselves. Because of this, the mutated cells continue to grow and divide indeterminately without dying, forming a collection of abnormal cells or a tumor. This tumor would eventually interfere with the normal function of the cells within the organ, organ system, and the entire body where it is located. In addition, these abnormal cells metastasize or spread to other parts of the body, unlike the healthy cells that simply stay in their organ of origin. They do this by acquiring access to the bloodstream and/or the lymphatic system. When the tumor has already attained the capability of "creating" other tumors in other areas through spreading, it is simply called a malignant tumor, or else cancer. [157]

Intestinal cancer, also called colorectal or simply colon cancer, is a cancer located in the large intestines. It is second to lung cancer in causing death. However, in females, it is third next to breast and lung cancer, and in males it is also the third, next to prostate and lung cancer. In the

United States about 140,000 new cases of colon cancer are diagnosed each year, and the risk of acquiring it is 2.5–5 percent.[158]

Formal studies of colon cancer manifestations in people suffering from celiac disease demonstrate a higher risk for cancer. These include a much higher susceptibility of developing *intestinal adenocarcinomas* and malignant neoplasms such as lymphomas than the general population.[159] However, there is still a lack of a large-scale systematic evaluation on this matter. This is the reason why further studies were conducted. One study, involving 12,000 subjects, found that the overall cancer risk for adult patients with celiac disease is higher than in the general population. For children and adolescents, there was no significant difference in the risk of having cancer for celiac and nonceliac patients. The researchers also supported other past studies, which claimed the risk of having lymphoma and intestinal cancer is higher in patients with celiac disease.[160]

Other experts also proved and summarized the association of celiac disease and cancer. As an example, researchers stated that celiac disease is indeed associated with lymphomas and other forms of cancer—especially in the intestines, the esophagus, the pharynx, and also extraintestinal in the liver, spleen, thyroid, skin, nasal sinus, and brain. Their report also maintains that a gluten-free diet gives protection against cancer development, especially in younger individuals.[161]

However, there are other studies that prove the opposite, in which the instance of colon cancer is very limited in patients with celiac disease. Instance of colon cancer has not increased in patients with celiac disease, especially those that were diagnosed with celiac disease at or above the age of 60. For this reason, one study hypothesized that untreated celiac disease (as in the case of adult patients diagnosed later in their lives) is protective *against* colon cancer, since dietary fat, hydrocarbons, and fat-soluble carcinogens are inadequately absorbed and quickly excreted in the gastrointestinal tract of patients with celiac disease.[162]

Some scientists disagree. This is because when colon adenomas were compared in celiac disease patients and healthy controls, results showed that 13 percent of celiac disease patients have at least one adenoma while 17 percent of healthy controls have at least one adenoma.[163] This may be because celiac disease patients have more proper health care attention than the healthy controls. Also, some celiac patients may have also undergone colonoscopy, which may also decrease the chance of having precancerous adenoma by removing it through the procedure. Whatever the reason may be for the increased or decreased risk of having colorectal cancer in celiac disease patients, conflicting results show that if ever there is indeed an increase in the risk of developing a cancer, it must be very small, for that would be the average considering the different results from the studies involving different sets of patients.

Infertility

There are many causes for why men and women are biologically unable to produce children; celiac disease may be one of them. Malabsorption of nutrients—such as iron, folic acid, and zinc, which play very important roles in early pregnancy—can affect reproduction.[164] Deficiency of certain nutrients can also affect female and male hormones, which in turn may cause the reduction of sperm count and may impair the ovulation process.[165] A study group composed of 99 couples that were being examined for infertility at the Department of Obstetrics and Gynecology of the University of Sassari, Italy, was observed from August 1997 to October 1998 for the prevalence of celiac disease. It was found that around 3 percent of the infertile women studied suffered from celiac disease.[166]

Diabetes

Diabetes is a chronic or lifelong disease in which the body cannot use carbohydrates or sugar properly. This is because this disease interferes with the way insulin, a hormone that regulates glucose levels in the blood, is made and used. In the United States, over 20 million people are affected by this disease.[167] Diabetes and celiac disease sometimes occur together, especially in people with Type 1 diabetes. For example, in the United States, the estimated rate of celiac disease in people with Type 1 diabetes is about 10–20 percent, while the estimated rate of celiac disease in the general population is about 1 percent. In a larger-scale study, the occurrence of celiac disease in children afflicted with Type 1 diabetes was found to be 1:6–1:103, while for adults the rate is 1:16–1:76. On this note, one can conclude that celiac disease is common in patients with Type 1 diabetes.[168] Additional reports suggest that the range of prevalence of celiac disease in patients with Type 1 diabetes is from 3 to 16 percent. The close association may be attributed to common genetic links and environmental factors such as gluten and viral infections, which play a role in the maturity of each disease.[169]

One proof for the genetic link between celiac disease and Type 1 diabetes is a study involving thousands of patients with Type 1 diabetes, thousands more with celiac disease, and thousands of healthy control subjects.[170] All the subjects' DNA samples were analyzed through geno-typing and statistics, and they were searched for the common allele that they share. Aside from the genes that both are associated with a specific chromosome, three celiac disease loci were also associated with Type 1 diabetes. One (plus an additional three previously discovered loci) Type 1 diabetes locus was also found to be associated with celiac disease. This finding brings the total number of loci associations between the two diseases to seven. This information implies that there may be common biological mechanisms, such as the tissue damage caused by autoimmu-nity, between these two. Results suggest there may also be environmental factors that could affect both diseases in a similar way.[171]

Now if ever a diabetes patient is unaware that he or she also has celiac disease and is taking medication for diabetes but not for the latter, the patient is expected to have an erratic glucose level in the blood. This is could be explained by taking into consideration the medication of diabet-ic patients, which is insulin. The reason is that the dose of insulin taken was designed to match the expected amount of carbohydrate to be ab-sorbed by the body. Since celiac disease will lessen the amount of nutri-ents to be absorbed, there would be a mismatch in the amount of insulin and the amount of carbohydrates. Fortunately, once the celiac disease gets treated, the expected/predicted glucose result would match the insu-lin dosage and would be absorbed by the body as needed.

The fact that both celiac disease and Type 1 diabetes involve an auto-immune process, in which the body's leukocytes that normally fight against infections attack their own healthy body cells, makes these two diseases more closely associated with each other. This is also one of the major reasons why there is a higher risk for acquiring one of the two diseases if already diagnosed previously with the other. Consequently, a person who has a preexisting autoimmune disease is more likely to devel-op another autoimmune disease due to the many genetic and environmen-tal reasons discussed previously. So as a preventive measure, regular autoimmune screening for patients with Type 1 diabetes (or celiac disease, or any other autoimmune disease for that matter) is suggested, even in the absence of symptoms. [172]

ANALYSIS

Celiac disease is an autoimmune disorder of the intestine that may be indirectly associated with the presence of other disorders. These include gastrointestinal manifestations such as dental enamel defects, thyroid, hepatobiliary and pancreatic disorders, inflammatory bowel disease, irritable bowel syndrome, diabetes, and cancer. In addition, skin disorders such as dermatitis herpetiformis, alopecia areata, chronic urticaria, psoriasis, eczema, acne and dry skin, and bacterial and viral manifestations may occur.

9

PAIN AND CELIAC DISEASE

Celiac disease is considered a silent source of pain that places patients in a very dangerous position regarding proper diagnosis. There are people who spend years without being diagnosed appropriately, and this is because celiac disease does not present itself with simple, identifiable pain that would allow a prompt diagnosis and/or easy recognition. By reading this chapter, celiac disease patients will realize that the specifics of celiac disease–related pain can be very intricate and complicated. Therefore, a thorough exploration of its roots and forms must be undertaken.

ROOTS OF PAIN IN CELIAC DISEASE

Pain is not the cornerstone of celiac disease, as in most adults the disease develops without ever presenting any symptoms or pain but a general feeling of discomfort. Nevertheless, when pain does manifest, it is due to the digestive problems and poor absorption that lead to the lack of vitamins and minerals that the body needs to function properly, compromising not only the digestive system but also other systems in the body. It is well known that when an organ such as the small intestine breaks down, the whole individual is compromised.[1] The disruptive process of celiac disease in the human body causes conditions that range from stomachaches to life-threatening ones that result in different levels of pain.

Children suffering from celiac disease have the disadvantage that they often cannot express well or properly describe their pain. They may not have a big appetite because eating may cause them discomfort. Therefore, parents tend to be very cautious and observant of them. So early diagnosis could be made when the general discomfort of gastrointestinal problems appears together with malnutrition derived from the malabsorption of any vitamin and/or mineral. However, the types of celiac disease developed in adulthood are sometimes asymptomatic, making early diagnosis very difficult, as pain or discomfort may not be present. That in turn makes it easier for other painful conditions to develop. However, not all symptoms from celiac disease—or conditions derived as a result of the damage caused by it—cause pain.

Bloating Pain

Celiac disease patients suffering from an excess of gas, diarrhea, or reflux experience degrees of bloating and, as a result, pain or discomfort that could go from mild to severe. Some describe it as an unbearable pain due to the stomach problems located in different places, ranging from the pit of the stomach to the lower stomach. It is also common that pain is felt only on one side of the stomach (left or right). This is described as a constant, severe pain coupled with extra waves of cramps. Lower back and leg pain are also related due to the cramping of the organs to give space to the inflamed intestine.[2]

Autoimmunity-Related Pain

The body mistakes local elements as foreign and targets them as malignant, and the antibodies sent to protect the body start to destroy themselves. The triggering of celiac disease can cause, in some cases, a second and/or even a third autoimmune disorder that in turn leads to a variety of painful symptoms. These conditions include, but are not limited to, the following:

thyroid disease, which causes muscle and joint pain
Sjögren's syndrome, which affects the glands that secrete tears and saliva, causing pain in the eyes and discomfort in the mouth as well as damage to lungs and kidneys
cardiomyopathy, which is an inflammatory heart disease that attacks the heart muscle; the most common type found in celiac disease

patients is dilated cardiomyopathy, in which the muscle weakens, and, as a result, the heart dilates and causes arrhythmia and even heart failure—mild chest pain is present as a general discomfort rheumatoid arthritis, which causes joint swelling, stiffness, and loss of joint function; relatives with an autoimmune disease have up to a 25 percent chance of having celiac disease[3]

Joint Pain

People with celiac disease have reported joint pain commonly located in the knees, back, hips, wrists, and shoulders; if there is a past injury, it could act up as well. How high the joint pain could go has not been medically researched; people have reported that it could go from mild discomfort to extreme pain known to be very similar to that of strong arthritis.[4] Joint pain may appear even before any digestive problems appear, if they appear at all, but like many of the other symptoms, it is not exclusively a symptom of celiac disease. As people get older, joint pain is more and more common, regardless of whether they suffer celiac disease. In celiac disease, joint pain is caused from malnutrition stemming from the lack of nutrients; another reason is due to the inflammation itself caused by ingesting gluten. There have been reported cases of rheumatoid arthritis diagnosed first and then celiac disease. Some studies show now that in some of these cases rheumatoid arthritis was in fact the underlying symptom for patients that suffer from celiac disease.

Neurological Pain

There are several neurological conditions that could develop from celiac disease, but not all of them develop into pain-related symptoms. The most common are headaches. In fact, nearly 40 percent of children and adolescents diagnosed with celiac disease have presented with chronic headaches.[5] Other high-risk, painful conditions include migraine, which is a chronic neurological disorder characterized by recurrent moderate-to-severe headaches often in association with a number of autonomic nervous system symptoms. These migraines could last up to seventy-two hours or more. Another condition is peripheral neuropathy, which is the result of nerve damage. The damage causes several symptoms with pain ranging from mild to severe. The levels of pain will depend on the af-

fected area and the severity of the damage. While the discomfort is generally described as tingling or prickling, some describe it as a burning and/
or freezing pain.[6] These neuropathies result in nerve damage in the peripheral nervous system. This condition only affects nerves outside of the
brain and spinal cord; this means that there is no damage to the central
nervous system. Seizures might also present, even though not all patients
that experience seizures report feeling any pain. Nevertheless, there have
been reports of some patients that have experienced headaches and even
back pain.[7]

RECOGNIZING PAIN IN CELIAC DISEASE

When someone has celiac disease and is not exactly asymptomatic, they
could recognize some of the pain that comes with the autoimmune reaction from the damaged tissues of the small intestine. To understand how
pain could be present, it is important to remember how the disease works.
Essentially, the body does not perceive that it is being attacked. It be-
lieves that it is attacking a foreign element that certain types of food
contain, making the organs destroy the same thing that is trying to protect
its integrity. This causes the villous atrophy (flattened villi) and the small,
crypt-like places where the cells that cover and protect the villi (crypt
hyperplasia), and an intense inflammatory reaction that causes severe or
mild pain. Unfortunately, the intestine will continue to suffer and be
damaged until the vicious cycle is broken and gluten is taken from the
diet.

Feeling pain and discomfort makes the individual somehow lucky, as
a battery of tests to rule out other conditions may reveal celiac disease,
but in asymptomatic patients they can go for years feeling terrible pain
and discomfort without being diagnosed because doctors focus on treating the conditions derived from the malabsorption of vitamins and minerals without uncovering celiac disease. In order to recognize the types of
pain, it is necessary to keep in mind that pain can spread from the gastrointestinal region to other areas of the body.

Painful heartburn and reflux are also present in most cases, causing the
bile to traverse from the duodenum to the stomach and then later to the
esophagus. This causes irritation and inflammation in celiac disease patients. Heartburn, as the name suggests, consists of the burning feeling

near the chest behind the breastbone and can radiate onto the neck, throat, and angle of the jaw.[8] Cramps that are very painful can interrupt normal activities due to the inflammation of the intestine. The pain is mostly located in the upper part of the small intestine, but some cases present with pain on one side of the abdomen. All the previous painful symptoms could be related to other diseases and could be easily confused as a result of reactions, making it difficult to suspect celiac disease. However, all of these symptoms could be developed after ingesting food containing gluten, and if there is a constant reaction to this type of food, one can suspect that celiac disease is the cause.

When the celiac disease itself is silent or latent, pain could come from other organs and conditions, which are presented in other chapters of this book. As every patient can develop different disorders depending on the lack of nutrients that the body is failing to absorb, it is possible to recognize specific and complicated types of pain. Usually, pain symptoms come from the autoimmune, neurological, and physical conditions typically presented as a result of celiac disease or that have helped develop it. If all that has been presented is collected, there are certain nongastrointestinal painful symptoms that can be identified:

joint pain
back pain
chest pain
headaches (up to migraines)
stomachache

Most of the time people who lack the trademark gastrointestinal pain of celiac disease are diagnosed on their other conditions first. Through the full battery of tests, they find they also have celiac disease as an underlying or primary condition. Moreover, damage in organs and tissue cannot be undone in most painful conditions and must be treated accordingly.

Even after following the doctor's indications and eliminating gluten from the diet, some celiac disease patients continue to present with pain or discomfort. There are medications that could help the patient with those lasting symptoms, but some of these remaining symptoms could be the result of other underlying conditions that have to be treated and are unrelated to gluten consumption but were already present in the patient. Some of these underlying conditions, which often cause pain and discomfort, are as follows:

- Patients could still be consuming gluten and might not know about it. As a result, they continue to suffer pain. It is important to check ingredients and labels when going grocery shopping.
- Lactose intolerance: Also called *lactase deficiency* or *hypolactasia*, this condition makes the body unable to digest lactose properly. Lactose is a type of sugar found in milk and to a lesser extent in some dairy products. Lactose intolerance cannot be categorized as a full-blown clinical disease, but more like a characteristic determined by genetics.[9] When the person consumes any milk or dairy product that contains lactose, the stomach will continue to bloat. Therefore, discomfort and pain could be present.
- Pancreatic insufficiency: Diarrhea is a common symptom, and the damage in the intestine can damage the pancreas, which produces hormones known to have roles in metabolism and sugar regulation. Once the intestine starts to heal, the pancreas starts to secrete the hormones and to work efficiently.
- Bacterial overgrowth: Some bacteria migrate from the colon to the intestine. Celiac disease patients that take too many antacids damage the protective walls of the intestine, allowing bacteria to prosper.
- Refractory sprue: With this condition, the damage continues even six months after following treatment. This condition has yet to be defined as a result of celiac disease or researched to see if it affects patients because of misdiagnosed celiac disease.[10] There is fear and lack of understanding if this condition is really connected to celiac disease or if it is just a cause of misdiagnosis or is a condition that parallels the latter. However, there are certain characteristics that researchers agree on: (1) the presence of persistently damaged villi in the small intestine that are not repaired after the gluten-free diet has been successfully initiated and/or maintained; (2) an increased presence of intraepithelial lymphocytes (IEL) in the small bowel; and (3) severe malabsorption.[11]
- Intestinal inflammation: This is the most common painful symptom caused by the inflammation of the intestine.

ADDRESSING THE PAIN

There are medications that can be used to placate the pain and discomfort associated with celiac disease. Prescribed pain medication is not exactly to prevent celiac disease. It is to help deal with the inflammation. In the event that the small intestine is severely damaged, doctors may recommend steroids to control inflammation.

General Pain from Inflammation

Steroids can help control and ease painful symptoms of celiac disease while the small intestine heals itself. These medications, known as *corticosteroids*, are heavily used to deal with a diverse range of conditions. They mimic the effects of hormones that the body produces naturally, and when these are prescribed they elevate the hormone levels just above what is needed to treat inflammation and to lower the severe pain. Corticosteroids can be administered by mouth, as an inhaler or spray, topically (through the skin), and by injection.[12] Corticosteroids are really a class of chemicals that include steroid hormones naturally produced in the adrenal cortex of vertebrates, and analogues of these hormones are routinely synthesized in controlled laboratories. Corticosteroids are heavily involved in a wide range of processes and reactions within the body, including response to stress, metabolism of carbohydrates, immune response, protein catabolism, levels of blood electrolytes, and human behavior.[13] The most common application form is oral, but that is also the form that may cause serious side effects, some of which can be painful. Side effect severity will depend on three basic factors:

1. *The type of corticosteroid steroid tablets*: Some types are more likely to cause side effects than inhalers or injections.
2. *The dosage*: The higher the dose, the greater the risk of developing side effects. In this case it will depend on the dose prescribed by the doctor to treat the inflammation.
3. *The time frame*: Prolonged use increases the risks. For example, it is highly likely that the celiac disease sufferer will develop more serious side effects if the medicine intake is prolonged. A minor side effect could be face swelling, while a serious and major side effect could be glaucoma.[14]

The risks seem high, but a patient can benefit from corticosteroids without elevating the risk of developing severe side effects by taking certain precautions, which, of course, need to be revised and approved by a health care professional. There are newer forms of corticosteroids that may vary in strength and length of action; it is recommended that one talk with a doctor and ask about the best course of action for the specific case and to review the opportunities to lower the dose. Corticosteroids that are inhaled for asthma, for example, would reach lung surfaces directly, reducing other organs' exposure to them and leading to fewer side effects. For inflammation of the intestine, this type of application does not act immediately; therefore, the treatment could take longer and is not recommended for celiac disease patients. Injected corticosteroids might also be an option.

Furthermore, making healthy choices during therapy is also important. When on corticosteroid medications for a prolonged period, patients could lessen risks by reducing calories in their diet and exercising more often. These simple activities will help maintain a balanced and healthy lifestyle that will lower the risk of developing major side effects brought on by corticosteroids. Celiac disease patients should also take care after therapy with corticosteroids is completed. The intake of oral corticosteroids for prolonged periods causes the adrenal glands to produce less of their natural steroid hormones. To give the adrenal glands time to recover their standard functions, doctors may reduce the dosage gradually. If the dosage is reduced too quickly, patients may experience fatigue, body aches, and lightheadedness, as is the case with any major withdrawal from medications.[15] Short-term side effects include high blood glucose levels and fluid retention. The mineralocorticoid properties of prednisone are relatively weak. Additional short-term side effects can include the following:

insomnia
euphoria (somewhat uncommon)
mania (i.e., bipolar disorder)
depression or depressive symptoms
anxiety in some individuals
face swelling
unusual fatigue or weakness
memory or attention dysfunction
black stool

hyperactivity
sensitive teeth
acne
nervousness

No matter the kind of pain celiac disease patients develop, if the pain persists, they must inform their doctor in order to be monitored and evaluate whether to discontinue the medication if side effects are too risky. There is a risk of dependency, causing the body to stop producing its own hormones after at least a week of administering prednisone and taking it away. Therefore, the medication cannot be abruptly stopped; it is recommended to gradually reduce dosage. Celiac disease sufferers should be careful and vigilant regarding any allergic reactions from ingesting corticosteroids for pain. While on medication, patients must avoid vaccinations, immunizations, or skin tests unless the doctor allows for it. If there is a history of ulcers or if patients are used to taking a considerable amount of aspirin, patients should limit the consumption of alcoholic beverages because the combination makes intestines more susceptible to the effects of both alcohol and aspirin. Patients can always report injuries or signs of painful infection. If a celiac disease sufferer has diabetes, the medication may increase blood sugar levels. Continuous monitoring of blood and/or urine glucose levels must be done, as directed by any doctor. Exercise plans and diet may also need to be adjusted.

Dermatitis Herpetiformis

Due to the itching and painful skin rash that sometimes comes with celiac disease, skin medication along with a gluten-free diet helps the overall situation of the patient. One of the most recommended medications to treat the rash is diaminodiphenyl sulfone (DDS), which is an antibacterial. Its role in the treatment of dermatitis hepertiformis, which is not necessarily caused exclusively by bacteria, is poorly understood. The exact mechanism of action is unknown, but it is thought to be related to the inhibition of neutrophil migration and function. Patients confirm an improvement of their symptoms within hours after initiating therapy. DDS could cause adverse side effects such as anemia, neuropathy, and agranulocytosis, so regular monitoring is required.[16] This medication cannot treat the physical damage in the intestine. That is why a gluten-free diet is needed in case of celiac disease. Ibuprofen is another safe option for treating the condition. [17]

POTENTIAL UNCONVENTIONAL THERAPIES AND DESIGNER DRUGS

Even though the only known *surefire* way to keep celiac disease at bay is by a gluten-free diet and corticosteroids for inflammation and pain, the field of medicine is evolving. There are potential therapies that could help prevent celiac disease from developing. Some of them are listed below:

Genetically modified wheat: Researchers may find the way to eradicate genetically the genes that disallow people with celiac disease to consume wheat.

Immunizations: This has been initially proven through the feeding of infants who are still breastfeeding by introducing gluten at this stage. In other countries, specifically Australia, a type of intestinal parasite is being used in adult patients suffering from celiac disease, tricking the body into raising its protective immune defenses.

Larazotide: This is a blocker that inhibits intestinal permeability. Studies still continue, but after phase two, patients presented fewer symptoms and even developed antibodies.

ANALYSIS

Pain itself will never be the one symptom that would identify or define celiac disease. In this disease, pain arrives through inflammation and, in some patients, through other conditions that can develop from the damaged intestine. There is a manageable solution for pain in most cases. That is yet another important point for patients and caregivers to understand when it comes to dealing with celiac disease.

Part IV

Treatment Options

10

NATURAL TREATMENTS AND DIET

Celiac disease is most common in Caucasians or those of European descent, and recently it has been discovered that approximately 1 percent of the population in the United States is diagnosed with the disease.[1] However, hope is not lost, for although no cure is available to entirely eliminate the problem, there are natural treatments available to suppress the harmful effects of this disease.

BENEFITS OF NATURAL TREATMENTS

There are two available choices for any patient to consider when thinking about undergoing treatment for celiac disease: natural treatment, or drug (conventional) treatment. Centuries before the breakthrough of pharmaceutical medication, natural or herbal treatments were the primary holders of attention in the field of healing. However, in the second half of the nineteenth century, drugs took over the spotlight. Since then, the majority of the human population has depended on drugs for practically every single problem that exists in the human body, and the once widely used natural treatments took a backseat as "alternative" medicine. In the United States alone, over $135 billion is spent on drug medications every year, and yet, to the astonishment of most, the rate of Americans acquiring diseases continues to rise.[2] This fact in itself speaks greatly of the efficiency of the use of drug medication; as a result, many are beginning to turn back to the practice of the "old days" when natural treatments once flourished in the world.

Before weighing the scale between the two available options, it is necessary to understand what qualifies as natural treatment or drug medication. A drug medication, often called synthetic or conventional, is defined as having a scheduled intake of a chemically formulated and processed artificial substance for medical reasons, such as the management, analysis, or avoidance of a particular disease or condition. A natural treatment, however, refers not only to the intake of natural substances, such as natural supplements, but also to a change in lifestyle to minimize the devastating effects of a certain disorder such as celiac disease, or to eradicate it altogether.

Drug medication has undeniably saved lives over the past centuries, but the benefits come with great expense. More often than not, side effects are known to manifest, temporarily fixing one part of the body while compromising the other areas. Consumers grow increasingly dependent on gulping down painkillers, unconsciously masking symptoms—they are in actuality very important in any diagnosis, for these are the primary bases that will name the condition, or warn the individual of any life-risking occurrences that may happen. When the condition is left undiagnosed for a time, it can be very precarious. Medicines contain these artificially processed chemicals that will take the body's much required energy to break down the substances for them to be of any use.

Also, conventional medicines are highly commercialized, so that a great portion of the price is allotted for the expense made to process, package, and advertise the product as a commercial commodity. Many perceive conventional medication as a needed method of treatment, most especially in major diseases that are seen as heights unreachable to simple and primitive herbal medicine. It may be true that drug medication is very much needed as a firsthand approach to complex diseases that involve the invasion of harmful antibodies that quickly replicate and therefore must immediately be halted, or to certain abnormalities that require surgery. When it comes to long-term treatment, the natural way is highly recommended, for the negative side effects of synthetic medicine can be downright life threatening if taken for such long periods of time.

Natural treatment, however, not only requires the intake of a special tablet or capsule but also actively involves the celiac disease patient's whole person in a process that helps understand the aspects of the body, and therefore enables one to consciously execute any necessary efforts to make the changes needed in order to develop a healthier body. Natural treatments are proven to be the most beneficial to those with celiac disease, basically because a change in lifestyle—most especially with food intake—is very much required to keep the detriments of the autoimmune disorder to a minimum.

One of the benefits of natural treatment is that it does not act as a hindrance to the body's natural body processes because it is in a form compatible with our own natural system, given that it is integrated into our own lifestyle and the usage of any herbal medicine is unprocessed synthetically. In fact, not only does it not hinder the body's healing processes, but it also enhances and accelerates the body's own way of healing itself. Conventional medicine does the following:

manipulates the body in ways to correct unusually low levels of hormones

affects the nervous system to alter a certain process

blocks signals from pain receptors

injects a certain agent similar to a specific germ or a germ itself that has been altered so as to condition the immune system on how to combat the particular antibody in the future

On the contrary, herbal medicine merely induces various glands to activate suitable hormones in order to maintain a balanced internal environment ideal to pave the way to recovery. Hormones are known to be the messengers that transmit distress signals to the appropriate parts of the body to stimulate *or* hamper particular body processes to boost healing.

Another benefit is that natural treatments target the celiac disease sufferer's very way of life—rest, diet, exercise—that work hand in hand with the intake of herbal medicine to further enhance the effectiveness of the herb by conditioning the body in such a way that it reacts to the treatment in the most desirable and efficient way. These changes in the way of life ultimately benefit the individual, for it trains the body to get into a healthy rhythm that will soon develop into a habit that will continue to exist even after recovery from a particular disease or ailment, thus greatly decreasing the possibility of repeating the same problems over and over again. As a result of an enhanced body system and a change in lifestyle, the immune system is significantly strengthened, consequently boosting the celiac disease patient's natural defenses against pathogens—

viruses, bacteria, or any other microorganisms capable of causing further harm.

Moreover, natural enhancements in the body lead to an improvement in metabolism, which will result in better absorption of nutrients obtained from one's diet. This is the main reason why natural treatment usually limits or prohibits the intake of food that contains too many fats or stimulants, such as junk foods and caffeine, respectively, for two known factors. First, fatty foods do not give the body its much-required amount or variety of nutrition. Second, stimulants hinder the function of the herbal medicine, therefore diminishing the effectiveness of the treatment.

METHODOLOGY

There are three basic natural treatment goals in trying to address celiac disease:

adapt to a gluten-free diet
stimulate the repair of the intestinal track
replenish the body with much-needed nutrients

It is important to have a plan on how to remedy celiac disease in order to stay on track. The first step is to stop the very source of agitation in the patient's body, which is gluten. Otherwise, stimulating repair of the intestinal track or replenishing one's body would be meaningless, for the already damaged small intestine will not be able to perform its function of absorbing the nutrients from any ingested food, or supplement, for that matter. A continued gluten diet would be very detrimental, for it can worsen the patient's condition with a gradual deterioration of the intestine, which can further result in malnutrition. The second step is to stimulate the repair of the intestinal tract in order to heal the symptoms that plague the patient. Once the small intestine is recovered enough to resume its vital function of digestion and absorption, it is time to replenish the deprived body of the nutrients it needs to continue functioning. Moreover, the inability to consume gluten-filled foods will also result in deficiencies in vitamins and minerals, since the needed nutrients found within those foods cannot be eaten. In loyally paying heed to these given steps, the road to recovery may be long and challenging, but all the effort will be of great worth in the end.

Living Gluten-Free

The protein called *gluten* is the main culprit in the degradation of the small intestine in patients inflicted with celiac disease, since the said disease is an abnormal response of the immune system against gluten most often found in wheat, barley, and rye. Therefore, avoiding the intake of any kind of food with gluten is a must, and this can be done by removing it from the diet regimen. These are not the only sources of gluten, however, for sources such as flour, beer, oats, soy sauce, and cake also contain the protein in question.

As part of the natural treatment for celiac disease, the advisable diet that a celiac patient can develop is one with limited (1) sugar, (2) alcohol, (3) mushrooms, (3) yeast, and (4) caffeine. All canned and/or processed meats and vegetables must be avoided, and organic food is the option that should be chosen as much as possible. Artificial sweeteners are proven to be detrimental to celiac patients, and therefore they must never use sugar substitutes. Instead, the use of honey is very much encouraged. A good diet will consist of supplemental fatty acids, especially the ones that turn into omega-3 during the process of digestion, such as the ones found in flaxseed oil. Omega-3 is at its best when consumed in combination with sulfur proteins, including yogurt, nuts, eggs, fish, sesame paste, cottage cheese, and garlic. A more elaborate list of what cannot be eaten follows:

any foods or ingredients that are wheat-derived or that have wheat
durum flour, self-rising flour, bromated flour, plain flour, phosphate
  flour, enriched flour, graham flour, and white flour
baked products such as bread, cakes, cookies, brownies, or muffins
pasta, pizza, bagels, crackers, couscous, tortillas, pastries, cereals,
  croutons
natural flavorings, emulsifiers, stabilizers, flavorings, coating mixes,
  baking powder, food starches
sauces with malted vinegar, gravy products, soy sauce, ketchup, mus-
  tards, oriental sauces
beer and instant coffee

Before consuming any beverage or food, the ingredients must be taken into careful examination in order to prevent any further damage to the body. Developing a new gluten-free diet is a great improvement, and, in addition to being accomplished through the avoidance of eating any foods known to contain gluten, it is also achieved by being certain that gluten-free products will not be contaminated. The contamination of gluten-free foods with foods containing this protein is called cross-contamination. Prevention of cross-contamination can be accomplished by having a gluten-free kitchen and by having utensils entirely dedicated to cooking food for people unable to tolerate gluten. The storage of food is also a possible avenue through which gluten-free foods can be contaminated; therefore, it is imperative to have a separate place for food intended solely for the celiac patient.

An individual with celiac disease should be very prepared when it comes to having food that is gluten-free at hand. In the modern industry of processed and packaged foods, it is recommended to have gluten-free food ready, in one's bag, purse, car, office—practically every possible place one may go. Additionally, it is highly advised that celiac patients keep a journal or diary to keep track of the different reactions or effects different foods have on them. This can be very helpful in remembering which ones are safe to eat and which ones trigger some sort of negative response.

Gluten-free food is the only treatment for celiac disease and the key to staying healthy. To be sure the diet is both gluten-free and healthy, one must ensure a few other things first. Learning about gluten-free foods is a giant step to living with celiac disease after diagnosis. Food items prepared with wheat, rye, oats, barley, and their derivatives are completely avoided in a strict gluten-free diet. There are many gluten-free grains and vegetables that are good sources of vitamins, minerals, protein, and fiber.[3] A basic list of naturally gluten-free foods includes butter, chicken, eggs, fish, fresh fruit and 100 percent fruit juices, fresh vegetables and 100 percent vegetable juices, honey, lentils, meats, milk, nuts, seeds, shellfish, and sugar.[4]

Alcohol was considered harmful for people with gluten intolerance and celiac disease until a few years back. Now, affected people can consume alcoholic drinks as long as they are distilled, even if they are made from wheat, rye, or barley.[5] All items containing gluten should be removed from the house, especially from the kitchen, and recently diagnosed celiac disease patients should ideally start from scratch. To live a symptom-free life, it is important to make sure that all shelves, crevices, and corners are thoroughly cleaned before stocking up on gluten-free items so as to prevent contamination with previously used items that contained gluten. It is not easy if patients are living with other family members. Therefore, it must be discussed with the others before deciding on which shelves and counter space will be gluten-free. The gluten-free area in the house is the safe zone for the person suffering from celiac disease, be it an adult or child. Household items as well as toiletries such as mouthwash and toothpaste also need to be gluten-free. It is also important that children in the family understand celiac disease and the importance of a gluten-free diet. Therefore, one should take enough time to communicate with them. In a celiac disease–safe kitchen, children can help adults obey the rules. It is advisable to always make sure there is a special place in the refrigerator to keep leftovers and mayonnaise, relish, mustard, and all other condiments in separate bottles with a sticker or marker. [6]

Natural Repair of the Intestinal Tract

The following are some of the most effective natural treatments that will help improve the health of the small intestine.

Apple pectin is known to be a type of fiber that can be found in practically all plant cell walls and tissues. All plants may contain pectin. However, a particularly high concentration is found in apples. Apple pectin gives numerous benefits, such as the supply of soluble fibers, and the improvement of the intestinal environment. Soluble fiber is a kind of fiber that can be readily spread or dispersed in water. Apple pectin is very rich in soluble fibers that contribute in the prevention and treatment of numerous diseases, most especially of digestive disorders, for it can regulate bowel movements. People suffering from diarrhea will benefit greatly from pectin, for it can make stools firm and decrease the inflammation correlated with loose stools. Additionally, it can aid people with constipation by helping the substances move along. Improving the intestinal environment can also be attributed to pectin, for it facilitates the bacteria found in the intestinal tract to make way for a good internal environment. Of note is the fact that the intestinal tract holds both good bacteria and bad bacteria, and the ideal situation would be the good ones outnumbering the bad bacteria. The function of good bacteria in the intestines is to aid in digestion and absorption, and to make sure that viruses and bad bacteria are in check. However, too much apple pectin can cause bloating since it has the tendency to absorb too much water from the intestines, which may further result in abdominal pain and cramps. To lessen the possibility of experiencing this side effect, introduce high-fiber foods gradually and drink plenty of water.

Marshmallow root is a demulcent herb known to be thick and slimy. It is used to sooth mucous membranes by moistening, thus giving relief to dehydrated areas. It is often used to treat digestive problems by treating internal inflammation, such as ulcers. This particular ability is possible because of the presence of polysaccharides that form a kind of protective layer over aggravated and inflamed mucosal tissue.

Aloe vera is recognized as the most nutritional plant on the surface of planet Earth, for it contains over 200 nutritional substances.[7] Aloe vera significantly strengthens the immune system and thus improves the body's general health. Now, it is important to take note that most of the problems that the immune system has to work on are the toxins found in the small intestine due to the intake of polluted food and water. This well-known plant is a powerful antioxidant, and it does well in cleaning up the mentioned toxins found in the small intestine. It also helps in relieving constipation by continually cleansing the small intestine, therefore regulating stool movement. The main component of aloe vera, which is called *aloin*, promotes the stabilizing of intestinal motor activity by decreasing the rate of the decay of protein and of the putrefactive processes, and thus supports the healing of the intestinal tract.

Paprika is a spice in powdered form, which is a dark red-orange in color and has a mildly heady flavor, prepared from dried ground fruits of particular varieties of sweet pepper. It contains high levels of vitamin C, and it is widely known as an antibacterial agent that boosts the immune system. Moreover, it helps digestion by increasing the production of digestive juices and saliva, as well as escalating peristaltic movement.

Dandelion is known to most people as a weed, but to some of those knowledgeable, it is an herb with many health benefits. It is used for treating loss of appetite, intestinal gas, upset stomach, and constipation by supporting digestion, motivating appetite, and harmonizing the naturally beneficial bacteria in the intestines, thus healing and nourishing the digestive tract.

Yogurt comes from milk and therefore provides protein. More importantly, it is known to be a rich source of probiotics. *Probiotics* is another term for the good bacteria discussed in the previous paragraphs, which must outnumber the bad bacteria if a positively ideal internal environment of the intestinal tract is to be achieved. Yogurt will help gastrointestinal ailments such as lactose intolerance, constipation, and diarrhea. Lactose is a particular type of natural sugar that can be found in milk and other dairy products. Lactose intolerance, therefore, is the inability to digest lactose, which may lead to diarrhea, nausea, or vomiting if significant amounts of lactose are consumed. Yogurt is helpful for lactose-intolerant people, not because it lacks lactose but because of the combination of a lesser amount of lactose with the presence of probiotics that aid in the digestion of lactose. People who are lactose intolerant may consider removing lactose from their diet altogether, as with the case of celiac patients. However, unlike gluten, lactose is an important ingredient that gives energy and improves the development and growth of certain functional bacteria in the intestines such as lactobacilli. Yogurt helps alleviate constipation and diarrhea because the good microorganisms existing in it condition the intestinal environment and enable the regulation of the movement and condition of stools.

Meadowsweet is known to be a mild, demulcent herb, which soothes inflammation because of the presence of tannin. It also has flowers and leaves that contain a type of compound called *salicylates*, which, if ingested, will be converted by the body into aspirin. It is very efficient in treating digestive problems, such as diarrhea, inflammation of the digestive tract, gastritis, and stomach ulcers.

Chamomile means "ground apples" in ancient Greek and is most beneficial to digestion. It contains essential oils that act as an anti-inflammatory, antispasmodic, and antiulcerative agent that heals the stomach lining when irritated and helps stimulate the natural production of digestive juices essential for proper digestion. If the celiac disease patient is suffering from acute conditions, chamomile is highly advised to be taken after every meal and right before bedtime. If otherwise, its consumption can be limited to two to three times a day. There are certain precautions and side effects that come along with the consumption of chamomile. It is generally considered safe. However, excessive doses may cause vomiting and could trigger allergic reactions. Allergic reactions toward the plant group that chamomile belongs to, daisies, are common. Therefore, one must be aware of any stimulus that may bring about these reactions, for unawareness of stimulants to one's allergies can be very dangerous and even life threatening. Chamomile is also considered a blood thinner that may worsen bleeding conditions due to the presence of coumarin. For pregnant women, chamomile must be avoided, because it can heighten the possibility of a miscarriage.

Slippery elm was once used as a last resort food supply in history. At present, it is often used as an alternative medicine for its health benefits. It contains sugar, iodine, calcium, amino acids, starch, bromine, zinc, and mucilage. Mucilage is the most abundant content in the bark of the slippery elm and is vital in the healing of internal mucosal tissues found in organs such as the intestinal tract.

Lemon balm leaf is a lasting herb in the mint family. It is used to treat problems in the digestive tract, such as bloating, vomiting, intestinal gas, and upset stomach. Lemon balm leaf is very rich in antioxidants; it contains caffeic acid and rosmarinic acid. It also contains eugonel, a natural anti-inflammatory substance that relives painful conditions. Lemon balm is not to be taken in high amounts in individuals using the thyroid medication thyroxine, and in breastfeeding and pregnant women.

Licorice root is typically used in flavoring and medicinal purposes. It contains compounds good for the body, such as plant sterols, glycosides, chalcones, asparagines, coumarins, flavonoids, anethole, and glycyrrhizic acid. Licorice root is known for its antibacterial, antispasmodic, and anti-inflammatory properties, which help with many digestive abnormalities. In particular, the healthy compounds found in the root, such as flavonoids and chalcones, can relieve discomfort as a result of the inflammation of the digestive system. It also regulates bowel movement by calming and soothing the digestion movement along the intestinal tract.

Peppermint leaf is a herb with a refreshing flavor that exudes a sharp menthol odor. It has strong antibacterial properties that are very potent against harmful organisms such as parasites. It has high value in treating gastrointestinal ailments, including functional dyspepsia, irritable bowel syndrome, and gastric emptying disorder.

Fennel seed belongs to the parsley family and is an aromatic herb with a sweet taste. Fennel seeds are used as antioxidants that are essential if the body is to eliminate dangerous free radicals. This is possibly due to quercetin and kaemoferol, which are the substances found in fennel seeds and are responsible for giving the seeds their antioxidant properties. Fennel seeds are also a good integration into one's daily meal, for they contain a fair amount of dietary fiber that improves digestion in the body by facilitating the opportune breakdown of food to be consumed by the cells. Despite their health benefits, it should be noted that fennel seeds are not to be consumed in large doses, for compounds found in fennel seeds may become dangerous to neurons when in high concentrations and may therefore result in seizures and hallucinations. Due to high levels of estrogen, they may worsen cancer conditions that are estrogen-receptor linked, such as ovarian, breast, and endometrial. Thus, pregnant women suffering from celiac disease are advised to avoid fennel seeds.

NUTRIENT REPLENISHMENT

Above all else, the small intestine is where most of the absorption of nutrients from the ingested food occurs. Therefore, a damaged small intestine will not be able to function, leading to the deprivation of important nutrients. Malnutrition is one of the major problems celiac patients experience as a result of this malady. Hence, it is recommended that the body be replenished with much-needed nutrients after adapting to a gluten-free diet regimen and after stimulating the repair of the small intestine.

Celiac disease patients often experience nutritional deficiencies in iron, calcium, vitamin D, zinc, vitamin B6, vitamin B12, and folate. They may need medically supervised vitamin and mineral supplementation until there is sufficient intestine recovery to absorb these nutrients. Gluten-free multivitamins are expected to deal with deficiencies. Multivitamins are usually recommended because many gluten-free foods on the market are unfortified. The following are among the most important nutrients celiac patients lack as a result of the removal of gluten from the diet and as well as from a damaged small intestine:

- Vitamin B12, also referred to as cobalamin, is a nutrient easily dissolved in water. It maintains the body's blood cells and neurons in good condition by aiding in DNA replication. Deficiency of this particular vitamin can cause weakness, weight loss, constipation, and megaloblastic anemia. It can often be found in foods such as clams and beef livers, poultry, fish, meat, eggs, breakfast cereals, milk, and other dairy products.
- Vitamin E is a potent antioxidant that minimizes the damage of body tissues caused by free radicals. It also boosts the immune system to keep antibodies out of the system. Vitamin E can be obtained from nuts, vegetable oils, green leafy vegetables, and

seeds. Too much vitamin E in food supplements may heighten the risk of bleeding and birth defects.

- Folic acid, also called vitamin B9, is important in many body functions, including cell division, synthesis and repair of DNA, and cell growth. It is especially beneficial to pregnant women, for it can promote proper fetal development. It can be found in beans, lentils, spinach, asparagus, lettuce, avocado, broccoli, oranges, and tropical fruits.
- Iron is involved in important molecular processes such as the production of red blood cells, which are responsible for carrying oxygen to the different cells. It is involved in the conversion of sugar in the blood into energy to be used by the body. It also aids in enzymatic reactions, such as the production of enzymes, which play an essential role in many body processes. It can often be found in red meat, raisins, bran flakes, prune juice, lettuce, and spinach.
- Carnitine is derived from an amino acid and is often used to reduce weight and raise energy levels. It plays a role in the energy production in the cell by moving lipids into the powerhouse of the cell, the mitochondria. Carbohydrates are immediate sources of energy, but when not readily available, lipids come in as energy reserves.
- Calcium is what basically makes up the hair, nails, and skin. It is also a very important component in bone and teeth formation. Good sources of calcium include yogurt, sardines, milk, sesame seeds, and spinach.

Contradictions are often found in the nutrition deficiencies and overconsumption in celiac patients. Too much intake of green leafy vegetables can cause indigestion, but, on the other hand, it is a much-needed factor to replenish a body lacking nutrients. It is therefore very important to achieve balance. Nutritional balance is the key to help celiac patients compensate for the nutrients lacking in their bodies without overdoing it to the extent of causing abnormalities within organs.

CHANGING THE SOCIAL AND LIVING ENVIRONMENT

People inflicted with celiac disease have difficulty in adjusting to the environment around them, as a new threat continually faces them: gluten.

What makes this most difficult is the fact that gluten is often found in foods lying around in the grocery store, primarily because a major portion of them are processed. Therefore, it is important to not rush when grocery shopping. Every single food item must be screened carefully for any possible traces of gluten. It is helpful to plan shopping and cooking ahead of time. A grocery checklist of what is gluten-free would certainly help, but no matter how confident one might be that a certain item is gluten-free, it is always best to recheck. Every minute of carefully examining the content label of the items bought is worth it.

Adjustments are not made by the celiac disease patient alone, however, for it is most certain that the people around the celiac disease sufferer must also change some of their habits so as not to invite more harm. A gluten-free kitchen is not the only factor that must be carefully observed, for several other things may pose a hazard to the celiac disease patient. One example would be the bathroom. There are many products found there that can also contain gluten, such as toothpaste, soap, shampoo or conditioner, lotion, and other possible items, and if gluten-infected products get in contact with the celiac patient, negative reactions, such as rashes, may occur. It is important to realize that gluten avoidance is not limited to food, but rather encompasses everything that might come into contact with the celiac disease patient. It would be best if everyone would adapt to a gluten-free bathroom by using products free from gluten so as to place everyone's mind in peace. If adapting to a gluten-free bathroom proves to be a hard task for family members, then perhaps an exclusive bathroom would help.

Celiac patients often encounter social anxieties, especially when trying to adapt to a gluten-free environment. Enormous peer pressure of constantly being tempted to eat what other people can, especially for children inflicted with celiac disease, is often experienced. For these children, the school administration must be informed of the current situation, for the assurance that the school is aware and therefore prepared for any events that may take place as a result of the child being inflicted with celiac disease would be a great help for both parties. In addition to teachers, friends who are closest to the patient should also be aware. It is easier for the inflicted individual to cope with all the responsibilities the disease gives if the ones closest to the person are showing their constant love and support. Informing friends is therefore very beneficial, for it removes the necessity of any pretenses. One should be very straightforward and picky

UNDERSTANDING CELIAC DISEASE

when it comes to what to eat and what not to eat, disregarding any negative opinions of other people who may not understand the current situation.

DIETS FOR PAIN RELIEF

Abdominal pain is pain or discomfort that a celiac disease patient may feel anywhere from the lower chest to the distal groin. Abdominal and chest pain are the two top reasons why people go to emergency rooms, according to the CDC.[8] If a person is not sure if the abdominal pain requires medical evaluation, it is recommended to speak with a doctor before using home remedies. A common diet that can be used as a home remedy to reduce the pain is the bananas-rice-applesauce-toast (BRAT) diet. The diet has just a couple of foods, and the only difference for a celiac patient is to find an alternative to the toast or use a bread based on a different type of flour that is not wheat, such as potato or rice.[9]

The BRAT diet is recommended for recovery from an upset stomach, vomiting, diarrhea, and nausea. It should be followed for a period of about 24 hours after diarrhea stops or as directed by the physician.[10] For any patient who has celiac disease or a gastrointestinal disorder, once pain is present there is another diet that can be followed. This diet is called the soft diet, and it can include creamed hot cereals that do not contain any gluten. The soft diet also includes gelatin; pudding; ice cream; sherbet; mashed or baked potatoes; pureed vegetables; creamed soups; baked turkey, chicken, or fish; meat loaf; milk; poached eggs; yogurt; and applesauce.[11]

Celiac patients following a soft diet due to abdominal pain will always have to take the same precautions to ensure that these foods do not contain gluten or are cross-contaminated. There are steps that can be taken in the diet to avoid abdominal pain, such as avoiding fatty or greasy foods, drinking plenty of water, eating small meals more frequently, exercising regularly, limiting foods that produce gas, and making sure that meals are well balanced and high in fiber. It is also advisable to regard fruits and vegetables as the main source of fiber.[12]

Abdominal Pain

When experiencing abdominal pain, a special diet can ease the symptoms the celiac disease patient is going through, such as bloating, pain, gas, diarrhea, or others. There are certain guidelines that can be followed to avoid different types of abdominal pain. Foods known to be too fatty may contain ingredients that can increase the amount of strength of intestinal contractions, which will result in cramping and will increase the pain felt by the patient. Eating small meals can also decrease intestinal contractions. When a person eats large meals, the digestive system is strained, and therefore it is best to eat small meals frequently throughout the day.

There are foods that produce more intestinal gas than others; these types of foods can contribute to cramping and abdominal pain. Most gas-producing foods tend to have high nutritional benefits, which makes avoiding them contradict a balanced diet. It is because of this that following an overly restrictive diet is often frowned upon. Whenever there is pain present in a person's digestive system, it is best to avoid these "gassy" foods, at least for that day. Gassy foods contain sugars such as fructose and lactose.[13] These cannot be digested by the stomach and end up traveling down the digestive system into the intestines, where bacteria break them down. Once broken down, they will result in the release of gas. It should also be mentioned that food is not the only cause for excessive intestinal gas. There are behaviors that can cause it, such as smoking or chewing gum, both of which allow air to be swallowed and result in painful belching and bloating over time.

Common dairy products that can cause those unwanted gasses can be cheese, ice cream, milk, and processed foods that contain milk. Certain whole grains can also result in excess gasses. Although whole grains are quite healthy, some of them can be made up with soluble fiber or other ingredients that can cause an increase in gas. An example is raffinose.

There are foods that will not be broken down by intestinal bacteria and will contribute to abdominal pain by creating gasses. Protein-containing foods that are fine for most celiac disease sufferers and are found in any regular diet are lean beef, fish, white turkey meat, and white chicken meat. Even though some vegetables are considered gassy foods, there are others that are not and are also nutritious, such as kale or spinach, green beans, lettuce, and tomatoes. There are also fruits that are usually recognized as less gassy, such as berries, grapes, and kiwi.

Stomach Pain

Any person that suffers from abdominal pain and discomfort, swelling, painful bowel movements, gas, or diarrhea should also note the diet being followed. The focus should be on the foods that seem to trigger discomfort and pain. A diet chart can be prepared to help the patient exclude these problem foods. The pain and discomfort can be controlled by improving the diet and eating habits. Another important recommendation is to drink the requisite amount of liquids in the form of water and fresh fruit juices to stay well hydrated, and liquids also improve digestion. Furthermore, it is recommended to eat slowly, taking the time to chew properly. Chewing properly will help with digestion and activate the movement of saliva in the mouth. This helps celiac patients since digestion is already somewhat of a burden for them. Fiber aids digestion and helps regularize bowel movements, thus reducing constipation and the consequent abdominal pain. Fiber intake should be increased and can be found in fresh fruits and vegetables. Too much fiber can also cause a problem, so it is wise not to overconsume these foods. Since food is one of the main triggers of stomach pain, a specific diet can be followed to control this ailment. A good diet for stomach pain will eliminate those foods that lead to flatulence, constipation, diarrhea, or inflammation.

The lists of common foods that cause stomach pain include fish, beef, mayonnaise, and alcohol. There are other foods that should be eliminated when it comes to stomach pain. Since tomatoes, citrus fruits, and juices contain high acidic levels, these foods can also be the cause of severe stomach pain. Processed foods and those made out of refined flour lead to constipation, which is why they can cause stomach and abdominal pain. Beyond causing stomach pain for a celiac disease patient, given that flour does contain gluten, there will also be damage to the small intestine, which will further create abdominal discomfort.

Caffeine is a stimulant; it does not allow the stomach muscles to relax, so anything containing it, such as coffee, teas, sodas, and hot chocolate, should be avoided. Milk is important for the body, but most people find it difficult to digest. The consumption of whole milk and other full-fat dairy products can cause stomach pain and cases of indigestion.

Some foods that are known to alleviate abdominal and stomach pain can be included in the diet to ease the pain. Garlic can be very beneficial to the whole body and is great for the digestive system. Cinnamon can help control several body conditions including indigestion and can help reduce acidity, and expel gas. Bananas can help alleviate stomach pain since they are an easily digestible fruit. Some health experts recommend eating one banana a day to fight stomach problems. Bananas can help heal wounds in the stomach and help overcome heartburn.

DIETS FOR INFLAMMATION AND THE IMMUNE SYSTEM

Digestion is considered one of the most important aspects of the human immune system and can have a very high influence regarding food allergies. Food allergies will flourish from the foods being consumed when the digestive system does not function the way it should. Having celiac disease does not make the situation any better. When toxins, bacteria, waste, or food particles enter the damaged lining in the small intestine, it will initiate a response from the immune system. The responses may appear in the form of gas, cramps, abdominal pain, and bloating. [14]

Probiotics are generally good bacteria that live in the intestines and help keep them in good health. These bacteria can be added to the regular diet since they compete with disease-causing bacteria for nutrients. Probiotics stimulate the enzymes and natural digestive juices that keep the digestive organs working properly, and since it is difficult for any celiac patient to digest foods, this will help the process immensely. The benefits of these bacteria are that they create a natural form of antibiotics in the body; this has been found true of the bacteria *L. acidophilus* through studies. The effects of this include the ability to defend against pathogens in the food that is ingested and the air that is breathed. [15]

The following are some of the other health benefits present when there is a daily serving of probiotics in the diet:

enhanced immune system response
healthy skin
increased ability to digest food
reduction in lactose intolerance
ability to assimilate nutrients in food
alleviation of constipation and diarrhea
an increase in the ability to synthesize vitamin B and also the ability to
    absorb calcium [16]

Studies have also shown that consuming probiotics increases the bio-availability of essential nutrients in the body such as zinc, iron, phosphorus, all of the B vitamins, calcium, copper, and magnesium. This is important for a celiac disease sufferer, since the digestion of food can be a challenge, and therefore nutrients might not be absorbed in the necessary quantities.[17] Live cultured yogurt is the most common and one of the most important probiotic foods, and it is best if it is handmade. The best type of yogurt is from goat's milk that has been infused with additional probiotics, such as lactobacillus or acidophilus. Goat derivatives such as cheese and milk are high in probiotics such as thermophillus, bifudus, bulgaricus, and acidophilus.

Another therapeutic approach uses microorganisms in breaking down gluten proteins. *Microbiome*, which is found in the upper gastrointestinal tract, is eyed as a favorable gluten-degrading enzyme. Gluten-degrading microorganisms, including the rothia bacteria, may aid in the digestion of immunogenic gluten proteins. A study was performed on these microorganisms involving isolation, identification, and functional characterization with regard to degradation capabilities.[18] The rothia enzyme source is an oral commensal bacterium within a human body, having a wide range of pH activity. The identified bacteria may be useful in the physiological degradation of gluten proteins that are harming celiac patients. However, a study on living organisms is yet to be done to test the full usefulness of these enzymes. It should be common practice for any celiac patient to read the ingredient lists on products, and when it comes to yogurt, there has to be enough awareness not to buy brands containing high fructose corn syrup or artificial sweeteners. Kefir is quite like yogurt; it is a fermented dairy product and based on goat's milk and the fermented kefir grains. This food is high in lactobacilli and bifudus bacteria and can be found in organic food stores.

A substitute for tofu as well as meat is tempeh. This is a fermented food rich in probiotics; it is a grain that is made from soybeans. Tempeh is an excellent source of vitamin B12. Besides discussing probiotics, there are other substances that should be added to a diet to strengthen the immune system, such as fiber. Fiber binds cholesterol and harmful toxins found in the digestive tract and removes them from the system. It provides the digestive tract with muscle contractions that help eliminate waste.[19]

Probiotics are beneficial digestive tract bacteria, and fiber helps them thrive. Probiotics can also help speed up digestion, changing the way nutrients and chemicals are absorbed by the body. Some types of fiber have the ability to absorb water located in the digestive tract and help avoid constipation. A healthy amount of fiber is considered to be around 40 grams a day for men and around 25 grams for women. Lentils, which are a member of the legume family, are a food that is really rich in fiber. This food has been cultivated since Neolithic times and is also a very good source of protein, B vitamins, iron, and other minerals.

Even though it is mentioned for other benefits, fruits and vegetables are also one of the best sources for soluble and insoluble fibers. Green peas, pears, and sweet potatoes are all considered rich in fiber as well as berries, apples, and also dried fruits such as dates. To make sure some of these will provide the most fiber, they should be consumed with the skin on when possible. There are several fruits that are rich in fiber; pears are considered fiber rich, just as others with edible skins. Pears that are consumed with their skin intact, which is very important for fiber, can contain about 5.5 grams of fiber. Berries are mostly sought after for their antioxidants, but they also contain lots of fiber. Since berries have large amounts of tiny seeds, their fiber content is higher than that of many other fruits.

Fiber can be found in corn, which, aside from the common yellow version, comes in a wide array of colors, including pink, blue, and black. Each variety has its own combination of antioxidant nutrients. Each ear of corn, which can be measured to a half cup of corn kernels, contains loads of fiber. Additionally, the flesh of an avocado is also a good source of fiber. An entire fruit contains about 10 grams of fiber, and a two-table-spoon serving contains about two grams of fiber. An artichoke contains approximately 10 grams of fiber when boiled, and about seven grams of fiber can be found in a small serving of artichoke hearts. Artichokes are also rich in silymarin, which is an antioxidant that can improve the liver health of the celiac disease sufferer. One ounce of seeds and nuts can provide a large contribution to the daily amount of fiber needed. Not only do nuts contain healthy fats and protein, but they are also an easy way to increase fiber consumption.

Glutamine is an amino acid that the human body produces, and it keeps the lining of the gastrointestinal tract, which is named mucosa, healthy. Glutamine also helps reduce infections and strengthens the immune system and can be consumed as a supplement when levels are low.[20] The glutamine blood level can lessen under different circumstances, such as surgery, trauma, infections, illnesses, and too much exercise. High-protein foods are a good source of glutamine. Even though glutamine is one of the amino acids that make up the gluten protein, it is not the same thing as gluten. The most important distinction is that the human body produces glutamine and does not produce gluten.

This amino acid is considered to be a building block for proteins, but it is also the main source of energy for cells that line the gastrointestinal tract, especially the small intestine, which is critical to celiac disease patients. Glutamine nourishes the cells in the intestinal lining, which in turn increases digestive health and immunity since the gastrointestinal tract lining is the first line of defense against pathogenic microorganisms.

Meat from animals and fish is a great source of protein. These can be broken down by the body to provide glutamine. Beef, chicken, turkey, and many species of fish are rich sources of glutamine and other amino acids. Fish and liver are the most bioavailable sources of glutamine. Glutamine can also come from other sources of protein derived from animals, including eggs, milk, yogurt, and cheese. When it comes to cheese, ricotta and cottage cheese are great sources of glutamine. All types of legumes are rich in protein and are considered good sources of glutamine. There are other vegetables that also contain glutamine, such as beets, kale, spinach, cabbage, and parsley. When considering vegetables, raw vegetables have higher amounts of glutamine than cooked vegetables.

A rotation diet can also help regulate the reactions of the digestive system to foods. It gives the digestive system time to recover from the reactions of a specific food before consuming it again, and it helps maintain immune and digestive tolerance. A person following this diet should allow at least four days before consuming the same food again.[21] The reason why four days should be allowed is that it takes approximately that amount of time for food to pass through the digestive system fully, and this way the person will not sensitize to that food. Rotation diets work by grouping foods into food families. Two foods from the same family can be eaten during the same day, but none of the foods from that family can be consumed for the next four days.

There are foods that should be avoided altogether when considering a healthy immune system and avoiding inflammation. It is always smart to check the labels for transfat, which can be listed as hydrogenated or partially hydrogenated oils. Transfats can induce inflammation by damaging the cells in the lining of blood vessels. Small amounts of transfats occur naturally in certain foods, but most are man-made, and that is the reason why the digestive system has difficulty breaking them down, which can trigger an inflammatory response.

Speaking of inflammation, white breads and pastas break down quickly into sugar and cause inflammation. These foods have been refined and processed into something that the human body does not need. For a celiac disease patient, these foods cannot be consumed anyway since they are wheat based. Animal fats have also shown an inflammatory response. A study traced how saturated fats, especially those from dairy products, can change the composition of naturally harmless bacteria in the digestive tract.[22] As the balance changes, it can cause an immune response that results in inflammation and tissue damage. This reveals how Western diets contribute to different types of digestive disorders.

Saturated fats can be difficult to break down, and the intestinal tract seeks help from sulfur-rich bile provided by the liver. Most bacteria cannot thrive under sulfur, but the *B. wadsworthia* bacteria can. As the digestive tract continues to grow sulfurous, this bacteria flourishes.[23] The presence of this triggers the immune system, initiating a state of inflammation and subsequent damage, not to mention that the bacteria's waste can compromise the intestine's wall, which is already weak in celiac patients.

Red meat contains a molecule called *Neu5GC* that the human body does not naturally produce on its own.[24] Once this is ingested, organs will develop antibodies for it, which can cause inflammatory responses. Animals who are grain fed with soy and corn can also be a cause for inflammation. These animals also gain excess fat and are injected with hormones and antibiotics. If meat must be added to the diet, it is best to opt for organic, free-range meats that have been fed natural diets.

When it comes to boosting the immune system naturally, most celiac disease patients will also benefit from a supplement that contains calcium and a considerable amount of magnesium. Too much magnesium causes diarrhea. Pyridoxal-5-phosphate (P-5-P) is a good choice in dealing with vitamin B6 deficiency. Vitamins A, C, D, and E supplements are advisable, along with a chelated zinc supplement. Vitamin K deficiency can be augmented by green food supplements, which contain essential nutrients. Two immune system boosters, echinacea and goldenseal, may help to speed up the process of healing the digestive tissues through their anti-inflammatory and antibacterial properties. These two are packaged together in a capsule, with the generic name Robert's formula.

The immune system can react to different sources of food in different ways, and when it comes to following a specific natural treatment such as diet, it would be best to consult with a dietician or doctor to see what is best from case to case. The experience gained from trial and error can be essential to determining what a celiac patient can and cannot consume, since even though a gluten-free diet can be followed, every immune system will react differently and can still become sensitive to certain foods. When taking care of the immune system, a celiac disease sufferer can often turn to common sense regarding what is "good" versus "bad." Foods found in natural form can be way more beneficial than anything that is man-made.

ANALYSIS

Natural treatments are currently the best options there are for an individual who has celiac disease. Studies and works of research are being undertaken by professionals in the field of medicine in an effort to address the needs of these individuals in a natural, chemical-free manner. Meanwhile, there are plenty of available supplements and herbal remedies, so that, if integrated into a healthy gluten-free lifestyle, recovery would not be far down the road.

11

SURGERY FOR CELIAC DISEASE

Whenever one has to undergo severe gastrointestinal surgery, for instance, having bariatric surgery in order to help the obese lose weight or having to go under the knife to remove part of one's stomach in order to treat an ulcer, celiac disease may be affected.[1] In general, however, celiac disease does not require an invasive surgical procedure as part of its treatment.

GASTROINTESTINAL SURGERY AND CELIAC DISEASE

Basically, gastrointestinal surgery is a comprehensive operation performed to treat any disease or control any health problem that occurs in the gastrointestinal section of the body, which includes cancer and benign conditions of the spleen, esophagus, liver, pancreas, bile ducts, stomach, and gallbladder. The technological advances in the field of surgical, imaging, pharmacology, and microbiology techniques and equipment, as well as the complex care in gastrointestinal surgery delivered by a team of experienced experts, may contribute to the improvement in gastrointestinal surgery, making it safer, more reliable, and faster than ever.[2] However, no matter how fast-forwarded technology is nowadays, there are still some unavoidable incidents that may result after gastrointestinal surgery. It is possible that celiac disease may be triggered or activated for the first time after undergoing gastrointestinal surgery. Even though the exact reason for the occurrence of celiac sprue as an acquired disease from the surgery is unclear and an official finding that directly correlates celiac disease as a consequence of gastrointestinal surgery has yet to be published, a study conducted by the National Center for Biotechnology Information (NCBI) evaluated the relationship between celiac disease and surgical abdominal pain.[3] According to this study, 3 percent of the patients who exhibited with unselected acute abdominal pain were diagnosed with celiac disease secondary to the trauma brought about by the surgery. It was also suspected that this acquired celiac disease was caused by the trauma that occurred during the surgery that may have led the body to release antibodies as an immune response against gluten. The investigatory team used immunoglobulins such as IgA/IgG antigliadin (AGA) and *endomysial antibodies (EMA)* to assess whether a particular patient had celiac disease initially. The researchers concluded that addressing patients with nonspecific abdominal pain (NSAP) or patients that exhibit other high-risk celiac symptoms or celiac-related disease might likely improve the diagnostic yield of the celiac disease. In addition, since undiagnosed or delayed detection of celiac sprue can lead to a multitude of long-term and permanent health problems, such as a high risk of osteoporosis, infertility, and even cancer, a more thorough and early detection of NSAP in relation to celiac disease and screening for celiac disease efficiently will be ideal.[4]

GASTROINTESTINAL SURGERY PREPARATION

Although no specific surgical procedure for celiac disease even exists, it is important to understand the general aspects of gastrointestinal surgery in light of the above paragraphs. Preoperative management in gastrointestinal surgery may include nutrition, medical history and clinical assessment, routine and advanced diagnostic tests, preoperative risk assessment, intake of some medication, and mechanical bowel preparation. Scientists drafted a comprehensive report regarding the usual perioperative management in gastrointestinal surgery.[5] It was indicated that the outcome of patients scheduled for gastrointestinal surgery is determined by several factors. Among the said factors are age and comorbidities of the patient as well as the complexity of the surgical procedure. Since the usual patients that are being referred for surgery are already in old age and suffer from multiple disorders, the close cooperation between the surgeons and the anesthesiologist, who is responsible for risk assessment, is very important for a successful surgery. Internists are also frequently involved to optimize the celiac disease patient's physical condition or medication.

Nutrition

Modern perioperative preparation has been improved in several ways over the last few years and nowadays is considered to be a highly multidisciplinary task.[6] Prior to elective (nonemergency surgery) or semielective surgery (semiurgent surgery), the nutritional state of the patient should be monitored and optimized. Malnutrition of a high degree can be controlled by enteral nutrition over a period of five to seven days.[7] Enteral nutrition, otherwise known as *tube feeding*, is special liquid food mixtures containing carbohydrates (sugars), protein, vitamins, minerals, and fats administered through a tube that is then inserted to the stomach or small bowel.[8] Potential problems with the patient's electrolytes should be corrected, and anemia should be treated by blood transfusion.[9]

Preoperative Assessment

Another point to consider in the preoperative management for gastrointestinal surgery is the medical history and clinical assessment. Acquiring a detailed clinical history and accurate medical assessment of the patient's physical as well as psychological condition is essential, since it may contribute to an efficient identification of patient risk factors. This is ideally completed before the patient is to be admitted to the hospital. On the flip side, in the case of an elective surgery, it is not advisable to conduct this medical history and clinical assessment listing, for it may delay the surgery.[10]

Routine Preoperative Tests

There are routine test results that should be available before the patient is referred to anesthesiology consultation.[11] These tests have different sections, including the laboratory, electrocardiography, and chest radiography. It is mandatory for all patients undergoing gastrointestinal surgery to have a preoperative laboratory test. The test should include a standard

complete blood count (CBC), international normalized ratio or prothrombin time (PT), and activated partial thromboplastin time (aPTT), along
with the concentrations of sodium, potassium, creatinine, and glucose.
The latest works of research have declared that an elevated preoperative
level of brain natriuretic peptide (BNP) is connected with increased cardiac morbidity after major surgery, but it remains to be seen whether this
level will be routinely determined for patients with cardiac risk factors. [12]
On the other hand, preoperative electrocardiography (ECG) allows for the
screening of undetected cardiac disorders and serves as a control should a
cardiac complication occur. ECG is mandatory for patients who are above
forty years of age; have significant cardiac disorders such as coronary
artery disease (CAD), heart insufficiency, heart rhythm disturbances or
any valve disorder; have a pacemaker (PM) or implanted cardioverter/
defibrillator (ICD); and have newly developed pulmonary or cardiac
symptoms, and those who are acquiring preoperative chemotherapy or
chemoradiotherapy. [13] Lastly, the chest radiography is important, since X-
ray images serve as a basis for comparison should perioperative complications occur, even though its sensitivity to detect pathophysiologic conditions in asymptomatic patients is relatively low. This examination is
necessary for patients who suffer from severe chronic obstructive pulmonary disease (COPD), who have unknown pulmonary or cardiac symptoms, and who have gastrointestinal malignancies to screen for pulmonary metastases.

Preoperative Risk Assessment

Advanced diagnostic tests may include echocardiography and carotid
doppler ultrasonography. Although these tests are not strictly indicated as
preoperative management on gastrointestinal surgery, these can help in
the assessment of potential risk, problems, and complications. The preoperative risk assessment is another factor to put into consideration in the
preoperative management of gastrointestinal surgery. Before the preoperative risk assessment is discussed, "high risk" should be defined. The
definition of being "high risk" for a poor outcome after surgery is nebu-
lous, as it is influenced by many variables that vary from patient to
patient and from one surgical procedure to another. [14] The surgeon and
anesthesiologist need to jointly evaluate the potential perioperative risk
for each patient and the intended procedure. Several scoring systems have
been developed that incorporate the patient's age and comorbidities and

the complexity of the surgical procedure to facilitate perioperative risk assessment. Well-known systems include (1) the Physiological and Operative Severity Score for the Enumeration of Mortality and (2) the Morbidity and the Estimation of Physiologic Ability and Surgical Stress Score.[15] Both systems indicate a general risk for complications but do not pinpoint any specific complication. In addition, the implementation of these systems into routine clinical practice has proven to be difficult. Data from our university medical center suggest that the subjective opinion otherwise known as "gut feeling" of the surgeon is a good predictor of postoperative outcome, especially in nonemergency gastrointestinal surgery.[16] All in all, gastrointestinal surgery is somehow related with a medium cardiac risk. Due to increasing incidence of coronary artery disease (CAD) and to an aging population as well as the increasing complexity of surgical procedures, postsurgical cardiac complications are now a leading cause of morbidity and mortality. Comorbidities that increase the cardiac risk for patients undergoing gastrointestinal surgery include first and foremost coronary artery disease, renal failure, diabetes mellitus, severe aortic stenosis, cerebrovascular insufficiency, peripheral artery disease, and heart insufficiency. Postoperative pulmonary complications, on the other hand, are the second-leading cause of morbidity and mortality after major surgery. Because of this, preoperative optimization of the patient's physical condition and medication is important.

Medication

Medication is another factor to consider before undergoing gastrointestinal surgery, since a sudden stop of the intake of a certain drug may cause adverse effects during the surgery. Therefore, a detailed medical history of patients' medication is essential. Cardiovascular medication such as beta-adrenergic blockers should be continued since these facilitate the balance of the supply-and-demand ratio of myocardial oxygen. Sudden discontinuation can cause unstable angina, tachyarrhythmia, myocardial infarction, and sudden death. The cardiovascular medication should be initiated at least one month before the procedure to allow for a dose adjustment if ever a patient who is scheduled for elective gastrointestinal surgery requires a new prescription.[17] The intake of clear liquids such as water or tea, but not milk, is permitted until two hours before anesthesia, and solid food intake is allowed for up to six hours prior to anesthesia, so continuing medication usually does not create problems. Diuretics should not be used on the day of surgery because this may increase the risk of *intraoperative hypovolemia*.[18] It is also recommended that the use of metformin, an oral antidiabetic drug, be stopped forty-eight hours prior to the surgery. Antiplatelet therapy (usually 100 mg of acetylsalicylic acid daily) is standard for most patients with coronary artery disease. Antiplatelet therapy, which usually consists of 100 milligrams of acetylsalicylic acid daily, is standard for most patients with coronary artery disease.

Other Factors to Consider

Other minor preoperative factors to consider include: avoidance of smoking, nutritional support, obesity, and chemotherapy or chemoradiotherapy. Discontinuation of smoking needs to happen several weeks before the surgery since smoking contributes to cardiac stress, therefore increasing the risk for perioperative complications.[19] Preoperative enteral and parenteral nutritional support has been recommended for malnourished patients since it is said that malnourished or poorly nourished patients are more prone to encounter postoperative complications as compared to well-nourished patients.[20] Obesity increases the chances of perioperative complications and increases morbidity and mortality after a colectomy.[21] It also poses a risk for postoperative intra-abdominal infection after a gastrectomy.[22] Doctors and surgeons should be aware of four common side effects of (1) frequently used chemotherapeutics such as anthracycline epirubicin, pyrimidine analogue 5-fluorouracil, and topoisomerase I inhibitor irinotecan, and (2) radiotherapy that poses threats to patients undergoing gastrointestinal surgery.[23] It is also recommended that patients with restricted pulmonary function perform some extended lung expansion exercises before the surgery.

SURGICAL PROCEDURES EXPLAINED

Not only is there no surgical treatment for celiac disease, but, in fact, medical procedures such as surgery may *cause* malabsorption or celiac disease, since foreign invaders may be introduced to the body, triggering the activation of celiac sprue.

Bowel Diversion Surgery

Bowel diversion surgeries include ileostomy, colostomy, ileoanal reservoir, and continent ileostomy. Bowel diversion surgery is done to allow waste to safely depart from the body when the large intestine is removed or requires additional time to heal. This procedure will divert the bowel to the abdomen, where a stoma (hole) is created. A stoma is formed by rolling the bowel and attaching it to the abdominal wall. Another way to perform bowel diversion surgery is to reroute the intestine after diseased portions are detached. Bowel diversion surgeries thus affect the large intestine, and often the small intestine as well. Semisolid waste flows out of the stoma and collects in an ostomy pouch, which must be emptied several times a day. An ileostomy bypasses the colon, rectum, and anus and has the fewest complications. A colostomy is similar to an ileostomy, but this time the colon itself is diverted to a stoma. During ileoanal reservoir surgery, the surgeon constructs a colon-like reservoir, called an ileoanal reservoir, from the last few inches of the ileum. In continent ileostomy, the large intestine is removed and a colon-like pouch is made from the end of the ileum. The surgeon attaches a Kock pouch to a stoma. The pouch needs to be drained every day by inserting a tube through the stoma.[24] Bowel surgery involves removing parts of one's bowel that have been affected by disease, such as cancer or inflammatory bowel disease. The exact procedure one will have will depend on the nature of one's condition and on how much of the patient's bowel is affected.

Colectomy

An operation to remove part of one's bowel is called a colectomy, which includes total colectomy, or removal of one's entire bowel; a proctolectomy, or removal of one's entire bowel, rectum, and anus; a hemicolectomy, or removal of either the left (descending) or the right (ascending) side of a person's bowel; a sigmoid colectomy, or removal of the part of one's bowel that is closest to a patient's rectum and anus; a transverse colectomy, or removal of the part of the patient's bowel that joins the left and right sides; and lastly, a protectomy, which is the removal of one's rectum and anus.[25]

Bariatric Surgery

Gastric bypass or malabsorptive surgery is a type of bariatric surgery or weight loss surgery that changes the process of digestion. Bariatric surgery functions in one of three ways, which includes limiting or totally restricting the amount of food intake by reducing the size of the stomach, limiting the absorption of foods in the intestinal tract of the celiac disease sufferer by "bypassing" a portion of the small intestine to varying degrees, or a combination of both restriction and malabsorption. [26]

POSTGASTROINTESTINAL SURGERY

Gastrointestinal surgery patients are more likely to experience surgical stress, nutritional depletion from inadequate nutritional intake, and the subsequent increase in metabolic rate. [27]

Surgical Stress

It is normal for a gastrointestinal patient to experience slight to extreme pain right after surgery. Therefore, it is important to address this pain properly since continuous pain may decrease the celiac disease patient's interest in staying in shape, and inability for mobilization interferes with the performance of lung exercise and restricts oral nutrition. [28] Modern principles of nonopioid-sparing or opioid-sparing analgesia as well as regional anesthetic techniques have been shown to reduce the rate of postoperative *paralytic ileus* and to accelerate postoperative recovery. [29]

Nutritional Depletion

A study by researchers on the struggles with food and eating after undergoing a major upper gastrointestinal cancer surgery concluded that the grieving that people experience suggests adjustment and coping fallacies similar to those of someone with a chronic illness. [30] Remodeling of health services is needed to ensure that the celiac disease patient group receives ongoing management and support. The research findings also showed that the physical symptoms and experiences of people differed among types of surgery, but the coping mechanisms remained the same.

The period of starvation or nil by mouth (NBM) is usually practiced after gastrointestinal surgery, during which an intestinal anastomosis or a surgical connection between two structures has been formed. The stomach is decompressed with a nasogastric tube and intravenous fluids are given, with oral feeding being introduced as gastric dysmotility resolves.[31] The reasoning behind the cessation of food consumption by mouth is to avoid postoperative nausea and vomiting and to provide time for the anastomosis to heal and protect it from mechanical stress from food consumption. However, it is not clear whether the deferral of enteral feeding is beneficial. This claim, on the other hand, is contraindicated by a study conducted by a team of scientists asserting that allowing patients to eat normal food at will from the first day after major upper GI surgery does not increase morbidity compared with traditional care with nil per os (also called nil by mouth) and enteral feeding.[32]

Increase in Metabolic Rate

The celiac disease patient's metabolic rate is usually increased by about 10 percent postoperatively.[33] The physiological stress of surgical trauma causes a sudden increase of sympathetic activity and an associated rise in catecholamine secretion. Excessive skeletal muscle proteolysis (protein breakdown) may occur if there is inadequate nutritional support at this point after undergoing surgery. Further depression of metabolism may continue to arise. Surgical trauma may also cause an increase in energy expenditure associated with a range of hormonal responses. The changes mentioned beforehand may not be of clinical relevance unless trauma or postoperative sepsis continues after surgery, but in relation to preoperative starvation, it results in a negative nitrogen balance.[34]

ANALYSIS

All things considered, there is no finding yet that places invasive surgical procedure as part of the treatment for celiac disease. However, there are several factors to consider when undergoing gastrointestinal surgery during the preoperational phase as well as postgastrointestinal procedure in order to avoid any celiac-related complications.

12

PHARMACOLOGICAL APPROACHES TO CELIAC DISEASE

There is currently no pharmacological cure for celiac disease, as a gluten-free diet is still the only proven treatment available. However, total rejection of gluten and its lifetime maintenance pose a challenge and health-related risks to patients. This fuels the need for an alternative solution to replace or, at least, supplement gluten-free diets. With the growing advances in technology, there is a higher possibility of producing drug medications to treat celiac disease. There is ongoing research for new treatments. Information campaigns are also being developed for doctors, patients, and the general public for a better understanding of this disease.

WHY THERE IS NO ABSOLUTE CURE FOR CELIAC DISEASE

Although the gluten-free diet is proven to eliminate the harmful effects and symptoms of celiac disease, this autoimmune disorder is really lifelong, and several studies support this claim. The University of Chicago Celiac Disease Center noted that recent research shows 60 percent of adult patients are not achieving complete small intestine healing, especially when the gluten-free diet is not strictly observed.[1] Investigational teams also conducted a study in 2009 on 465 celiac disease patients before and during a gluten-free diet.[2] The study assessed the factors affecting the histological outcome of a gluten-free diet. Only 8 percent experienced histological normalization after a median 16 months on a gluten-free diet. This implies that their gut tissues were restored to normal. They pointed out the exceptionally rare occurrence of complete normalization of duodenal lesions in adult patients even with compliance with the diet. The authors also observed a lessened amount of persistent intraepithelial lymphocytes, which are responsible for killing infected target cells. The lack of these lymphocytes in turn causes gut inflammation, associated with several health problems, including cancer.

In 2009, small intestine biopsies were taken from 45 children with celiac disease. These were compared to 18 clinical controls.[3] An increased presence of inflammatory markers, T-cells, was observed in patients who were already given proper treatment. This is an indication of possible epithelial stress due to constant attack. It is important to note that these patients did not experience the symptoms anymore, but the medical findings showed unlikely results. Furthermore, a 2010 experiment involved more than 380 biopsy-proven adult patients to estimate mucosal recovery rate and to assess implications of continual mucosal damage after complying with gluten-free treatment.[4] Among the biopsy-proven celiac disease patients who were subjected to diagnosis and follow-up biopsy, nearly 35 percent exhibited mucosal recovery after two years of diagnosis and gluten avoidance. At five years, the rate reached just over 65 percent. The authors concluded an absence of mucosal recovery after a gluten-free diet treatment. Another study was conducted in 2008 on 18 symptom-free celiac disease patients. It was observed that even after two years of gluten avoidance, gut inflammation markers continued to increase.[5]

Solid clinical research regarding the effects on celiac and nonceliac intestinal mucosa and intestinal cell lines has been completed.[6] Noting how zonulin protein initiates a "leaky gut," the experts emphasized that zonulin production on celiac disease patients on a two-year gluten-free diet is 30 times more than that of nonceliacs who were not gluten-free. Consequently, threefold more leakiness was observed for the patients compared to the nonceliacs. These imply a possibility of other elements besides gluten causing zonulin production in celiacs. In 2008, a leaky gut test was done on 22 celiac disease patients who were gluten-free for one year.[7] Compared to healthy control subjects, the patients were still found to have more gut leaks despite being gluten-free. In conclusion, the authors stated that there was no complete recovery, but there was persistent inflammation. This research shows a high inflammation rate, poor nutrition uptake, and persistent leaky guts. It can be asserted that a gluten-free diet, which is the only available treatment for celiac disease, does not provide a complete cure.

More Possible Reasons

One plausible reason why patients still suffer symptoms and continuous intestinal damage is unintentional gluten exposure. As gluten is in almost every food ingredient, it is almost completely unavoidable. No matter how much the patients try to completely avoid gluten, exposure to minimal amounts of gluten could still happen, especially outside the patient's household. It may be small enough not to cause symptoms to appear, but even a tiny amount of gluten can be enough to cause intestinal damage in the longer term. A patient's age is reported to be one contributing factor to a body's response to the gluten-free diet. The duration of gluten exposure also leads to continuous intestinal damage despite a gluten-free diet. Genetic features are not to be excluded as a contributor to how receptive the body is to gluten-free meals.

Researchers from the Mayo Clinic conducted a study in 2010 to find reasons for the increase of celiac disease.[8] In their investigations, blood tests were done on well-preserved blood samples taken from airmen 50 years ago and compared to recently collected blood samples from airmen. The research team assumed that the old blood samples would show the same rate of celiac disease as that of the current, which is 1 percent. There were way fewer positive results. This suggests that celiac disease was not as common as today. Younger men are 4.5 times more likely to have celiac disease. The lead scientist suggested that something has happened from an environmental perspective. He also advised proper diagnosis, treatment, and medical follow-ups.[9]

Special Note

Celiac disease was considered a condition in children that could be totally treated by gluten avoidance. This has been a long-term misconception that has gone on for decades and has hindered the pharmaceutical research industry from having its way. As of this time, no prescription medication is available specifically for celiac disease. The gluten-free diet is even known to be inadequate. Its challenges would include adherence, convenience, cost, risks of contaminations, inappropriate food labels, and foodstuff testing. The list could go on. There is a constant fear and worry about taking in gluten unknowingly. Moreover, the persistence of symptoms and lack of healing despite going gluten-free fuels the need for pharmaceutical therapy. For severe symptoms of celiac disease, doctors may prescribe prescription medicines, not for the disease but to help deal with the symptoms.

Special precautions must be considered when taking prescription medications or supplements for celiac disease. Proper dosage and time, as directed by the physician, must be observed. They should be taken continuously and should not be stopped without the physician's advice. Prescriptions may vary from patient to patient, so they should not be shared. It is necessary to be aware of the effects and side effects and be open about these with the doctor. Drug interactions must also be analyzed, particularly when more than one drug is being taken. When all is taken into consideration, one can see why there is currently no absolute cure for celiac disease.

ANTI-INFLAMMATORY AND IMMUNE SYSTEM APPROACHES

Azathioprine

This drug belongs to a class called immunosuppressants, which could be helpful for celiac disease patients as far as inflammation and/or immune responses are concerned. Azathioprine is prescribed to treat patients with rheumatoid arthritis that is severe and those who do not respond well to other medication such as ibuprofen. It is also prescribed to prevent a new kidney from a transplant from being rejected by the body, and it weakens the body's immune system so it will not be resistant to the new kidney. Other conditions that it can treat are other organ transplants, ulcerative colitis, and Crohn's disease that is not receptive to the usual treatment. It is also used to treat autoimmune diseases. Side effects include stomach and intestinal symptoms such as loss of appetite, nausea, vomiting, and diarrhea. It is best for the celiac disease sufferer to inform the doctor about all other medications, supplements, or herbal products that are currently being consumed.[10]

Cyclophosphamide

The standard therapy for remission induction from patients with severe ANCA-associated vasculitis (inflammation of blood vessels) has been cyclophosphamide.[11] ANCA is the abbreviation for anti-neutrophil cytoplasmic antibody. Once this drug combination was tested, disease control and temporary remission became possible instead of sudden death. However, not all patients were receptive to this treatment, and remission for them was not achieved. Those who did had disease flare-ups and needed repeated treatment. Side effects of cyclophosphamide are infertility, cytopenias (reduced number of blood cells—either platelet or red and white blood counts), infections, bladder injury, cancer, and other conditions that might come up after lengthy use of this drug. These side effects are the major causes of chronic (long-term) disease and even death.

Mycophenolate

This drug comes in a liquid, capsule, tablet, or delayed-release tablet. It must be taken orally. It belongs to the immunosuppressant class of medications, and it is used to treat systemic lupus erythematosus (SLE). It weakens the body's immune system so that transplanted organs such as liver, heart, or kidney will not be rejected by the body. After months of study, scientists reported that mycophenolate mofetil showed greater and faster positive results than azathioprine in maintaining the kidney's reaction to treatment and in preventing relapse or deterioration in patients with active lupus who underwent induction therapy.[12] Azathioprine now comes in second to mycophenolate mofetil in alleviating lupus.

Tacrolimus

This pharmacological drug comes in capsule or in injection form. It was initially approved by the Food and Drug Administration as an immunosuppressant for liver transplants. Presently, it is also prescribed in other organ transplants, such as those of the heart, lung, kidney, pancreas, bone

marrow, limb, trachea, cornea, skin, and small bowel. After transplantation, it is normally prescribed together with steroids. Using this drug
together with sirolimus is not recommended for heart and liver transplants. Celiac disease patients must not drink grapefruit juice while taking
this drug. It is also contraindicated to use tacrolimus and hydrogenated
castor oil at once. Possible side effects include risk for more infection,
such as bacterial, fungal, viral, and protozoal; new inception of diabetes
after transplant; elevated levels of potassium; thickening of the heart
muscle; anemia; and kidney toxin. For nursing mothers suffering from
celiac disease, it is advisable to discontinue breastfeeding. [13]

BENEFITS AND DRAWBACKS OF
PHARMACOLOGICAL APPROACHES

While potential pharmaceutical treatments for celiac disease are considered promising and provide hope for patients, there are drawbacks and
medical risks for these treatments.

Benefits

The benefits of using pharmacological approaches for treating celiac disease may be summarized as ease and compliance, better quality of life,
and a hope of complete recovery. Maintaining a lifelong gluten-free diet
can be challenging and expensive. Gluten is a very common food ingredient. It is even unlabeled in some countries. There is no vast availability of
gluten-free products on the market, and when they *are* available, they are
usually more expensive than their counterparts. Total compliance with a
gluten-free diet is therefore not exactly practical. This outstanding fact
makes pharmacological approaches favorable and beneficial.

Patients with celiac disease would possibly have improvements in
their way of living if drug treatments were available, giving them the
chance to take in even minimal amounts of gluten. This would allow them
to have a much freer lifestyle and provide a greater chance for them to
travel and join social events without any medical inhibitions, knowing
that they are protected and could obtain intermittent treatment from a
specific drug. Pharmacological approaches may allow low-to-moderate
amounts of gluten intake, protecting them from what is called "hidden

gluten," including cross-contamination and cross contact with other gluten-filled foods in processing, especially in commercial kitchens.

Therapeutic agents being developed aim to enhance the restoration of full intestinal function in celiac disease patients, especially for those who did not experience recovery through a gluten-free diet. Pharmacological treatments would also provide an excellent support to a gluten-free diet, particularly in cases in which patients still suffer from celiac disease symptoms despite strict adherence to nutritional recommendations.

Drawbacks

Pharmacological approaches for celiac disease treatment show promising results, but they cannot be considered a total replacement for a gluten-free diet. These types of therapies only permit minimal to, at most, moderate amounts of gluten intake—hence they should still be used in a gluten-controlled environment.

Even though alternative therapies are highly called for in celiac disease management, they still need to be proven safe. They should neither produce side effects nor just mask the symptoms while damage is actually occurring in the body. This would bring about a misleading feeling of being well because of the lack of symptoms, when in fact they are experiencing ongoing damage. Such a result would be proven through a Phase 3 clinical trial, and no drug treatment is on this stage as of yet. Some pharmaceutical treatments also seem to have possible side effects. Steroids, for instance, could create short-term side effects, including slow wound healing, indigestion, nausea or vomiting, diarrhea, headache, and extreme change in appetite (gain or loss) leading to weight gain or loss. Its long-term side effects include sluggish growth for young patients, acne, glaucoma, cataracts, diabetes, skin thinning, and osteoporosis. Some pharmacological approaches could even lead to death. These potential drug treatment side effects suppress the potency of others.

ANALYSIS

It is exciting to note that 10 or 15 years from now, there probably will be a treatment that could potentially replace the gluten-free diet entirely. As hope is turned into reality, celiac disease patients must learn to explore the pharmaceutical industry and the regulatory science field, for in such cases, knowledge plus action is indeed power.

13

CELIAC DISEASE AND EXERCISE

Since celiac disease is an autoimmune disorder that affects genetically predisposed individuals in whom the body produces an immune reaction to gluten, it significantly narrows the diet range for affected persons and causes physiological and even neurological symptoms that hinder physical activity.[1] The affected populace usually experiences fatigue, anemia, weight loss, and some varying degrees of discomfort and/or pain. Although physical activity can counter some of the more chronic symptoms, unfortunately many of the symptoms themselves deter the ability or the will of a celiac disease patient to exercise.[2]

SIGNIFICANCE

Exercise is normally recommended for healthy bowel movements, especially among postoperative patients. The muscle movements, particularly ones that have an effect on the abdominal area, are promoted to stimulate bowel movement after the effects of surgical anesthetics have worn off. However, in cases of patients with celiac disease, exercising may require a great amount of time and motivation on the part of the patient and the caregiver, since the mental symptoms of the condition have an effect on the person's psyche and overall motivation. Celiac disease is not heavily debilitating in comparison to other chronic illnesses, and it is usually easily treated with lifestyle changes and diet restrictions. Included in those lifestyle changes are certain exercises that a celiac disease patient may carry out to improve living conditions. Also included will be particular forms or methods of exercise that do not benefit but rather exacerbate the signs and symptoms of a chronic sufferer and deter the celiac disease patient's coping and healing process.

Exercise is usually underrated when it comes to benefiting the body in a holistic manner. In fact, it is one of the most essential ways to take care of the celiac disease sufferer's body. Exercise has the ability to cause the intestinal tract to move more easily, toning the muscles, improving cell nourishment, and maintaining a healthy weight. As the human physiology ages, muscles begin to naturally degenerate—even more so if they are left unused. This may cause weakness and some degree of immobility during old age, making the elderly more prone to physical injuries resulting from accidents that are related to impaired bodily movement as a result of the wasting away of unused muscle mass.[3]

EXERCISING THE RIGHT WAY

- *Wear proper clothing*: Wearing the right clothes is very important so as not to confine one's movements or hinder blood flow. The celiac disease patient should remember to never wear clothes that are too tight. It would be much better to wear ones made of a particular material that breathes well, given that one would unavoidably sweat in doing numerous procedures of different exercises. Fortunately, there are many clothes specifically designed for exercising that are available in many stores.
- *Wear the right footwear*: It is advisable to wear supportive footwear that has as much shock absorbency as possible. The celiac disease patient can acquire the ones that fit conveniently and are particularly designed for the type of activity that one intends to participate in.
- *Replenishment*: It is very important to drink lots of water before exercising. Water is essential to help one's muscles to work efficiently.
- *Warm up*: Doing warmup exercises will prepare one's muscles for exercise by gradually introducing them to the intense workouts one will do later by doing less intense versions so as not to "surprise" the muscles. Preparing for exercise by warming up will certainly help to reduce sudden strains and therefore aid in the prevention of injury. Also, it will help to condition the heart beforehand, for a sudden,

significant change in heartbeat could cause the celiac disease sufferer to tire more quickly.

- *Cool down*: This simply means to gradually slow down the level of activity occurring within the body after exercising. It helps to get one's heart rate (and therefore breathing) to eventually go back to normal resting levels. This is especially important because it helps prevent dizziness, or worse, fainting, that could result from blood pooling within the large leg muscles when intense activity is suddenly brought to a halt. Additionally, certain waste products could build up in the muscles after strenuous activities, and cooling down helps remove these toxic substances. It would be best for the individual with celiac disease to end the exercise by preparing for the next session through a proper cool down.

- *Consult a physician*: Having certain physical conditions requires a physician's advice before doing any forms of exercise so as to prevent any further complications. It is important to note that there are corresponding exercises to particular conditions, and it is essential to understand which ones to avoid. For patients with respiratory problems such as asthma, heart diseases, kidney problems, liver impediments, arthritis, or diabetes, consulting a doctor before beginning any exercise regimen is of absolute importance. The physician can recommend a more efficient exercise regimen that could best meet one's goals.

EXERCISES FOR THE DIGESTIVE TRACT

Exercise affects the digestive system in more ways than one can imagine, both positively and negatively. Moreover, different kinds of exercises have their respective goals, and, therefore, effects on the system. If certain intestinal problems exist, it may be wise to consult a formal caregiver such as a physician before attempting to commit to any exercise programs to confirm whether certain exercises would do no damage to tissues. Exercise not only helps improve the effectiveness of the digestive system but also aids in speeding up the digestive process, and thus it supports one in maintaining a healthy body weight. Specific types of exercises each have their own results. For instance, light exercises that simply increase one's breathing and heart rate can help the celiac disease sufferer to have more effective bowel movements. However, exercises that are extremely intense would have negative effects on the digestive system overall.

Aerobics

Although this form of exercise is similar to cardiovascular exercises in that it increases, and therefore improves, blood flow, it is different in that it is done at a much lower intensity and for a longer period of time.

- *Jump rope*: Many children love playing jump rope, probably not realizing that it actually is an excellent workout. It works the core muscles, including the arms and legs, and thus improves balance.
- *Climbing stairs*: This is a great aerobic exercise to get the heart rate going. This can refer to climbing real, actual stairs, but one could also opt for the stair machine at the local gym. This improves the leg muscles of the celiac disease sufferer.
- *Jogging and speed walking*: These are gentle exercises that are especially beneficial to those with knee problems. An hour a day of walking can maintain weight on a long-term scale and reduce the risks of acquiring particular conditions such as obesity and hypertension.
- *Cycling*: If the office is beyond walking distance, why not try biking? Biking is a very accessible and very efficient way of exercising. It works most muscles in the body, and it gets the heart rate up. Stationary bikes are certainly great alternatives for those who would prefer staying at home.
- *Jumping jacks*: This type of exercise is a fast way of getting the heart rate up. It is done first at a starting position, standing with legs together and arms at the sides, then proceeding to jump with the legs far apart and the arms raised above the head and the hands clapping. A few of these and the patient can hear his or her heartbeat booming in the chest.
- *Swimming*: This activity is a fun way to exercise. Swimming will get muscles working, but exactly which type of muscles depends on the style of swimming one does. This type of exercise is often recommended for celiac disease patients who are considerably overweight, since swimming burns numerous calories.

Yoga

- *Seated twisting*: There are two methods of seated twisting, but all give the same results common to that of the lying twist stance. However, this one has an added advantage for pregnant women, for those who have spinal injuries, and for those who are overweight. The first version includes sitting with the back erect and the legs stretched straight in front. The idea is to lift the left foot and place it over the right knee, then twist the entire upper spine to the left. The second version includes the first step as sitting in Indian position. Next, the right knee is bent over the left leg and placed next to the left thigh as close as possible, with the left leg still in the same position as it was in the previous step.
- *Forward folding*: This stance provides fresh oxygen to the organs and helps increase the rate of blood flow that aids digestion. The key is to begin in a standing position. Then the person slowly bends forward, with the back and the legs straight as far as possible, ideally until the chin is aligned with the knees, while one extends the arms backward until they can be clasped together. The trainee should maintain that position for at least 15 seconds and then repeat it twice after relaxing between attempts.
- *Bridge pose*: This unique pose will help improve one's blood flow. To do this, the celiac disease patient must first lie flat on the floor, with hands at the sides. Next, the knees are bent while the arms and feet are kept on the floor. The hips are lifted up to resemble the form of a right triangle.
- *Lying twist*: There are many benefits one can gain from such an exercise—in fact, from all twist stances. One of these is the improvement of the blood flow to the areas of digestion, an enhancement in mobility, a decrease in inflammation, and a reduction in pain. This stance is particularly valuable to those with back pain problems, as this does not exert pressure on the mentioned affected area. The exerciser begins by laying down on a mat with legs straight, perpendicular to the arms, which are stretched straight sideward, resembling the letter T. Inhalation and exhalation follows; then the person brings the knees close to the chest. Once the individual is steady, he or she then twists the lower spine along with the knees to the left side. It is best to hold the position for 15 seconds, and then relax.

Tai Chi

This is a well-known art originating in ancient China. Tai chi focuses on both the mind and the body with relatively slow-paced stances, which can surprisingly burn more calories than activities such as surfing. Not only that, but tai chi also improves flexibility, mental precision, strength, and, above all, the health of the celiac disease sufferer. This practice prioritizes the concept so important to the Chinese, called *chi*. Chi is said to be the physically imperceptible life force, or energy. In actual scientific studies, tai chi has been proven to help improve several conditions such as cardiovascular and muscle problems.[4]

First of all, one should prepare by warming up with proper breathing and by tapping into chi in order to wake the potential asleep within. Then the person must focus on each part of the body, a careful step at a time. This can be a good way to release tension from every single area of the body. Afterward, the exerciser is stabilized by rooting the consciousness to where one "is at present."

Then, from a wide array of styles available, the person selects the one that fits most comfortably. Chen style is a kind of style that plays with the tempo, often starting off slowly, then suddenly shifting to one that is fast. Yang style is the most well-known style of tai chi. It has a consistent tempo, and it commonly uses huge frame movements and thus can easily be imitated. Wu style is a style contrary to the large frame movements of the Yang style, and this one can be too difficult for a novice. It may be quick to learn, but it is very challenging to master. There is intense focus on the potent flow of inner energy that explains why the movements are very unhurried and deliberate. Hao style is probably the most mysterious, for it is relatively unknown.

If possible, the celiac disease sufferer should hire an experienced mentor in order to properly learn the art of this ancient practice. Once mastered, one can apply the concepts learned in stressful situations to remain balanced and calm. This is a perfect way to maintain mental stability, thus paving the way to physical improvement.

EXERCISES FOR CELIAC DISEASE–RELATED PAIN

Exercise has proven to be an excellent diversionary activity that not only distracts celiac disease patients from pain and discomfort but also improves coping and overall fitness. However, pain experienced by most patients causes them to opt not to exercise at all. It is a generally known fact that the presence of pain has always been an important occurrence in human wellness and survival. Pain is the impulse or signal that indicates that something is amiss within the body. It calls attention to the need to fix a problem area within the body. Pain, after the initial occurrence and as it continues, is what usually motivates an individual to avoid any more damaging activities and give organs the time to heal and to avoid similar instances that produce the same type of pain in the future.[5] In many medical conditions such as celiac disease, pain is a significant symptom and has a tendency to affect a person's quality of life and general function.[6] Mostly, the sedentary lifestyle can be attributed to the fear of worsening the experienced pain. In cases of pain related to the digestive tract, exercise is hampered by the fear of suddenly having to go to the bathroom in an undesirable setting or situation, such as in the middle of a jog, where bathrooms may not be readily available.

Nevertheless, exercise remains an essential part of coping with most types of pain, including those involving the digestive system and/or celiac disease. There are only certain types of exercise that prove to be particularly beneficial to the improvement and coping of a person suffering from pain, and certain specific methods and practices on how and when best to do them. Even in cases of chronic pain, it has been found that the possibility of damaging or further injuring the pain-producing structures is not as probable as usually imagined. In fact, exercise may even have a two-fold benefit when it comes to patients suffering from chronic pain, such that it improves and maintains a healthy muscular structure after correcting any physical complications that arise from the lack of mobility. Thus, exercise eliminates an unwanted cycle of pain-inactivity-pain.[7]

Exercise also plays a vital role in the overall mental health and wellness of a pain sufferer. Usually, patients with chronic pain experience a diminished motivation for social activities and increased tendencies for depression. When this happens, the idea of exercise becomes even more unlikely due to the usual lethargy brought about by feelings of hopelessness and absence of purpose or drive. Ironically, this inactivity resulting from a degeneration of energy may just be remedied by activity itself. It has been found that exercise or any form of routine physical activity increases energy levels and diminishes the severity of depression since it gives patients a form of stimulation and involvement in an activity that yields positive rewards, such as being able to cover a longer distance during a jog, or being able to do more laps in the pool. Consequently, after the physical gains produced by exercise for chronic pain sufferers, physical activity has also been found to provide later relaxation and to improve the quality of sleep since it is an effective avenue for the release of tension.[8] Considering that fact, although there may be therapeutic benefits to some forms of physical activity for most medical disorders such as celiac disease, pain has a tendency to interfere with mobility and an individual's will to do most forms of physical activity, since pain signals the body to refrain from any activity that may be potentially further damaging to the involved bodily structures.

Walking or ambulation is a staple physical activity for a healthy life. It is one of the simplest and most recommended forms of exercise available to just about anyone with well-functioning lower extremities. It is greatly recommended that postoperative patients induce colon movement after the effects of anesthesia have subsided. It is also advised by obstetricians during labor to stimulate uterine contractions and promote cervical dilatation. It is most suggested by dieticians and fitness doctors as a primary activity to counteract the effects of a sedentary lifestyle brought about by a sitting job or simply the lack of motivation to move around at home.

In a more routine setting, walking is said to produce vast benefits for individuals who are consistent with their ambulation. Steady, sharp movements such as those found in walking can improve a person's stamina, energy levels, life span, weight management, and mental well-being by reducing stress, improving memory, managing depression, and increasing confidence. Long-term physical benefits of walking include the management and/or prevention of dreaded diseases such as hypertension, heart disease, diabetes, osteoporosis, and even some forms of cancer, such as cancer of the colon.[9]

Another form of exercise that is suggested for most pain sufferers is swimming. It is primarily, like walking, an aerobic exercise, since it involves long stretches of exercise time, which require more oxygenation to the muscles.[10] Due to its highly aerobic quality, it has the ability to reduce stress, and the required movements also improve bodily posture.

This particular exercise is ideal for chronic pain patients because it basically involves minimal to no sharp impacts on the body to cause it to react with a pain stimulus. This unique characteristic of this exercise is why it is highly advised for patients suffering from bone and joint problems and for the fragile elderly. Aside from all the other benefits that can be had from other forms of aerobic exercise such as endurance and fitness, swimming grants all those benefits without the impact that can be harmful for some.

A relatively new form of exercise that can be advisable for individuals who suffer pain, especially that which involves the back and shoulders, is Pilates. It was developed in the early twentieth century by Joseph Pilates and is steadily gaining popularity in parts of Europe and the United States.[11] The aim is to routinely condition endurance, strength, and flexibility in parts such as the legs, arms, hips, back, and even the abdominal muscles.[12] Pilates programs are favored, since they are modifiable in terms of range of difficulty. A celiac disease sufferer may start at a beginner level and increase the strain to a more advanced level over time as the body develops to adapt to the workout.

Strength building is another form of physical activity that can be counteractive for conditions involving chronic pain. The newly acquired strength from this form of exercise and its routine aids the individual to physically cope with the conditions resulting from the continuing pain stimuli. Weights have a typical involvement in strength training and usually begin mildly, gradually increasing the load as strength improves. In fact, strength training is even recommended for people in rehabilitation or with an acquired infirmity, such as that from a stroke or a musculoskeletal debility, to hasten recuperation.[13] Other than that, strength training is highly beneficial and therefore widely practiced even for celiac disease sufferers without physical disability since it is found to be an effective weight-loss program. It is also very well known to be effective in building and sculpting muscles.

Generally doing almost any form of exercise requires a proper warm-up prequel, and stretching is an excellent preparation in a structured exercise routine. It involves literally stretching or flexing muscles and tendons to achieve a desirable perceived elasticity or tone of the muscles.[14] The main and most well-known purpose for stretching is to avoid injuries. A study of soccer players showed that a group of players who did static stretches suffered fewer knee injuries when compared to those who did not warm up.[15] Also, a review showed that there are a good number of beneficial stretches that improve the range of motion for athletes, especially runners.[16] Proper and consistent stretching has a vast range of benefits, including improved muscle and tendon elasticity, a decrease in physical and sports-related injuries that arise from tightened muscles, and increased flexibility.

EXERCISE AND INFLAMMATION

Consistent physical activity is said to decrease signs and symptoms or markers that indicate inflammation.[17] This information, however, has not fully been established as consistent and concise, revealing results with varied differentials. It has also been found that certain intensities of physical activity have contrasting effects on an individual who is suffering from chronic or acute inflammation.

Regular physical activity is well accredited to offer protection from a wide range of causes for mortality, primarily that of cardiovascular disease and Type 2 diabetes mellitus. These two illnesses have been associated with low-grade systemic or whole-body inflammation as shown by a marked increase in levels of cytokines, which are produced by immune cells in response to inflammation. Fatty tissues are held responsible for the production of chemicals that account for problems such as insulin resistance and dyslipidemia.[18]

Exercise, then, both eliminates a good number of fatty tissues if done constantly and has an effect on substances that stimulate the activation of anti-inflammatory cytokines and inhibits the production of pro-inflammatory cytokines. Above all that, the substances stimulated by regular physical activity augment the turnover of fats by encouraging lipolysis or the breakdown of fat as well as its oxidation. It is found that long-term exercise may aid in the reduction of chronic low-grade inflammation, while low-intensity exercises prove to be more efficient in lowering resting inflammatory markers as opposed to exercises of moderate to high intensity.[19]

ANALYSIS

Physical activity plays a major role in the health and wellness of individuals, especially those with conditions such as celiac disease. Despite conditions that pose as hindrances to exercise, there may still be methods that provide safe and effective delivery of an exercise regimen for such individuals.

Part V

Personal Quest

14

MOTIVATION AND CELIAC DISEASE

Going through checkups, surgery, and nonmedical treatments such as exercise and maintenance of proper digestive health are answers to treating celiac disease. However, the first giant leap toward achieving all these should be accompanied with a very vital approach—having the motivation to comply with whatever is expected in a patient with celiac disease. Given that celiac disease is considered curable, and that there have been a number of worldwide clinical advances on the ailment, people who have it have every reason to be optimistic.

Aside from the fact that one needs to get well from celiac disease, there are other reasons why it is important to be motivated as a patient, which also means having to sacrifice the life one has been used to. Given that having celiac disease has effects on other body systems, the mental system for one, there is a need to counterattack whatever additional disorder it may bring to a patient. It is a necessity that patients, being affected emotionally and mentally by the disease, have the right amount of determination or they may be at risk of aggravated effects or, in some cases, death.

MOTIVATION ROADBLOCKS

Still, a lot of patients with celiac disease are not at all motivated or adherent when it comes to treatment—in following a gluten-free diet, for instance. This is especially true because celiac disease is a lifelong commitment, particularly given that the social and mental aspects of lives are already affected. Removing gluten from one's diet is one of the cures for celiac disease, as the said ailment occurs due to sensitivity to food with gluten such as wheat, rye, and barley, mostly found in breads and cereals. Yet, in one research study, the scientists admit that failure to adhere to the diet is a common scenario for celiac disease patients, who say that it is restrictive and difficult to observe.[1] Their study on adult celiac patients in the northeastern part of England showed that, out of 287 respondents, 115 (or 40 percent) intentionally ate foods with gluten. Some 155 (54 percent) had demonstrated at least one identified refusal to diet, while 82 (29 percent) cited consuming gluten either on purpose or mistakenly, forgetting about the diet. This led to a conclusion that low self-worth, perceptions of tolerance to gluten, and intention lead to deliberate gluten consumption.[2]

Experts believe that noncompliance can be measured by dietary history and the measurement of serum antibodies, and also invasively, by the use of genetic/biological standards. They note that hindrances to compliance are the usual psychological troubles, such as depression and anxiety brought about by celiac disease and the confusing food-labeling practices and purported tastelessness of foods free of gluten.[3] In relation to this, one study showed that celiac disease patients with psychological outcomes were less compliant or motivated, particularly in maintaining a strict gluten-free diet despite positive intentions.[4]

Indeed, noncompliance or lack of motivation is often a problem with celiac disease patients worldwide. In the United Kingdom, low compliance has been accounted for in teenagers and adults, while less than 50 percent of all adults with celiac disease in France and Belgium followed a strict diet for more than a year. Other reasons cited for noncompliance are the nonavailability of gluten-free foods, nonexistent symptoms during diagnosis, lack of initial dietary counseling, and insufficient dietary information from resources such as the Internet.[5] Another fact is that wheat and other wheat-based products such as sandwiches, toast, and muffins are staple foods, especially in North America. Furthermore, it is reported that specialized gluten-free foods cost more than those with gluten, adding to the personal stress of keeping up with a gluten-free diet.[6]

Age is also one factor considered a deterrent in conformity with a gluten-free diet. From a celiac disease study at Tampere University Hospital in Finland, clinical investigators found that younger age, being a teenager, and current symptoms of the disease had something to do with neglect of the required diet.[7] There was not even a connection between the following:

nonconformity by gender
place of diagnosis
smoking
severity of symptoms before detection
family history of celiac disease
disease composition
presence of comorbidities (additional disorders)
self-effort for the diet
lack of follow-up length of diet
use of oats

Thus, experts deem it important that patients with possible celiac disease should have themselves diagnosed at a younger age, and routine checkups should be made for efficient celiac management.[8] The same goes for seeing a doctor at the onset of suspected celiac disease symptoms. As the saying goes, prevention is better than cure. Another roadblock is that there are several hidden sources of gluten in selected foods.[9]

With regard to patient adherence in all kinds of diseases, having mistaken beliefs is viewed as a determinant for lack of motivation. A study on effective patient adherence in general stated that some health practitioners are not even able to detect why patients do not adhere to their prescriptions.[10] It has been proven that race, gender, age, marital status, educational level, socioeconomic status, and religion are all regarded as factors for adherence, although they are not exactly representative of the celiac disease patient population in general.[11]

Other possible causes of nonadherence are the characteristics of the disease and its severity, although it could also happen that patients are more likely to adhere if the situations are more severe. With these findings, it is suggested that conformance is relative to individual diversity rather than variables attributed to patients as a group. Moreover, studies have found that the more patients need to change their lifestyle and other personal habits/choices, the less likely they are to get well. The easier the prescriptions, the more they are motivated to respond to treatment.[12] In this case, given the fact that some celiac disease sufferers already have mental impacts, there is no other way but to remain positive. It will just be a matter of effectively convincing these patients to get motivated to seek treatment.

DRIVING FORCES

There are a lot of ways to combat all the mentioned causes of nonmotivation in celiac disease patients. Another registered dietician says that successful management of celiac disease needs an individual approach that would include staying away from foods with gluten, going under other kinds of treatment, accepting the kind of life expected as well as understanding life's worth, and practicing a healthy lifestyle in general. It would also be useful to find motivation by having a team approach with the help of other external factors such as the family, support group, doctor, and dietician. The good news is that there have been initiatives by health food stores and gluten-less specialty companies to promote awareness of celiac disease and to increase the number of patients receiving education and training on celiac disease and gluten-free meals. [13]

Motivation to Resist Gluten

Since gluten is the main source of celiac disease, starting to avoid it at an early age creates an impact for efficient motivation. This can be practiced by getting children with celiac disease used to identifying which products have gluten or are gluten-free. That, in a way, leads them to decide which foods to avoid. Dieticians share that parents should teach their children to read labels that contain wheat. Doing so puts the blame on the food items and not on the parent, thereby making the child learn to be independent when it comes to food choices when not at home. Another way of making it fun is by engaging children in the planning and preparation of meals, including the selecting and buying of ingredients and the collection of recipes, which would be good quality time for the family and at the same time a learning opportunity for the kids. Role-playing by teaching children what to say when offered a suspicious or look-alike food is also suggested, as well as keeping the whole household free from gluten. With the latter, children with celiac disease need not feel bad if they see others eating foods with gluten, and at the same time, families will have to spend less compared to buying gluten-containing wheat bread and the like. [14]

Nowadays, there are many ways in which food companies entice consumers to eat foods without gluten, and patients with celiac disease can take advantage of them. Foods that children and even adults usually enjoy, such as pizza, candies, pastas, cereals, and cookies, are now offered without gluten.[15] It is also up to the parents to be creative, not just in preparing or cooking the right foods but also in how they can make their children eat them. Since the cost of a gluten-free diet can be a problem, there are ways in which patients can budget their money without compromising their health. The Beth Deaconess Medical Center recommends that instead of buying commercially packaged gluten-free rice, hot cereal, or other grain mixes, one can buy labeled gluten-free grains in packages and make his or her own cereal or side dish. Celiac disease patients can bake their own bread and other goods using labeled gluten-free flours. Natural and healthier gluten-free foods such as root vegetables can also be an option that actually lasts longer.[16]

Support Groups

Since low self-efficacy is one of the causes of low motivation among celiac disease patients, by uplifting one's self-esteem, patients are inspired not just to watch a gluten-free diet but also, and more importantly, to think positively—to believe that there is still hope and treatment for their situation. This can be attained by joining support groups for effective management of the disease. Experts say that by being active members of a local or national support group, more patients with celiac disease are, more often than not, adherent and more well informed about the diet.[17] Because of social and moral support, patients, feeling comfortable, can compare notes, making them more adept about the features of their ailment and giving them more insights on what they can do to improve themselves.

Experts also share that several people with celiac disease are consoled just by the thought that they are not alone in facing so many challenges because they can talk to others who are in the same situation about what and where to buy gluten-free foods as well as how to deal with other obstacles that come their way. There are many local and national support groups as well as websites that help families who have members with celiac disease, especially kids. Some of these groups offer coupons and recipe ideas.[18]

Celiac support groups do not just cater to those diagnosed with the disease—they also reach out to those who have early symptoms or are suspected to have it but lack the motivation to seek treatment. The Celiac Disease Foundation, for one, has a mission to diagnose and treat celiac disease at an early stage as well as participate in advocacy groups, awareness campaigns, and advance research, catering to patients and also to their families. The Center for Celiac Disease at the Children's Hospital in Philadelphia supports more than 1,000 kids with celiac disease and their families every year. The team is composed of medical experts from different fields and social workers. To make it easier for some clients, there is an online support group for the patient's queries and other concerns. The center conducts an annual education day for families, giving them gluten-free foods and inviting speakers to talk more about the disease. Kids get to participate in different kinds of activities.

Psychological support is also very beneficial, especially with celiac disease patients that have asymptomatic conditions such as anxiety and depression. This can be attested to by a study of 66 celiac disease patients with depression and anxiety.[19] Divided into two groups, the first was given psychological support at the start of their gluten-free diet, while the second got none. After follow-ups every two weeks for six months, while no difference was seen in both groups in terms of anxiety, a considerable decrease in depression was seen in the first group (15 percent) compared to the second group (around 80 percent). In the next follow-up, significantly lower compliance with the gluten-free diet was seen in the second group (about 40 percent versus roughly 9 percent). Apart from lessening affective disorders brought on by celiac disease, psychological counseling aids in the motivation to eat a gluten-free diet. In order to achieve consistent and updated information, the investigators proposed a need for collaboration of support groups that are spreading the needed information to patients, health professionals, and the media, as well as a concerted effort to lobby the government for more complete food-labeling guidelines so that all gluten sources are properly acknowledged, giving consumers and more particularly celiac disease patients an informed choice.

What Others Can Do: Schools and Parents

Other external factors aid in boosting a celiac disease patient's morale and outlook on life. Support from other organizations such as schools and the community can contribute in inspiring celiac disease patients to move on, with additional support, of course, from parents. Having an agreement and pursuing consistent meetings with school officials will lessen the possibility of "cheating" during mealtime. In Italy, 204 patients with celiac disease ages 13 years and above were subject to medical tests and were interviewed on their observance of a gluten-free diet as well as social interaction, academic performance, smoking habits, and family integration. The result: nearly 74 percent of them did not have diet lapses, while 54, or 27 percent, had occasional-to-repeated dietary transgressions. Meanwhile, it was found that 30 out of 54 poor compliers ate 0.001 to one gram of gluten, 14 ate gluten in the amount of one to five grams, and 11 ate more than five grams a day. Height was below the third percentile in 19 of the 204 patients, and weight was below the ninth percentile in 20. Clinical reports suggest that motivation to comply with a prescribed diet does not appear to have an effect on height and weight.[20] Moreover, most of the patients had good social relationships, school performance, and family integration. On the other hand, 54 percent admitted they had some restraints when it came to social life. Still, the researchers concluded that school integration is a factor for excellent diet compliance for celiac disease patients, while a better perception by the school of the ailment could also aid in improved gluten-free diet compliance.[21]

Experts recommend school survival tips such as the following: giving the school a list of gluten-free foods that the child prefers; making sure that the child with celiac disease is given gluten-free food when a classmate celebrates birthdays, at which time pastries such as cupcakes, cake, and other foods with gluten are distributed; and making a "survival box" available in times of unplanned events. By also volunteering as a room parent, it can make the latter aware of class activities such as those that involve playing with craft-making materials such as flour, which children could ingest.[22]

There are gluten-free foods that can be packed for lunch and field trips, camps, and parties that children can enjoy, such as yogurt, potato chips, fruit snacks, and pudding cups. The Gluten Intolerance Group offers camps specifically for children with celiac disease.[23]

When youngsters suffering from celiac disease reach college, it is also important that food choices in universities are kept in mind. It is helpful for the parent and student to meet with whomever is in charge of the college cafeteria menus to check on the food list and to see if there can be other substitutes for foods with gluten. Constant contact should also be made. This also does not mean that parents cannot show their support while their children are away. Parents can surprise their children with homemade gluten-free treats.

Parents of celiac disease patients indeed have a special role in motivating their children. This was determined in research done on approximately 40 children in Israel, where the attitudes, dietary activities, and awareness of parents of nonresistant patients were matched with those of resistant patients. [24] Aside from having discovered that parents of compliant patients are more educated and sophisticated, it was found that they are sufficiently knowledgeable about celiac disease and can choose gluten-free foods from a menu, though objective information about the disease was the same in each subject. Moreover, parents of compliant patients are less bothered about health as a whole. What worries them more are the potential undesirable effects of celiac disease their children might have to face in the future. Parents of both groups do not differ much when it comes to being well informed about hindrances to compliance, social support, diet, or use of medical care. Still, it was recommended that parents improve their personal assessment of their own understanding of celiac disease, develop their skills in managing a menu, and be more concerned about possible future effects of the disease in order to boost dietary compliance. [25] Parents maintaining a positive attitude (even if they have to pretend) also helps children with celiac disease to do the same. [26]

Health Experts as Driving Forces

Medical professionals also play a role in motivating a celiac disease patient. Aside from being a patient's right, education provided by the health attendant about the patient's situation, including the negative consequences of untreated celiac disease, is contributory in making the latter diligent about what has to be observed in order to get well. By making the right information available to a patient, confusion is limited. Experts say that a large number of doctors are really not familiar enough about specific diets to guide patients. [27] Hence, in order to give information, professional caregivers should make sure they are well informed first. Registered dieticians should also be taught how to assess patients and counsel them on how to strictly follow a gluten-free diet, giving healthy alternatives to gluten. This would consist of meal planning and supporting the change in diet. However, things should not stop there. When a relationship is established between the dietician and the patient, there should be constant monitoring.[28]

Dieticians also recommend the empowering of children by enlightening them about celiac disease at a young age. There are many available books on celiac disease for children that parents can read to them for fun, which are proven to make kids assertive in playing their roles toward wellness. It is also the dietician's role to recommend support groups to their patients not just for compliance or to avert other complications but also to improve the overall quality of their lives.[29]

Physicians, on the other hand, should maintain a positive approach and push the importance of a gluten-free diet for life. It is their responsibility to instantly recommend an experienced dietician, because delaying this could result in patients resorting to incorrect and obsolete information from the Internet, friends, health food stores, or alternative health practitioners and other questionable sources. Although it is the patient or the parent who will manage continuous treatment such as food preparation, it is still the duty of dieticians to give information on the role of food on nutrition therapy and find solutions to psychological, economic, and educational factors influencing food behaviors.[30]

On top of this, in order to achieve reinforcement it is important that health experts give comprehensible and unbiased information and make sure the patient understands what is being said. Poor communication is one of the most significant aspects for lack of patient adherence. The manner of communication (in a nonthreatening way, for instance) and contentment of the patient have been connected with higher levels of adherence. Aside from this, it would help if health professionals do the following:

show concern to patients
build trust
make them feel at ease
involve them in decision making
find a way for the patient to cooperate by giving him/her freedom of
    choice
have an open relationship and listen to their concerns, feelings, or
    limitations without judging them

It is also suggested that the health practitioner and the patient have a good working relationship and a mutual agreement.[31] Patient education is still different from patient teaching, which is making sure the patient applies what he or she has learned. Teaching aims to involve the patient and the family to handle and deal with the whole situation and prevent complications from occurring. It should be patient centered and not disease centered, focusing on the individual's needs, as each celiac disease sufferer differs in values, thinking, view of quality of life, and preference.

As evidence that patient education and teaching increases compliance and motivation, of the 584 individuals with celiac disease in a study who were told to answer a questionnaire that aimed to assess their knowledge of the disease and compliance to a gluten-free diet, a higher percentage of correct answers were noted. Examples are that 90.4 percent knew that the disease is permanent, 97 percent responded that they have to totally remove gluten from their diet, 67 percent answered that gluten is a protein, and 92.1 percent said protein is seen in rye, barley, wheat, and oat. It was concluded that the more patients know about their condition, the easier it is for them to comply with their diet.[32]

Theories of Motivation

There are six general theories of motivation that can be considered and applied to health teaching and learning situations. The first is the theory of reinforcements, which is related to motivation in that behaviors that were reinforced in the past are most likely to be reinforced again. In this instance, if there is consistency or follow-up in the treatment of a celiac disease patient, then he or she is more inclined to repeat the same procedure and retain the expected lifestyle.[33]

The second theory speaks of needs. Individuals differ in the levels at which they give value to needs such as food, shelter, maintenance of self-esteem, and love. Meeting the need to maintain positive self-esteem, for example, increases the chances of self-motivation, while too much control and lack of connectedness interrupt motivation and sustained learning. Next is the cognitive dissonance theory, which explains that a person feels anxious or pressured when a deeply held value or behavior is tested by a psychologically conflicting behavior or idea. The patient may change the behavior that he has gotten used to in order to resolve the pressure.[34] Thus, in celiac disease sufferers, this theory can be applied to adhere to a change in eating lifestyle.[35]

Attribution, the fourth theory, says that it is innate in humans to look for reasons for why some things happen to them. This act of attribution is said to have a controlling effect on psychological behavior, adjustment, and morbidity (rate of sickness). Thinking about why a patient has celiac disease will prompt him or her into reasonable self-management of the disease. Hence, it is always important to know the patient's belief about the cause of the disorder because that is what patient behavior will some-what depend on.[36]

The fifth talks about depending one's approach on the personality of the patient. There is a general inclination for a person to struggle for success or social connection. However, there are some who feel that they will fail no matter what. This kind of thinking is said to be caused by erratic use of rewards and punishments by teachers. To avoid this, celiac disease patients should be rewarded for motivation, offered positive comments right away, and given constant expectations and follow-up. Coping styles may be also a component of personality. Patients cope physiologically, psychologically, and behaviorally when the information they get is patterned to their way of coping. It is also important to note, though, that there are some persons who are watchful and who seek information from all sources on hand. If they find something wrong in this information, they tend to feel anxious. Others actually want *little* information to avoid stress. Some check the environment for possible threatening information and go over the threats, while some patients cope with aversive health information through distraction.[37]

The last theory, expectancy, implies that motivation is dependent on the chances of success and how much value the person gives to it. If the celiac disease sufferer is given the assurance that he or she will recover from illness by going through a certain treatment, then motivation will be more likely. Self-efficacy is also believed to be strongly related to satisfactory performance. How people see the ability to create and control happenings in their lives affects their motivation, emotion, behavior, and judgment. Those who think they will not be able to survive their illness settle on their personal deficiency and imagine that possible problems will arise more often. Self-efficacy boosts significantly when one acquires new abilities to manage threatening activities and when a person's experience contradicts their fears. It is also important to know that lower self-efficacy is caused by frequent failures. Judgment on self-efficacy is influenced by the following sources of information: observing another's performance, verbal persuasion and other social influences, and psychological condition and performance attainments. Therefore, it will help if patients are shown concrete examples of other patients who went through the same treatment and exited successfully. Making achievable subgoals on top of major goals will also help a patient into self-efficacy.[38]

Other Incidences

Aside from the above-mentioned factors, there are others based on experience that need to be taken into consideration in finding motivation. Out of 70 celiac disease study subjects who were children, dietary compliance was better in smaller families because maintaining an expensive gluten-free diet is not easy.[39] Forty-five percent of celiac children complain that their teachers are not well informed about the nature of the ailment.[40] Special attention should also be given to minorities with celiac disease. Being foreign in a country, celiac disease patients do not feel confident in seeking treatment because of the lack of support and people to turn to. By way of an experiment on celiac disease in African Americans, it was learned that dietary compliance among them is low. For example, Caucasians are said to be more compliant compared to minority populations such as South Asians. The latter do not usually join support groups or go to dietetic clinics, and are not contented with information from health practitioners, and so more support is needed for them in the long run.[41]

ANALYSIS

It is still up to the patient to allow himself to be pushed into fighting the disease, if he or she has the will to recover. The idea of being readmitted to the hospital, getting worse, acquiring celiac disease–related ailments, or spending more money should prompt him or her to summon the discipline for continuous recovery.

15

CONCLUSION

Albeit rare, being born with a lifelong disease can be difficult. Not being able to eat the things one wants from time to time—because eating them might result in serious conditions—is not something anyone would want. Continually watching out for gluten in everything one buys and eats is a tedious task that a person with celiac disease unfortunately must suffer. Moreover, gluten-free food is pretty expensive.

HOPE DESPITE THE INJURIOUS NATURE OF CELIAC DISEASE

Celiac disease is an abnormal reaction of the immune system to the presence of the protein gluten. It is said to be abnormal, as gluten is naturally found in many grains—wheat, rye, barley, and rice.[1] Gluten is used to make dough firm, add chewiness to food, and produce imitation meat eaten by vegetarians.[2] Though it has much use in creating the texture of food, the injuries that can be caused by the immune system to the small intestine far outweigh the benefits gluten can offer. With the intent of helping people with gluten intolerance, many steps for the standardization of food labeling and preparation have been made for those with intolerances to gluten and other food allergies. This is one way in which hope is present in spite of the ordeals that celiac disease sufferers have to go through.

FDA Initiatives

In August 2013, the Food and Drug Administration, or FDA, released a press announcement stating that they had initiated a move to standardize the labels "gluten-free," "no gluten," and "without gluten" in all food products that it mandates. The move is aimed to help people with celiac disease to manage their diet. The law only allows products to be labeled "gluten-free" if they do not contain (1) any raw materials with gluten, (2) grains that contain gluten, (3) any ingredient derived from raw materials with gluten, or (4) any ingredient that has more than 20 parts per million (ppm) of gluten or 20 micrograms of gluten per one gram of food. In short, products mandated by the FDA that are labeled "gluten-free" contain less than 20 parts per million of gluten, or no gluten at all.[3]

This is hopeful news for celiac disease patients, as the typical threshold of gluten a patient can tolerate, although it greatly varies from patient to patient, is 50 milligrams per day.[4] A demographic report from the U.S. Department of Agriculture, or USDA, states that the average American citizen consumes about 200 pounds of grain every year, or about .55 pounds a day, including products derived from grains.[5] Hypothetically, if a patient eats .55 pounds or 249 grams of grains that are up to the "gluten-free" standard of the FDA, then a person would only be eating a maximum of five milligrams of gluten. It is just 0.1 percent of the average gluten threshold for celiac disease patients—very minimal for the average tolerance of celiac disease patients. This step in the standardization of food products that are advertised as "gluten-free" is a great source of hope for those who suffer from this disease.

Codex Alimentarius Commission on Gluten-Free Labeling

The codex alimentarius is a set of standards on all kinds of food that are recognized by the international community as a reference in settling disputes relating to consumer protection and food safety.[6] This codex was created to harmonize the standards on food safety, which also happen to include standards on food labeling.[7] An international commission adopted a standard, codex standard 118-1979, on foods for special dietary use by gluten-intolerant persons in 1979, and it was amended in 1983 and again in 2008, the most current revision of the standard.[8]

The codex states that for a food item to be considered gluten-free, it must not exceed 20 milligrams of gluten per kilogram, and the preparation of the food must comply with certain manufacturing practices in order to avoid, if not limit, harm from gluten.[9] A person would have to eat at least two-and-a-half kilograms of a gluten-free food that complies with this standard before he or she experiences any adverse effect of the disease. This, theoretically, would not happen in a normal daily diet, as a typical U.S. citizen consumes .55 pounds or around half of a kilogram. The codex is not mandatory for all member nations or other international organizations; instead, it is a set of recommended standards that subsequently provide hope for celiac disease patients around the world. If there are any disputes at the international level, the codex can stand as a very valid reference.[10]

Hope beyond Home

Dining out at a restaurant has become a part of everyday life, but it is also becoming a major component of a healthy interpersonal relationship. When dining out, the focus is on the time spent together eating rather than the food itself. This holds true for many families and in business relationships. Celiac disease patients, however, can now actually dine in fast food restaurants because there are some venues that offer gluten-free menus for those with very special diet needs. This might have been done to keep a large number of their customers—children. The prevalence of celiac disease in children in Finland is 1 in 99.[11]

If a celiac patient gets to eat in a restaurant, he or she may tell the server about the intolerance to gluten, and that any trace amounts of wheat, rye, and barley will make him or her sick. Many restaurants will be more than happy to change their dishes or the way they prepare the food just for him or her. Of course, if the server is not familiar with gluten intolerance, the celiac disease patient might need to spend a lot of time explaining. Experts recommend bringing a preprinted or prewritten card that can be given to the server.[12]

Permanent Relief May Be Close at Hand

Although the movement of the FDA is already a huge help for celiac disease patients, experts in the medical field are continually researching a possible cure for this autoimmune response by the body that would fully relieve the patients of all negative physiological reactions to gluten. A recent experiment has found the root cause of this disease, and scientists are very hopeful that a treatment—a permanent one—for celiac disease is close at hand.[13] Soon, people with celiac disease will be able to eat and nourish themselves with the needed food that in turn will result in perfect harmony inside their body. They will become stronger than ever and will be able to grow well physically and emotionally. They will "feel good" about themselves: being healthy and strong, and capable of working while helping others. They will become physically capable of living a life they want, as they will no longer be limited by their physical incapability.[14]

Joining Others on the Road to Hope

Becoming strong and willed to live and pursuing everything they have dreamed will inspire others to continue pushing through the barriers that their illness has created. It is when the celiac disease sufferer exceeds what he or she is capable of doing, and in doing what normally cannot be done, that things turn for the better. Patients can inspire other patients who are suffering from the same adversities. They can tell stories of how they manage to live normally, or even succeed professionally and personally in life.

PATIENCE AND CONFIDENCE

Celiac disease has been dubbed a jigsaw puzzle in the medical field, for it has daunted scientists and doctors alike.[15] For now, experts only have the pieces completed on one side of the full puzzle. Finding a cure for any medical disorder takes time. That is why patience is an important virtue when approaching celiac disease.

Continuously explaining one's condition is relatively discouraging. Aside from that, living with celiac disease can be a tiring routine task. It makes a person feel as if there is no one in the world who can understand them, and without patience, things can get worse. When dealing with any kind of disease, whether celiac disease or another, a person must be patient. In a sense, the general public has already realized the prevalence and the difficulty of having celiac disease. There are many celiac disease awareness groups that are spawning, even on the Internet. Some even have organizations that help these people financially. [16]

A celiac disease patient should always feel confident. Patients are individuals who play or will be playing a significant role in society, and therefore they should never be discouraged by differences. They should know that they are not alone, that there are other people out there who experience the same struggles. They should know that although they suffer from celiac disease, there are always other people who are more than willing to help. Taking all of the above into consideration will undoubtedly boost the confidence of the celiac disease sufferer in the long run. Additionally, a research paper states that confidence in one's abilities generally improves life, and that confidence is a valuable asset for those with dwindling willpower. [17] This goes to show that confidence is vital to a person's professional and personal life. Experts have concluded that self-esteem, a concept very close to self-confidence, has a significant positive influence on academic performance. High self-esteem has high value in making people continue to strive in the face of failure. [18]

That is how important confidence is for individuals suffering from celiac disease. A person's state of mind is very important when it comes to getting treated for a disease. The gluten-free diet takes care of the physical part of treatment, while mind-set, self-confidence, and self-esteem will take care of the state of mind that in turn encourages faster healing of the body. Patients should talk more to people—especially to those who do not know what celiac disease is. They could explain it to them concisely, because extraversion is linked to self-confidence. [19] The more outgoing a person is, the more he or she can be regarded as a confident individual.

IMPORTANCE OF SEEING A DOCTOR

Being a celiac disease patient requires a great deal of personal and professional help. This is a disease yet to be fully understood and cured. It is not yet fully comprehensible even to experts of modern-day science and medicine. [20] If people in the medical field are sailing in the mist, then those who are not well versed in medicine will be walking through a dense fog. Doctors often try to keep themselves up to date with the newest research results. They are the first to know whether the previous diagnosis is a failure, a success, or something that could worsen the patient's condition. They know the myths and facts that surround celiac disease. Celiac disease patients should understand that health care professionals are often trained to be considerate of a patient's religious beliefs and personal preferences when prescribing medications. A report published by the University of Washington School of Medicine states that many nurses and physicians believe that the religious practices of patients have significant effects on the latters' experiences when facing death. [21]

Another point is that every doctor has some kind of specialization within the broad field of medicine. A doctor of the heart may not be proficient at treating celiac disease. This means that getting aid and advice from doctors of different specialties helps greatly. The bottom line: people with celiac disease should consult with a dietician, physician, and gastrointestinal specialist. It is also important not to ignore the emotional side of celiac disease. The patient can ask for help from a family member and, if necessary, a psychologist. Complex medical situations such as those seen with celiac disease are treated in this way. [22]

Most of the time, two or more heads are better than one. The more scientists agree on an opinion and/or theory, the more the theory becomes reliable. The scientific community is a peer-reviewed world in which the practitioners within the field criticize each other's work for the betterment of all. This ensures that the celiac disease research is unbiased and is up to the standards of factual science. The practice ensures the truthfulness of all the information that circulates in the community. This all equates to reliability. Doctors are normally up to date with research as well as other technological advancements in their own specific field. [23] In turn, celiac disease sufferers can trust professional caregivers when it comes to their medical condition and can protect themselves from hearsay that usually arises from superstitious beliefs—which are somewhat unreliable when symptoms turn serious.

Unfortunately, many people self-medicate and self-diagnose. With the dawn of new technology, people tend to "research" their symptoms online and simply choose (from a long list) a disease that is somehow associated with the symptoms they are experiencing. When people are too stubborn to get medical advice, they might mistakenly diagnose themselves with a certain disorder when they truly have a different disease. Herein lays the problem of self-diagnosis and self-medication. [24]

The World Health Organization does not deny the importance of self-medication in health care, and they have even published a report on the pros and cons of self-medication. [25] Self-medication may only be applicable for first aid, but if the condition turns out to be much more than a simple stomachache, then a painkiller will not only be insufficient but also result in worsening of the case. It is of vital importance that the problem be identified as early as possible and as accurately as possible. This will pave the way to (1) the timely treatment of the celiac disease and (2) prevention of further complications. [26]

ANALYSIS

In the final analysis, celiac disease patients and caregivers should know that although the disease may not be considered as threatening as a more severe situation such as cancer, celiac disease should not be taken lightly. The disease primarily affects the digestive system, but it can have an impact on other organs and body systems as well.

APPENDIX A

Celiac-Disease-Related Links

Advanced Clinical Research, http://www.acr-research.com/study-137-Celiac-Disease-(SLC)
American Family Physician, http://www.aafp.org/afp/2007/1215/p1795.html
American Journal of Gastroenterology, http://www.nature.com/ajg
Association of European Coeliac Studies, http://www.aoecs.org
Bellingham Gluten Information Group, http://www.glutenfreeway.info
Boston Children's Hospital, http://www.childrenshospital.org/centers-and-services
Canadian Medical Association, http://www.cmaj.ca
Celiac.com, http://www.celiac.com
Celiac Community Foundation of Northern California, http://www.celiaccommunity.org/
    celiac-disease
Celiac Disease & Gluten Sensitivity, about.com, http://celiacdisease.about.com
Celiac Disease Awareness Campaign, http://www.celiac.nih.gov
Celiac Disease Center at Columbia University Medical Center, http://www.celiacdiseasecenter.
    org
Celiac Disease Foundation, http://www.celiac.org
Celiac Society, http://www.celiacsociety.com
Celiac Support Association, http://www.csaceliacs.info
Children's Hospital Colorado, http://www.childrenscolorado.org/departments/digestive/
    programs
Children's Hospital of Philadelphia, http://www.chop.edu/service/center-for-celiac-disease/
    home.html
Coeliac Australia, http://www.coeliac.org.au
Coeliac New Zealand, http://www.coeliac.org.nz
Coeliac Society of Ireland, http://www.coeliac.ie
Coeliac UK, http://www.coeliac.org.uk
Gluten-Free Living, http://www.glutenfreeliving.com
Gluten Intolerance Group, http://www.glutenfreerestaurants.org/
Healthy Villi, http://www.healthyvilli.org
Informa Healthcare, http://www.informahealthcare.com
JAMA Pediatrics, http://archpedi.jamanetwork.com/journal.aspx
Jefferson University Hospitals, http://www.jeffersonhospital.org
KidsHealth.org, http://www.kidshealth.org/teen/diseases_conditions/digestive/celiac.html

LaJolla Institute for Allergy and Immunology, http://www.liai.org/pages/celiac-disease-research

MassGeneral Hospital for Children, http://www.massgeneral.org/children/services/treatmentprograms.aspx?id=1723

Mayo Clinic, http://www.mayo.edu/research/discoverys-edge/celiac-disease-rise

Medline Plus, http://www.nlm.nih.gov/medlineplus/celiacdisease.html

National Digestive Diseases Information Clearinghouse, http://www.digestive.niddk.nih.gov/ddiseases/pubs/celiac

National Foundation for Celiac Awareness, http://www.celiaccentral.org/research-news

National Health Service UK, http://www.nhs.uk/Conditions/Coeliac-disease/Pages/Introduction.aspx

Nationwide Children's, http://www.nationwidechildrens.org/celiac-disease

Netherlands Genomic Initiative, http://www.genomics.nl/Research/GenomicsCentres/Celiac.aspx

New England Journal of Medicine, http://www.nejm.org

New York-Presbyterian, http://nyp.org/services/digestive/celiac-disease.html

Prevent Celiac Disease, http://www.preventceliacdisease.com/startpagina

Prometheus Therapeutics & Diagnostics, http://www.celiacplus.com

Rush University Medical Center, http://www.rush.edu/rumc/page-1175113041252.html

San Gabriel Valley Celiac Support Group, http://www.sgvceliac.org

Sheffield Children's NHS Foundation Trust, http://www.sheffieldchildrens.nhs.uk/patients-and-parents/coeliac-disease.htm

The Patient Celiac, http://www.thepatientceliac.com/tag/celiac-disease

Ultimate Gluten Free, http://ultimateglutenfree.com

UCLA Health, http://www.gastro.ucla.edu

University of Chicago Celiac Disease Center, http://www.cureceliacdisease.org

University of Chicago Medical Center, http://www.uchospitals.edu

University of Iowa Hospitals & Clinics, https://www.uihealthcare.org/celiacdisease

University of Maryland School of Medicine, http://www.medschool.umaryland.edu/celiac

Victoria Celiac, http://www.victoriaceliac.org

Wake Research, http://www.wakeresearch.com

WebMD, Celiac Disease Health Center, http://www.webmd.com/digestive-disorders/celiac-disease

Wm. K. Warren Medical Research Center for Celiac Disease, http://celiaccenter.ucsd.edu/

Women's Health.gov, http://www.womenshealth.gov

APPENDIX B

Celiac Disease Research and Training

ACR Idaho
2950 E. Magic View Drive, Suite 182
Boise, ID 83642
(208) 377-8653
Fax: (208) 377-8659

ACR Utah
3590 West 9000 South, Suite 300
West Jordan, UT 84088
(801) 542-8190
Fax: (801) 542-8197

Adult Celiac Disease Program
Rush University Medical Center
1725 W. Harrison Street, Suite 207
Chicago, IL 60612
(312) 942-8570
http://www.rush.edu

Alfred I. DuPont Hospital for Children
Pediatric GI Division
1600 Rockland Road
Wilmington, DE 19803
(302) 651-4200
http://www.nemours.org

Allegheny Center for Digestive Health
1307 Federal Street, Suite 301
Pittsburgh, PA 15212
(412) 359-8956
Fax: (412) 359-8977

http://www.pittsburghceliac.org

American College of Gastroenterology
6400 Goldsboro Road, Suite 200
Bethesda, MD 20817
(301) 263-9000
info@acg.gi.org
http://www.gi.org

Beth Israel Deaconess Medical Center
330 Brookline Avenue
Boston, MA 02215
(617) 667-7000
http://www.bidmc.org/

Boston Children's Hospital
Celiac Disease Program
300 Longwood Avenue
Boston, MA 02115
http://www.childrenshospital.org

The Celiac Center at Paoli Hospital
255 West Lancaster Avenue
Paoli, PA 19301
(484) 565-1000
http://www.mainlinehealth.org/

Celiac Disease and Gluten Sensitivity Center
Stony Brook Children's Hospital
4 Technology Drive
East Setauket, NY 11733

(631) 444-8115
Fax: (631) 444-6045
http://www.stonybrookchildrens.org

Celiac Disease Awareness Campaign
National Digestive Diseases Information
   Clearinghouse
2 Information Way
Bethesda, MD 20892
(800) 891-5389
celiac@info.niddk.nih.gov
http://www.celiac.nih.gov

Celiac Disease Center
Beth Israel Deaconess Medical Center
330 Brookline Avenue
Boston, MA 02215
(617) 667-1272
http://www.bidmc.harvard.edu/celiaccenter

Celiac Disease Center at Columbia University
Harkness Pavilion
180 Fort Washington Avenue, Suite 936
New York, NY 10032
(212) 342-4529
cb2280@columbia.edu
http://www.celiacdiseasecenter.org

Celiac Disease Consortium
c/o Leiden University
P.O. Box 9600
2300 RC Leiden
The Netherlands
+31 71 526 5266

Celiac Disease Research Program
Mayo Clinic
200 First Street
Rochester, MN 55905
(507) 284-2511
http://www.mayoclinic.org/celiac-disease

Celiac Disease Study Group
Biokatu 10, 3rd Floor
FI-33520 Tampere, Finland
+358 3 3551 8400
Fax: +358 3 3551 8402
http://www.celiacresearch.eu

Celiac Sprue Research Foundation
P.O. Box 1506
Healdsburg, CA 95448

http://www.celiacsprue.org

The Center for Celiac Disease at Children's
   Hospital of Colorado
13123 East 16th Avenue
Aurora, CO 80045
(800) 624-6553
http://www.childrenscolorado.org

Center for Celiac Research & Treatment
Yawkey Center for Outpatient Care
55 Fruit Street, Suite 6B
Boston, MA 02114
(617) 724-8476
Fax: 617-643-2384

Children's Hospital of Los Angeles
Gastroenterology Division
4650 W. Sunset Boulevard
Los Angeles, CA 90027
(323) 361-7336

The Children's Hospital of Philadelphia
Center for Celiac Disease
34th Street and Civic Center Boulevard
Philadelphia, PA 19104
(215) 590-3076
http://www.chop.edu

Children's Hospital of Wisconsin
Bonnie Mechanic Celiac Disease Clinic
9000 W. Wisconsin Avenue
Wauwautosa, WI 53226
(877) 607-5280
http://www.chw.org/

Digestive Disease Research Institute
Kargar Shomali Avenue
Tehran, 14117-13135, Iran
Fax: +98-21-82415400
info@ddri.ir
http://www.ddri.ir

Jefferson Celiac Center
Thomas Jefferson University Hospital
132 South 10th Street
Philadelphia, PA 19107
(800) 533-3669
http://www.jeffersonhospital.org

La Jolla Institute for Allergy & Immunology
9420 Athena Circle
La Jolla, CA 92037

(858) 752-6500
contact@liai.org
http://www.liai.org

Stanford Celiac Sprue Clinic
Stanford University Medical Center
300 Pasteur Drive
Stanford, CA 94305
(650) 732-6961
http://www.stanfordhospital.com

UCLA Santa Monica Gastroenterology
1223 16th Street, Suite 3100
Santa Monica, CA 90404
(310) 582-6240

University of Chicago Celiac Disease Center
5841 S. Maryland Avenue
Chicago, IL 60637
(773) 702-7593
Fax: (773) 702-0666
http://www.cureceliacdisease.org

University of Iowa Celiac Disease and In-
    flammatory Bowel Disease Center
200 Hawkins Drive
Iowa City, IA 52242
(800) 777-8442
https://www.uihealthcare.org/

University of Maryland Center for Celiac Re-
    search
655 West Baltimore Street
Baltimore, MD 21201
(410) 328-6749
orpedsgi@peds.umaryland.edu
http://www.medschool.umaryland.edu/celiac

University of Tennessee Medical Center
Celiac Center
1924 Alcoa Highway

Knoxville, TN 37920
(877) 882-2737
http://www.utmedicalcenter.org/

University of Virginia Digestive Health
Center of Excellence: Celiac Disease
P.O. Box 800708
Charlottesville, VA 22908
(434) 924-2959
http://www.healthsystem.virginia.edu

U.S. National Library of Medicine
8600 Rockville Pike
Bethesda, MD 20894
(301) 594-5983
Fax: (301) 402-1384
http://www.nlm.nih.gov/

Wake Research
3100 Duraleigh Road, Suite 304
Raleigh, NC 27612
(919) 781-2514
Fax: (919) 420-6067
http://www.wakeresearch.com

Walter and Eliza Hall Institute of Medical
    Research
1G Royal Parade
Parkville ,Victoria 3052, Australia
+61 3 9345 2555
Fax: +61 3 9347 085
communityrelations@wehi.edu.au
http://www.wehi.edu.au

Wm. K. Warren Medical Research Center for
    Celiac Disease
9500 Gilman Drive
La Jolla, CA 92093
(858) 822-1022
celiaccenter@ucsd.edu
http://celiaccenter.ucsd.edu/

APPENDIX C

Celiac Disease and Related Organizations

American Celiac Disease Alliance
2504 Duxbury Place
Alexandria, VA 22308
(703) 622-3331
info@americanceliac.org
http://www.americanceliac.org

American Celiac Society
P.O. Box 23455
New Orleans, LA 70183
(504) 737-3293
americanceliacsociety@yahoo.com
http://www.americanceliacsociety.org

American Gastroenterological Association
4930 Del Ray Avenue
Bethesda, MD 20814
(301) 654-2055
Fax: (301) 654-5920
http://www.gastro.org

Bi-State Celiac Support Group
P.O. Box 410707
Creve Coeur, MO 63141
http://www.bscsgonline.org

Canadian Digestive Health Foundation
1500 Upper Middle Road
P.O. Box 76059
Oakville, ON L6M 3H5
(905) 829-3949

http://www.cdhf.ca

Celiac Community Foundation of Northern
  California
P.O. Box 1506
Healdsburg, CA 95448
(707) 579-9683
info@celiaccommunity.org
http://www.celiaccommunity.org

Celiac Disease Foundation
20350 Ventura Boulevard, Suite 240
Woodland Hills, CA 91364
(818) 716-1513
Fax: (818) 267-5577
http://www.celiac.org

Celiac Disease Resource, Inc.
P.O. Box 621
Glenmont, NY 12077
(518) 461-7065
UpstateCeliacs@yahoo.com
http://www.celiacresource.org

Celiac Society for Delhi
Capital Trust House 47
Friends Colony, New Delhi 110025
(011) 4162-7007
celiacsocietyindia@gmail.com
http://www.celiacsocietyindia.com

Celiac Support Association
1941 S. 42nd Street, Suite 522
Omaha, NE 68105
(877) 272-4272
Fax: (402) 558-0600
http://www.csaceliacs.info

Children's Digestive Health and Nutrition
  Foundation
1501 Bethlehem Pike
P.O. Box 6
Flourtown, PA 19031
(215) 233-0808
cdhnf@cdhnf.org
http://cdhnfsite.wms.cdgsolutions.com/
  wmspage.cfm?parm1=14

Coeliac Australia
P.O. Box 271
Wahroonga, NSW 2076
+ 02 9487-5088
Fax: (02) 9487-5177
http://www.coeliac.org.au

Coeliac New Zealand
P.O. Box 35724
Browns Bay, Auckland 0753
(09) 820-5157
Fax: (09) 414-7468
http://www.coeliac.org.nz

Coeliac Society of Ireland
Carmichael House
4 North Brunswick Street
Dublin 7
+353 (1) 872-1471
info@coeliac.ie
http://www.coeliac.ie

Digestive Disease National Coalition
507 Capitol Court, NE, Suite 200
Washington, DC 20002
(202) 544-7497
Fax: (202) 546-7105
http://www.ddnc.org

Gastrointestinal Research Foundation
70 East Lake Street, Suite 1015
Chicago, IL 60601
(312) 332-1350
Fax: (312) 332-4757
girf@earthlink.net
http://www.girf.org

Gluten Intolerance Group of North America
31214 124th Avenue
Auburn, WA 98092
(253) 833-6655
Fax: (253) 833-6675
info@gluten.net
http://www.gluten.net

International Foundation for Functional
Gastrointestinal Disorders
700 W. Virginia Street, #201
Milwaukee, WI 53204
(414) 964-1799
Fax: (414) 964-7176
iffgd@iffgd.org
http://www.iffgd.org

Kicking 4 Celiac Foundation
34 Audrey Avenue, 3rd Floor
Oyster Bay, NY 11771
info@kicking4celiac.org
http://www.kicking4celiac.org

National Foundation for Celiac Awareness
P.O. Box 544
Ambler, PA 19002
(215) 325-1306
Fax: (215) 643-1707
http://www.celiaccentral.org

National Organization for Rare Disorders
55 Kenosia Avenue
Danbury, CT 06810
(203) 744-0100
Fax: (203) 798-2291
http://www.rarediseases.org

North American Society for Pediatric Gastroenterology, Hepatology, and Nutrition
P.O. Box 6
Flourtown, PA 19031
(215) 233-0808
Fax: (215) 233-3918
naspghan@naspghan.org
http://www.naspghan.org

Raising Our Celiac Kids (ROCK)
4927 Sonoma Highway, Suite C
Santa Rosa, CA 95409
(707) 509-4528
Fax: (707) 324-6060
http://www.celiac.com

Teens Living with Celiac
1191 Edgewater Avenue
Ridgefield, NJ 07657
(201) 563-1211
info@teenslivingwithceliac.org
http://www.teenslivingwithceliac.org

Westchester Celiac Sprue Support Group
P.O. Box 66
Montrose, NY 10548

info@WestchesterCeliacs.org
http://www.westchesterceliacs.org

World Gastroenterology Organisation
555 East Wells Street, Suite 1100
Milwaukee, WI 53202
(414) 918-9798
Fax: +1 (414) 276-3349
info@worldgastroenterology.org
http://www.worldgastroenterology.org

APPENDIX D
Nationally Recognized Celiac Disease Clinics

Adult Celiac Disease Program
Rush University Medical Center
1653 W. Congress Parkway
Chicago, IL 60612
(312) 942-5861
http://www.rush.edu/rumc

Akron Digestive Disease Consultants, Inc.
570 White Pond Drive
Suite 100
Akron, OH 44320
(330) 869-0124
http://www.addc.myohiogi.com

Alegent Creighton Clinic
601 North 30th Street, Suite 5730
Omaha, NE 68131
(402) 449-4692
Fax: (402) 449-5926
http://www.alegentcreighton.com

Allegheney Center for Digestive Health
   Multi-Disciplinary Celiac Sprue Clinic
1307 Federal Street, Suite 301
Pittsburgh, PA 15212
(412) 359-8956
Fax: (412) 359-8977
http://www.pittsburghceliac.org

Arizona Center for Advanced Medicine
8841 East Bell Road

Scottsdale, AZ 85260
(480) 240-2600
Fax: (480) 240-2601
http://www.arizonaadvancedmedicine.com

Atlanta Gastroenterology Associates Pediatric and Adolescent Division
5445 Meridian Mark Road, Suite 490
Atlanta, GA 30342
(404) 843-6320
http://www.atlantagastro.com

Atlantic Gastroenterology Associates
3205 Fire Road
Egg Harbor Township, NJ 08234
(609) 407-1220
Fax: (609) 407-0220
http://www.atlanticgastro.com

Austin Gastroenterology
4310 James Casey Street #4A
Austin, TX 78745
(512) 454-4588
http://www.austingastro.com

Bay Area Surgicare Center
502 Medical Center Boulevard
Webster, TX 77598
(281) 332-2433
http://www.bayareasurgicare.com

Baylor University Medical Center
3500 Gaston Avenue
Dallas, TX 75246
(214) 820-0111
http://www.baylorhealth.com

Bonnie Lynn Mechanic Celiac Disease Clinic
9000 West Wisconsin Avenue
Wauwatosa, WI 53226
(414) 607-5280
http://www.chw.org

Brenner Children's Hospital
Medical Center Boulevard
Winston-Salem, NC 27157
(336) 713-4500
http://www.brennerchildrens.org

Brooklyn Gastroenterology and Endoscopy
2211 Emmons Avenue
Brooklyn, NY 11235
(718) 368-2960
Fax: (718) 368-2249
http://www.nygicare.com

California Pacific Medical Center
3700 California Street
San Francisco, CA 94118
(415) 600-6000
http://www.cpmc.org

The Celiac Center, Arnold Palmer Hospital
  for Children
92 West Miller Street
Orlando, FL 32806
(321) 841-3338
http://www.orlandohealth.com/
  arnoldpalmerhospital

Celiac Sprue Clinic
Stanford University Medical Center
300 Pasteur Drive
Stanford, CA 94305
(650) 723-4000
http://www.stanfordhospital.com

Center for Advanced Digestive Care, Duke
  Raleigh Hospital
3400 Wake Forest Road
Raleigh, NC 27609
(855) 278-7418
Fax: (919) 954-3916
http://www.dukeraleighhospital.org

Center for Advanced Digestive Care, Weill
  Cornell Medical Center
525 East 68th Street
New York, NY 10065
(877) 902-2232
http://cadc.nyp.org/

Center for Advanced Medicine, GI Center
4921 Parkview Place
Suite C, Floor 8
St. Louis, MO 63110
(314) 747-2066
http://wuphysicians.wustl.edu/page.aspx?
  pageID=917

Cleveland Clinic
9500 Euclid Avenue
Cleveland, OH 44195
(800) 223-2273
http://my.clevelandclinic.org/default.aspx

The Digestive Disease Center of the Hudson
  Valley
400 Westage Business Center Drive, Suite
  209
Fishkill, NY 12524
(845) 896-0736
Fax: (845) 896-5196
http://www.digestivediseaseny.com

Digestive Disease Services: The Mount Sinai
  Hospital
One Gustave L. Levy Place
New York, NY 10029
(212) 241-6500
http://www.mountsinai.org

Fletcher Allen Health Care
111 Colchester Avenue
Burlington, VT 05401
(802) 847-0000
http://www.fletcherallen.org

Floating Hospital for Children
755 Washington Street
Boston, MA 02111
(617) 636-5000
http://www.floatinghospital.org

Gastroenterology Center of Connecticut
Spring Glen Medical Center
2200 Whitney Avenue, Suite 360
Hamden, CT 06518

(203) 281-4463
Fax: (203) 287-2930
http://www.gastrocenter.org/celiac-center

Gastroenterology Clinic: University of Colorado
1665 Aurora Court, Second Floor
Aurora, CO 80045
(720) 848-2777
http://www.uch.edu

Gastroenterology Practice Associates
301 Highlander Boulevard, Suite 121
Arlington, TX 76018
(817) 468-1162
Fax: (817) 468-7201
http://www.gpagastropractice.com

Hill Park Medical Center
616 Petaluma Boulevard, Suite C
Petaluma, CA 94952
(707) 778-3171
Fax: (707) 778-6744
http://www.hillparkmedicalcenter.com

IBS Treatment Center
1301 Pinehurst Way
Seattle, WA 98125
(206) 264-1111
http://www.ibstreatmentcenter.com

Kogan Celiac Center, Saint Barnabas
Ambulatory Care Center
95 Old Short Hills Road
West Orange, NJ 07052
(973) 322-7272
http://www.barnabashealth.org

Levine Children's Specialty Center
1001 Blythe Boulevard, Suite 200-E
Charlotte, NC 28203
(704) 381-8840
http://www.carolinashealthcare.org/levine-childrens-specialty-center-lch

Lurie Children's Hospital
225 East Chicago Avenue
Chicago, IL 60611
(312) 227-4000
http://www.luriechildrens.org

Manhattan Gastroenterology
170 East 78th Street

New York, NY 10075
(212) 427-8761
http://www.manhattangastroenterology.com

Marin Gastroenterology
1350 South Eliseo Drive, Suite 130
Greenbrae, CA 94904
(415) 925-6900
Fax: (415) 925-6919
http://www.maringastro.com

Medical University of South Carolina
Digestive Disease Center
25 Courtenay Drive
Charleston, SC 29425
(843) 792-6999
http://www.ddc.musc.edu

Nebraska Medical Center
987400 Nebraska Medical Center
Omaha, NE 68198
(402) 552-3344
http://www.nebraskamed.com

Northern California Gastroenterology Consultants, Inc.
2089 Vale Road #33
San Pablo, CA 94806
(510) 234-5012
http://www.norcalgi.com

Ohio State University Wexner Medical Center
410 West 10th Avenue
Columbus, OH 43210
(614) 293-8652
http://www.medicalcenter.osu.edu

Palm Beach Gastroenterology Consultants
1157 South State Road 7
Wellington, FL 33414
(561) 795-3330
http://www.gitrip.com

Park Central Surgical Center
12200 Park Central Drive, 3rd Floor
Dallas, TX 75251
(972) 661-0505
http://www.parkcentralsurgicalcenter.com

Pediatric Celiac Center
Englewood Hospital and Medical Center
350 Engle Street

Englewood, NJ 07631
(201) 894-3690
http://www.englewoodhospital.com/ms_
    pediatrics_celiac.asp

Pediatric Gastroenterology Associates
2577 Samaritan Drive, Suite 815
San Jose, CA 95124
(408) 358-3573
Fax: (408) 356-2888
http://www.pediatricgisanjose.com

Penn State Hershey Medical Center
500 University Drive
Hershey, PA 17033
(800) 243-1455
http://www.pennstatehershey.org

Rady Children's Specialists
8110 Birmingham Way
Building 28, 2nd Floor
San Diego, CA 92123
(858) 966-4003
Fax: (858) 560-6798
http://www.rchsd.org

Robert Wood Johnson University Hospital
One Robert Wood Johnson Place
New Brunswick, NJ 08901
(732) 828-3000
http://www.rwjuh.edu

Rocky Mountain Health Centers Pediatrics
15101 East Iliff Avenue, Suite 140
Aurora, CO 80014
(303) 996-9601
Fax: (303) 369-2605
http://www.rmhcpeds.com

St. Vincent Health
10330 N. Meridian Street
Indianapolis, IN 46290
(317) 338-2273
http://www.stvincent.org

Salem Gastroenterology Associates
1830 South Hawthorne Road
Winston-Salem, NC 27103
(336) 765-0463
Fax: (336) 768-9452
http://www.salemgi.com/

South Florida Gastroenterology Associates,
    P.A.
1325 South Congress Avenue, Suite 211
Boynton Beach, FL 33426
(561) 732-2900
Fax: (561) 738-7055
http://www.sfgastro.net

Texas Children's Hospital
6621 Fannin Street
Houston, TX 77030
(832) 822-3131
http://www.texaschildrens.org

Tufts Medical Center
800 Washington Street
Boston, MA 02111
(617) 636-5000
http://www.tuftsmedicalcenter.org

Tulane Gastroenterology Clinic
1415 Tulane Avenue, 6th Floor
New Orleans, LA 70112
(504) 988-5110
http://www.tulane.edu

University of Alabama at Birmingham
500 22nd Street
South Birmingham, AL 35233
(800) 822-8816
http://www.uabmedicine.org

UCLA Celiac Disease Program
10920 Wilshire Boulevard, Suite 400
Los Angeles, CA 90095
(310) 794-0500
http://www.gastro.ucla.edu

University of California San Francisco Medi-
    cal Center
505 Parnassus Avenue
San Francisco, CA 94131
(415) 476-1000
http://www.ucsfhealth.org

University of Chicago Celiac Disease Center
5841 South Maryland Avenue
Chicago, IL 60637
(773) 702-7593
Fax: (773) 702-0666
http://www.cureceliacdisease.org

University of Colorado Hospital
Anschutz Inpatient Pavilion
12605 East 16th Avenue
Aurora, CO 80045
(720) 330-3921
http://www.uch.edu/locations/get-care/um-anschutz/

University of Maryland Center for Celiac Research
20 Penn Street, S303B
Baltimore, MD 21201
(410) 706-8021
http://www.umm.edu/programs/celiac-research

University of Minnesota
Amplatz Children's Hospital
2450 Riverside Avenue
Minneapolis, MN 55454
(612) 365-6777
http://www.uofmchildrenshospital.org

University of Minnesota Medical Center, Fairview
2450 Riverside Avenue

Minneapolis, MN 55454
(612) 624-9708
http://www.uofmmedicalcenter.org

University of Rochester Medical Center
601 Elmwood Avenue
Rochester, NY 14642
(585) 275-8762
http://www.urmc.rochester.edu

University of Southern California
Department of Pediatrics
Keck School of Medicine
4650 Sunset Boulevard
Los Angeles, CA 90027
(323) 361-2303
Fax: (323) 361-3719
http://keck.usc.edu/

University of Virginia Health System,
The Digestive Health Center of Excellence
P.O. Box 800708
Charlottesville, VA 22908
(434) 924-2959
http://www.medicine.virginia.edu

APPENDIX E
For Further Reading

Acton, Ashton. *Celiac Disease: New Insights for the Healthcare Professional.* Atlanta, GA: Scholarly Editions, 2013.

Alpers, David, Anthony Kalloo, Neil Kaplowitz, Chung Owyang, and Don Powell. *Textbook of Gastroenterology.* 5th ed. Edited by Tadataka Yamada. Oxford: Wiley-Blackwell, 2008.

Banerjee, Bhaskar. *Nutritional Management of Digestive Disorders.* Boca Raton, FL: CRC Press, 2011.

Bishop, Warren. *Pediatric Practice Gastroenterology.* New York: McGraw-Hill, 2010.

Bower, Sylvia, and Mary Sharrett. *Celiac Disease: A Guide to Living with Gluten Intolerance.* New York: Demos Health Publishing, 2006.

Braly, James, and Ron Hoggan. *Dangerous Grains: Why Gluten Cereal Grains May Be Hazardous to Your Health.* New York: Avery Trade, 2002.

Buchman, Alan. *Clinical Nutrition in Gastrointestinal Disease.* Thorofare, NJ: Slack, 2006.

Burns, David. *100 Questions & Answers about Celiac Disease and Sprue.* Sudbury, MA: Jones & Bartlett Learning, 2007.

Coulston, Ann M., Carol J. Boushey, and Mario Ferruzzi. *Nutrition in the Prevention and Treatment of Disease.* 3rd ed. San Diego: Academic Press, 2013.

Dennis, Melinda, and Daniel Leffler. *Real Life with Celiac Disease: Troubleshooting and Thriving Gluten Free.* Bethesda, MD: AGA Press, 2010.

Duggan, John M., and Anne E. Duggan. *The Epidemiology of Alimentary Diseases.* Dordrecht, the Netherlands: Springer, 2006.

Edwards, Matthew. *Celiac Disease: Etiology, Diagnosis, and Treatment.* New York: Nova Science Publishers, 2010.

Fasano, Alessio, Riccardo Troncone, and David Branski. *Frontiers in Celiac Disease.* Basel, Switzerland: Karger Medical and Scientific Publishers, 2008.

Feldman, Mark, Lawrence S. Friedman, and Lawrence J. Brandt. *Sleisenger and Fordtran's Gastrointestinal and Liver Disease: Pathophysiology/Diagnosis/Management.* 9th ed. Philadelphia: Saunders, 2010.

Ferri, Fred. *Ferri's Practical Guide, 9th Edition: Fast Facts for Patient Care.* Philadelphia: Saunders Elsevier, 2014.

Floch, Martin, and Neil Floch. *Netter's Gastroenterology.* 2nd ed. Philadelphia: Saunders Elsevier, 2010.

Greenberger, Norton, Richard Blumberg, and Robert Burakoff. *Current Diagnosis & Treatment Gastroenterology, Hepatology, & Endoscopy.* 2nd ed. New York: McGraw-Hill, 2011.

Griffiths, Helen. *Coeliac Disease: Nursing Care and Management.* West Sussex, UK: John Wiley & Sons, 2008.

Guandalini, Stephen. *Textbook of Pediatric Gastroenterology and Nutrition.* London: Taylor & Francis, 2005.

Helferich, William, and Carl K. Winter. *Food Toxicology.* Boca Raton, FL: CRC Press, 2001.

Holmes, Geoffrey, Carlo Catassi, and Alessio Fasano. *Fast Facts: Celiac Disease.* Abingdon, Oxford: Health Press, 2009.

Jackson, Patricia, Judith A. Vessey, and Naomi Schapiro. *Primary Care of the Child with a Chronic Condition.* 5th ed. Philadelphia: Saunders Elsevier, 2010.

Kliegman, Robert, Bonita Stanton, Joseph St. Geme III, Nina Schor, and Richard Behrman. *Nelson Textbook of Pediatrics.* 19th ed. Philadelphia: Saunders Elsevier, 2011.

Kohlstadht, Ingrid. *Advancing Medicine with Food and Nutrients.* 2nd ed. Boca Raton, FL: CRC Press, 2012.

Korn, Danna. *Kids with Celiac Disease: A Family Guide to Raising Happy, Healthy, Gluten-Free Children.* Bethesda, MD: Woodbine House, 2001.

Kumar, Vinay, Abul Abbas, Nelson Fausto, Jon Aster, and James Perkins. *Robbins and Cotran Pathologic Basis of Disease.* 8th ed. Philadelphia: Saunders Elsevier, 2010.

Lebwohl, Benjamin, and Peter Green. *Celiac Disease: An Issue of Gastrointestinal Endoscopy Clinics.* Philadelphia: Saunders Elsevier, 2012.

Lifschitz, Carlos H. *Pediatric Gastroenterology and Nutrition in Clinical Practice.* New York: Marcel Dekker, 2002.

Longo, Dan, and Anthony Fauci. *Harrison's Gastroenterology and Hepatology.* New York: McGraw-Hill, 2010.

Maconi, Giovanni, and Gabriele Bianchi Porro. *Ultrasound of the Gastrointestinal Tract.* Berlin: Springer, 2007.

Marsh, Michael N. *Celiac Disease: Methods and Protocols.* Totowa, NJ: Humana Press, 2000.

McPherson, Richard, and Matthew R. Pincus. *Henry's Clinical Diagnosis and Management by Laboratory Methods.* 22nd ed. Philadelphia: Saunders Elsevier, 2011.

Mullin, Gerald E., Laura E. Matarese, and Melissa Palmer. *Gastrointestinal and Liver Disease Nutrition Desk Reference.* Boca Raton, FL: CRC Press, 2012.

Pizzorno, Joseph Jr., and Michael T. Murray. *Textbook of Natural Medicine.* 4th ed. Philadelphia: Saunders Elsevier, 2013.

Prousky, Jonathan. *Principles & Practices of Naturopathic Clinical Nutrition.* Toronto: CCNM Press, 2008.

Rampertab, S. Devi, and Gerard E. Mullin. *Celiac Disease.* Totowa, NJ: Humana Press, 2014.

Ross, Catherine A., Benjamin Caballero, Robert J. Cousins, Katherine L. Tucker, and Thomas R. Ziegler. *Modern Nutrition in Health and Disease.* 11th ed. Philadelphia: Lippincott Williams & Wilkins, 2012.

Segal, Isidor, C. Pitchumoni, and Joseph Sung. *Gastroenterology and Hepatology Manual: A Clinician's Guide to a Global Phenomenon.* New York: McGraw-Hill, 2011.

Shepard, Jules. *The First Year: Celiac Disease and Living Gluten-Free: An Essential Guide for the Newly Diagnosed.* Cambridge, MA: Da Capo Lifelong Books, 2008.

Talley, Nicholas, and Eric G. Tangalos. *Gastroenterology in the Elderly: An Issue of Gastroenterology Clinics.* Philadelphia: Saunders Elsevier, 2009.

Wangen, Stephen. *Healthier without Wheat: A New Understanding of Wheat Allergies, Celiac Disease, and Non-Celiac Gluten Intolerance.* Seattle: Innate Health Publishing, 2009.

Wong, John L. H., Iain Murray, S. Hyder Hussaini, and Harry R. Dalton. *Clinical Handbook of Gastroenterology.* Boca Raton, FL: CRC Press, 2002.

Wyllie, Robert, and Jeffrey S. Hyams. *Pediatric Gastrointestinal and Liver Disease.* 4th ed. Philadelphia: Saunders Elsevier, 2011.

GLOSSARY

Addison's disease. A medical disorder caused by a damaged adrenal
cortex found in the adrenal glands. It is mainly the result of the
insufficiency of the glucocorticoid hormones, mineralocorticoid
hormones, and sex hormones—which are produced by the adrenal
cortex.

agranulocytosis. Lower amount of granulocytes (a type of cell) in the
blood.

antiendomysial antibodies. Refers to testing for specific IgA antibodies characteristic of celiac disease.

aphtous stomatitis. Commonly known as a mouth ulcer or canker
sore, this is a painful break on the mouth's membrane caused by
acidic food, biting, or by hormonal imbalance.

arthritide. A medical condition that causes irregularity of the joints
manifested by inflammation, pain, or dysfunctionality.

auscultation. Medical procedure to check the circulatory and respiratory system of a patient. The doctor listens to the sounds of the
heart, lungs, and intestines. It is usually done using a stethoscope.

autohemolysin. Produced by the immune system, it is an antibody
that attacks or destroys the red blood cells or erythrocytes of an
organism.

autoimmune enteropathy. Usually described by weight loss, bodily
membrane inflammation, excessive fluid loss, and skin rashes, this
is a medical condition in which the digestive system of the body is
attacked by its own immune system.

bicarbonates. These are the intermediate anions of carbonic acid caused by the removal of protons from the carbonic acid molecule.

bifidobacteria. Important for digestion and boosting of the immune system, these bacteria are the major constituents of the bacterial flora inside mammals. They do not need oxygen during biological processes and they exhibit violet stains during the Gram staining procedure.

borborygmi. The plural form of borborygmus, they are commonly associated with the sound heard when someone is hungry. The moving gases inside the stomach cause this rumbling sound.

brush border. The surface of epithelium, which has both cubelike cells and columnar cells covered by hairlike structures.

celiac disease. Disorder that disables the body's process of digesting the protein called gluten.

celiac sprue. Caused by the intolerance of gliadin, this is a medical disorder in which certain nutrients from food will not be absorbed by the body.

cerebral perfusion. Related to the average blood pressure of an individual and inversely to the supply of blood to the brain over a given duration of time, it is described as the blood flow to the brain.

chronic ischemia. Condition that has a long-term effect in cellular metabolism caused by the shortage of glucose and oxygen. This happens when the blood supply to the blood vessels is impeded.

cold hemoglobinuria. Kind of autoimmune anemia caused by the attack of antibodies to the red blood cells when the temperature changes from cold to warm, or vice versa.

collagenous sprue. Observed as a mucosal abnormality on the intestinal tissue resulting in the nonabsorption of nutrients and vitamins.

Crohn's disease. Disease caused by environmental and bacterial factors. It affects the intestinal tract, and is characterized by irregularity of bowel movements and pain in the abdominal tract and vomiting.

crypts of Lieberkuhn. Gland that secretes enzymes such as sucrase and lactase. It is located in the small intestine and colon, specifically embedded in the epithelial lining of the digestive organs.

cytoplasmic vacuole. A cavity in the cell that contains nutrients and waste products.

deamidated gliadin peptide (DGP). Important synthesized gliadin peptide used in medical tests to diagnose celiac disease. It has high specificity and sensitivity.

demulcent herb. Herb used to relieve pain and inflammation of a bodily mucous membrane.

double-blind experiment. A procedure in conducting experiments in which the facilitator and the subject have no idea of the experiment's critical background or aim. This is done to avoid biases, especially for the implications of the placebo effect.

elastase. Enzyme that helps in determining the strength of connective tissue by breaking down the elastic fiber called *elastin*.

endomysial antibodies. Antibodies originating within the muscles.

enterocytes. Cells that are found in the intestinal track, colon, and appendix. They are "simple columnar" in structure and are classified as epithelial cells.

enteropathy associated T-cell lymphoma. Type of blood cancer attacking the T-cells in the small intestine.

eosinophilic gastroenteritis. Treatable disease in the stomach and intestine caused by the increase of parasite-combatting white blood cells.

extraintestinal. Region or environment outside the intestine.

farinaceous food. Food group that is a good source of starch, usually characterized by a powdery appearance or texture.

gastric antrum. Part of the stomach that is a closed cavity lined by mucous membrane. It is the portion between the stomach and duodenum.

gastrointestinal tract. Region of the digestive system that extends from the stomach to the intestines. It is sometimes called the alimentary canal and is commonly known as the gut.

giardiasis. Diarrhea-causing parasitic disease caused by a parasitic protozoan, *G. lamblia.*

gliadin. A class of protein that is involved in bread making/baking, specifically in the proofing or the rising of the dough bread. Commonly found in wheat seeds.

graft versus host disease (GVHD). Disease caused by complications after a bone marrow or stem cell transplant in which the cells of the patient are attacked by the foreign transplanted cells.

gram-negative. Red-colored stain observed after the application of Gram staining.

gram-positive. Observed as a violet stain during the bacterial identification method of Gram staining.

histocompatibility leukocyte antigen. Immune system's antigen that can differentiate foreign cells from the recipient's cells, which is important in the transplant of stem cells.

hyperperfusion. Pumping of blood to an organ is excessively increased.

hypoalbuminemia. Disorder characterized by low levels of albumin (a protein) in the blood.

hypoperfusion. Pumping of blood to an organ is critically lowered.

immunoreactive epitopes. Biologically active part of an antigen (foreign particle) recognized by the immune system.

infiltrative duodenosis. Inflammation or disease of the duodenum that may spread to other organs.

intestinal adenocarcinomas. Cancer originating from the epithelial tissue of the intestine, usually from the glandular tissue. It is commonly diagnosed as a malignant cancer.

intraepithelial lymphocyte infiltration. Permeation or spread of white blood cells throughout a region of epithelial tissue or a surface of an organ.

intraoperative hypovolemia. Condition encountered during surgery in which the circulation of blood is critically deferred, resulting in a reduced amount of blood plasma.

lactobacillus acidophilus. Probiotic that converts sugars to lactic acid. This species of bacteria is found in the mouth and generally in the gastrointestinal tract.

lamina propria. Constitutes the mucous membrane with the epithelium. It is usually characterized as loose connective tissue and contains capillaries.

lichtleiter. Basic form of a medical device used to check or to examine the inside of an organ that has a space or that is hollow. Organs examined are anus, ears, mouth, nose, and abdomen.

Marsh classification. Anatomical study of the degree of severity of a celiac disease case through the examination of the duodenum. Blunting of villi is usually observed.

mean corpuscular hemoglobin concentration (MCHC). The abundance of hemoglobin per volume of erythrocytes or red blood cells.

mean corpuscular volume (MCV). Size of red blood cells computed from hematocrit and number of erythrocytes.

megaloblastic anemia. Decrease in amount of red blood cells due to the impairment of DNA synthesis or to the deferral of cell growth during the production of red blood cells.

mesenteric lymph node cavitation syndrome. A combination of symptoms leading to the death of cells in the lymph nodes located at the layers of mesentery. Usually caused by the inability to digest a nongluten diet and can come with coeliac diseases.

natural killer cells. White blood cells that attack cells that are either virally affected or tumor forming.

nil per os (NPO). Medical protocol in which the patient is not allowed to take in food or liquid through the mouth.

organismal. Standards specified as the level of or relating to each of the individual living things or organisms.

packed cell volume (PCV). Amount of red blood cells in contrast to the total amount of blood.

paralytic ileus. Impairment of the ability of the gastrointestinal tract to produce movements.

pathogenesis. Process of production or progression of a disease.

peptic. Describes body parts that have an acidic inside structure of an artery, intestine, or a cellular component.

polymeric binder molecules. Uniform layer of polymeric molecules that holds protein or any biological substance together.

primary biliary cirrhosis. Autoimmune disease that slowly degrades and destroys the tubelike structures, called the bile ducts, of the liver.

primary sclerosing cholangitis. The irritation and swelling of the bile ducts that cause the impediment of these tubular structures due to the immune system's reaction.

puerperium. Stage experienced by a woman right after giving birth extending to the first two months until the return of the uterus to normal size.

refractory celiac disease. Disease resulting from the failure of the small intestine to recover and heal because of the degradation of villi.

refractory sprue. Described as an autoimmune disorder that is resilient or indifferent to treatment under a no-gluten diet.

Sjögren's syndrome. Autoimmune disease in which the glands secreting saliva and tears are destroyed by white blood cells.

tissue transglutaminase. Enzyme responsible in indirectly determining and diagnosing celiac diseases. It only acts with the presence of calcium.

transglutaminase. Enzyme that aids in the formation reaction of the covalent bond in the side chain of a protein-bound glutamine.

villi. Nutriment-absorbing hairlike structure on the mucous membrane of the small intestine.

Zollinger-Ellison syndrome. Medical condition that causes a breach in the mucous membrane due to the excessive production of gastric acid from the pancreas.

NOTES

PREFACE

1. R. Presutti, J. Cangemi, H. Cassidy, and D. Hill, "Celiac Disease," *American Family Physician* 76, no. 12 (2007): 1795–1802; "Coeliac Disease," National Health Service, accessed December 17, 2013, http://www.nhs.uk.
2. "Coeliac Disease," National Health Service.
3. "Coeliac Disease," National Health Service.
4. "Coeliac Disease," National Health Service.
5. "Coeliac Disease," National Health Service.
6. D. Schuppan and K. Zimmer, "The Diagnosis and Treatment of Celiac Disease," *Deutsches Arzteblatt International* 110, no. 49 (2013): 835–46.

I. HISTORY OF CELIAC DISEASE

1. G. Capaccio, *Digestive Disorders* (Salt Lake City: Benchmark Books, 2010).
2. J. Nunn, *Ancient Egyptian Medicine* (London: British Museum Press, 1996).
3. M. Gilger, MA, "Gastroenterologic Endoscopy in Children: Past, Present and Future," *Current Opinion in Pediatrics* 13, no. 5 (2001): 429–34.
4. P. Rathert, W. Lutzeyer, and W. Goddwin, "Philipp Bozzini (1773–1809) and the Lichtleiter," *Urology* 3, no. 1 (1974): 113–18.
5. Rathert, Lutzeyer, and Goddwin, "Philipp Bozzini (1773–1809) and the Lichtleiter."

6. S. Scheinin and P. Wells, "Esophageal Perforation in a Sword Swallower," *Texas Heart Institute Journal* 28, no. 1 (2001): 65–68.

7. W. Wolff and H. Shinya, "Colonofiberoscopy," *Journal of the American Medical Association* 217, no. 11 (1971): 1509–12.

8. J. Jennette and R. Falk, "The Rise and Fall of Horror Autotoxicus and Forbidden Clones," *Kidney International* 78, no. 6 (2010): 533–35.

9. I. Mackay, "Travels and Travails of Autoimmunity: A Historical Journey from Discovery to Rediscovery," *Autoimmunity Reviews* 9, no. 5 (2010): A251–58.

10. U. Bertram and P. Halberg, "Organ Antibodies in Sjögren's Syndrome," *Acta Allergolica* 20, no. 6 (1965): 472–83.

11. A. Sundermann and U. Mey, "Animal Experimental Studies of the Formation of Anti-Erythrocyte Autoantibodies," *Folia Haemotologica* 84, no. 4 (1965): 387–401.

12. A. Puxeddu, A. Colonna, G. Nenci, and E. Del Piano, "On a Rare Case of Hemolytic Anemia Autoimmune Caused by Influenza B Virus [Article in Italian]," *Haematologica* 50, no. 12 (1965): 1073–92.

13. J. Michalski, T. Daniels, N. Talal, and H. Grey, "Beta2 Mocroglobulin and Lymphocytic Infiltration in Sjögren's Syndrome," *New England Journal of Medicine* 293, no. 24 (1975): 1228–31.

14. P. Bastenie, "Autoimmunity and Aging," *Bulletin et Memoires de l'Academie Royale de Medicine de Belgique* 20, no. 130 (1975): 517–26; E. Wachsmuth and U. Born, "Alpha-Haemolytic Streptococcus Causing Lethal Autoallergic Heart Disease," *British Medical Journal* 3, no. 5827 (1972): 623.

15. S. Guandalini, "A Brief History of Celiac Disease," University of Chicago Celiac Disease Center, *Impact* 7, no. 3 (2007): 1–3.

16. B. Dowd and J. Walker-Smith, "Samuel Gee, Aretaeus, and the Coeliac Affection," *British Medical Journal* 2, no. 5905 (1974): 45–47.

17. Dowd and Walker-Smith, "Samuel Gee, Aretaeus, and the Coeliac Affection."

18. A. McNeish, H. Harms, J. Rey, D. Shmerling, J. Visakorpi, and J. Walker-Smith, "The Diagnosis of Coeliac Disease. A Commentary on the Current Practices of Members of the European Society for Paediatric Gastroenterology and Nutrition (ESPGAN)," *Archives of Disease in Childhood* 54, no. 10 (1979): 783–86.

19. D. Schuppan, "Current Concepts of Celiac Disease Pathogenesis," *Gastroenterology* 119, no. 1 (2000): 234–42.

20. Guandalini, "A Brief History of Celiac Disease."

21. A. Fasano, "Zonulin and Its Regulation of Intestinal Barrier Function: The Biological Door to Inflammation, Autoimmunity, and Cancer," *Physiological Reviews* 91 no. 1 (2011): 151–75.

22. Cathryn Delude, "Celiac Disease Timeline: A Glutinous History," Proto Massachusetts General Hospital, Winter 2010, accessed February 24, 2014, http://protomag.com/assets/celiac-disease-timeline-a-glutinous-history.

23. M. Losowsky, "A History of Coeliac Disease," *Digestive Diseases* 26, no. 2 (2008): 112–20; F. Adams, *On the Coeliac Affection: The Extant Works of Aretaeus, The Cappadocian* (London: Sydenham Society, 1856), 350–51.

24. Adams, *On the Coeliac Affection*; Losowsky, "A History of Coeliac Disease."

25. Guandalini, "A Brief History of Celiac Disease."

26. "Celebrities with Celiac Disease; See Who Is on the List and Discuss How They Promote Awareness!" accessed April 1, 2014, http://www.gluten-free-for-life.com/celebrities-with-celiac.html.

27. Glutenista.com, "Gluten-Free Celebrity List," accessed April 1, 2014, http://www.glutenista.com/gluten-free-celebrity-list.html.

28. "Celebrities with Celiac Disease."

29. "Celebrities with Celiac Disease."

30. J. Adams, "Mom Helps Novak Djokovic Stick to Gluten-Free Diet," Celiac.com, April 25, 3013, accessed April 1, 2014, http://www.celiac.com/articles/23252/1/Mom-Helps-Novak-Djokovic-Stick-to-Gluten-free-Diet/Page1.html.

31. "Celebrities Suffer from Gluten Allergies—You're Not Alone!" Probiotics.org, accessed April 1, 2014, http://probiotics.org/gluten-celebs/.

32. "Celebrities Suffer from Gluten Allergies—You're Not Alone!"

33. Samantha Wallad, "Top Ten Gluten-Free Celebrities," TheCelebrityCafe.com, April 27, 2011, accessed April 1, 2014, http://thecelebritycafe.com/feature/top-ten-gluten-free-celebrities-04-27-2011.

34. HealthResearchFunding.org, "Famous People with Celiac Disease," December 17, 2013, accessed April 1, 2014, http://healthresearchfunding.org/famous-people-celiac-disease.

35. "Gluten-Free . . . for Medical Reasons," CeliacCentral.org, August 20, 2010, accessed April 1, 2014, http://www.celiaccentral.org/News/NFCA-Blogs/Did-You-Hear/Did-You-Hear-Gluten-Free-in-the-Mainstream/389/month--201008/search--celebrities/vobid--3583/.

36. "Celebrities with Celiac Disease."

2. ANATOMY AND PHYSIOLOGY OF CELIAC DISEASE

1. H. J. Freeman, A. Chopra, M. T. Clandinin, and A. B. Thomson, "Recent Advances in Celiac Disease," *World Journal of Gastroenterology* 17, no. 18 (2011): 2259–72; P. Green, "The Many Faces of Celiac Disease: Clinical Presen-

tation of Celiac Disease in the Adult Population," *Gastroenterology* 128, no. 4 (2005): S74–S78; D. Schuppan, M. Dennis, and C. P. Kelly, "Celiac Disease: Epidemiology, Pathogenesis, Diagnosis, and Nutritional Management," *Nutrition in Clinical Care* 8, no. 2 (2005): 54–69.

2. C. Cellier, C. Flobert, C. Cormier, C. Roux, and J. Schmitz, "Severe Osteopenia in Symptom-Free Adults with a Childhood Diagnosis of Coeliac Disease," *Lancet* 355, no. 9206 (2000): 806; H. Vasquez, R. Mazure, D. Gonzalez, D. Flores, S. Pedreira, S. Niveloni, E. Smecuol, E. Mauriño, and J. Bai, "Risk of Fractures in Celiac Disease Patients: A Cross-Sectional, Case-Control Study," *American Journal of Gastroenterology* 95, no. 1 (2000): 183–89; R. Ransford, M. Hayes, M. Palmer, and M. Hall, "A Controlled, Prospective Screening Study of Celiac Disease Presenting as Iron Deficiency Anemia," *Journal of Clinical Gastroenterology* 35, no. 3 (2002): 228–33; D. Leffler, S. Saha, and R. J. Farrell, "Celiac Disease," *AJMC: American Journal of Managed Care* 9, no. 12 (2003): 825–31.

3. "The Digestive System," Boundless.com, accessed October 20, 2013, http://www.boundless.com/physiology/the-digestive-system.

4. H. Gray, "The Pharynx–Splanchnology," in *Anatomy of the Human Body*, 20th ed. (Philadelphia: Lea & Febiger, 1918).

5. T. Taylor, "Stomach," InnerBody.com, accessed October 21, 2013, http://www.innerbody.com/image_digeov/dige11-new.html.

6. T. Taylor, "Duodenum," InnerBody.com, accessed October 21, 2013, http://www.innerbody.com/image_digeov/dige11-new.html.

7. Gray, "The Small Intestine–Splanchnology."

8. M. Ventura, S. O'Flaherty, M. Claesson, F. Turroni, T. Klaenhammer, D. van Sinderen, and P. W. O'Toole, " Genome-Scale Analyses of Health-Promoting Bacteria: Probiogenomics," *Nature Reviews Microbiology* 7, no. 1 (2009): 61–67; F. Backhed, R. Ley, J. L. Sonnenburg, D. Peterson, and J. I. Gordon, "Host-Bacterial 415 Mutualism in the Human Intestine," *Science* 307, no. 5717 (2005): 1915–20.

9. M. Molyneaux, "Digestive Health and Immunity," FoodProductDesign.com, April 15, 2011, accessed October 20, 2013, www.foodproductdesign.com/articles/2011/03/digestive-health-and-immunity.aspx.

10. G. R. Gibson, "From Probiotics to Prebiotics and a Healthy Digestive System," *Journal of Food Science* 69, no. 5 (2006): M141–M143.

11. S. Rabot, J. Rafter, G. Rijkers, B. Watzl, and J. Antoine, "Guidance for Substantiating the Evidence for Beneficial Effects of Probiotics: Impact of Probiotics on Digestive System Metabolism," *Journal of Nutrition* 140, no. 3 (2010): 677S–689S.

12. Ventura et al., " Genome-Scale Analyses of Health-Promoting Bacteria: Probiogenomics."

13. R. E. Ley, D. A. Peterson, and J. I. Gordon, "Ecological and Evolutionary Forces Shaping Microbial Diversity in the Human Intestine," *Cell* 124, no. 4 (2006): 837–48.

14. E. S. Wintergerst, S. Maggini, and D. H. Hornig, "Contribution of Selected Vitamins and Trace Elements to Immune Function," *Annals of Nutrition and Metabolism* 51, no. 4 (2007): 301–23.

15. J. Holmgren and C. Czerkinsky, "Mucosal Immunity and Vaccines," *Nature Medicine* 11, no. 4 (2005): 545–53.

16. L. Mayer, "Mucosal Immunity," *Pediatrics* 111, no. 3 (2003): 1595–1600.

17. F. Lucas, "Promoting a Healthy Digestive Tract: Healthy Digestion Is the Highway to Health . . . Bad Digestion Can Be the Road to Ruin," Nupro.net, accessed October 20, 2013, http://nupro.net/promoting-a-healthy-digestive-tract.

18. E. Lipski, *Digestive Wellness: Strengthen the Immune System and Prevent Disease Through Healthy Digestion*, 4th ed. (New York: McGraw-Hill, 2012).

19. J. L. Groff, S. Gropper, and J. L. Smith, *Advanced Nutrition and Human Metabolism* (New York: West Publishing Company, 1995).

20. E. N. Marieb, *Human Anatomy & Physiology*, 6th ed. (San Francisco: Pearson, 2004).

21. T. W. Nichols and N. Faass, *Optimal Digestive Health: A Complete Guide* (Rochester, VT: Inner Traditions/Bear, 2011).

22. S. Govind, A. Lapenna, P. O. Lang, and R. Aspinall, "Immunotherapy of Immunosenesence; Who, How and When?" *Open Longevity Science* 6 (2012): 56–63.

23. "Chapter 48: The Digestive System," in *Biology*, 8th ed., edited by P. Raven, G. Johnson, K. A. Mason, L. Losos, and S. Singer (Columbus, OH: McGraw-Hill, 2008): 963–82.

24. E. T. Champagne, "Low Gastric Hydrochloric Acid Secretion and Mineral Bioavailability," *Advances in Experimental Medicine and Biology* 249 (1989): 173–84.

25. Champagne, "Low Gastric Hydrochloric Acid Secretion and Mineral Bioavailability."

26. Lucas, "Promoting a Healthy Digestive Tract."

27. Ventura et al., " Genome-Scale Analyses of Health-Promoting Bacteria: Probiogenomics."

28. E. Hilton, H. Isenberg, P. Alperstein, K. France, and M Borenstein, "Ingestion of Yogurt Containing Lactobacillus Acidophilus as Prophylaxis for Candidal Vaginitis," *Annals of Internal Medicine* 116, no. 5 (1992): 353–57; M. E. Falagas, G. I. Betsi, and S. Athansiou, "Probiotics for Prevention of Recurrent Vulvovaginal Candidiasis: A Review," *Journal of Antimicrobial Chemotherapy* 58, no. 2 (2006): 266–72; M. Clements, M. Levine, R. Black, R. Robins-Browne, L. A. Cisneros, G. L. Drusano, C. F. Lanata, and A. J. Saah, "Lactobacillus

Prophylaxis for Diarrhea Due to Enterotoxigenic *Escherichia coli*," *Antimicrobial Agents and Chemotherapy* 20, no. 1 (1891): 104–8; I. Sakamoto, M. Igarashi, K. Kimura, A. Takagi, T. Miwa, and Y. Koga, "Suppressive Effect of Lactobacillus Gasseri OLL 2716 (LG21) on Helicobacter Pylori Infection in Humans," *Journal of Antimicrobial Chemotherapy* 47, no. 5 (2002): 709–10; P. Michetti, G. Dorta, P. Wiesel, D. Brassart, E. Verdu, M. Herranz, C. Felley, N. Porta, M. Rouvet, A. Blum, and I. Corthesy-Theulaz, "Effect of Whey-Based Culture Supernatant of Lactobacillus Acidophilus (Johnsonii) La1 on *Helicobacter pylori* Infection in Humans," *Digestion* 60, no. 3 (1999): 203–9; A. Ravael, Z. Heshmati, T. Salehl, I. Tamal, M. Ghane, and J. Derakhshan, "Evaluation of Antimicrobial Activity of Three Lactobacillus spp. Against Antibiotic Resistance *Salmonella typhimurium*," *Advanced Studies in Biology* 5, no. 2 (2013): 61–70.

29. L. O'Mahony, J. McCarthy, P. Kelly, G. Hurley, F. Luo, K. Chen, G. O'Sullivan, B. Kiely, and E. M. Quigley, "Lactobacillus and Bifidobacterium in Irritable Bowel Syndrome: Symptom Responses and Relationship to Cytokine Profiles," *Gastroenterology* 128, no. 3 (2005): 541–51.

30. Lipski, *Digestive Wellness*.

31. Gibson, "From Probiotics to Prebiotics and a Healthy Digestive System."

32. D. Brambilla, C. Mancuso, M. Scuderi, P. Bosco, G. Cantarella, L. Lempereur, G. Benedetto, S. Pezzino, and R. Bernardini, "The Role of Antioxidant Supplement in Immune System, Neoplastic, and Neurodegenerative Disorders: A Point of View for an Assessment of the Risk/Benefit Profile," *Nutrition Journal* 7 (2008) 7: 1–9.

33. S. Zelenay, M. Moraes Fontes, C. Fesel, J. Demengeot, and A. Coutinho, "Physiopathology of Natural Auto-Antibodies: The Case for Regulation," *Journal of Autoimmunity* 29, no. 4 (2007): 229–35; Brambilla et al., "The Role of Antioxidant Supplement in Immune System, Neoplastic, and Neurodegenerative Disorders."

34. J. Barker and E. Liu, "Celiac Disease: Pathophysiology, Clinical Manifestations and Associated Autoimmune Conditions," *Advances in Pediatrics* 55 (2008): 349–65.

35. K. Erb, "Helminths, Allergic Disorders and IgE-Mediated Immune Responses: Where Do We Stand?" *European Journal of Immunology* 37, no. 5 (2007): 1170–73; H. Gould, B. Sutton, A. Beavil, R. Beavil, N. McCloskey, H. Coker, D. Fear, and L. Smurthwaite, "The Biology of IGE and the Basis of Allergic Disease," *Annual Review of Immunology* 21 (2003): 579–628.

36. Y. van de Wal, Y. Kooy, P. van Veelen, W. Vader, F. Koning, and S. Pena, "Coeliac Disease: It Takes Three to Tango!" *Gut* 46, no. 5 (2000): 734–37.

37. M. Marsh, "The Natural History of Gluten Sensitivity: Defining, Refining and Re-Defining," *QJM: An International Journal of Medicine* 88, no. 1 (1995): 9–13.

38. Schuppan, Dennis, and Kelly, "Celiac Disease: Epidemiology, Pathogenesis, Diagnosis, and Nutritional Management."

39. NIH Consensus Development Conference on Celiac Disease, *NIH Consensus and State-of-the-Science Statements* 21, no. 1 (2004): 1–16.

3. CAUSES OF CELIAC DISEASE

1. M. Dennis and D. Leffler, *Real Life with Celiac Disease: Troubleshooting and Thriving Gluten Free* (Bethesda, MD: American Gastroenterological Association [AGA] Press, 2010).

2. A. Scaramuzza, C. Mantegazza, A. Bosetti, and G. Zuccotti, "Type 1 Diabetes and Celiac Disease: The Effects of Gluten-Free Diet on Metabolic Control," *World Journal of Diabetes* 4, no. 4 (2013): 130–34.

3. J. Shepard, *The First Year: Celiac Disease and Living Gluten-Free: An Essential Guide for the Newly Diagnosed* (Cambridge, MA: Da Capo Press, 2008).

4. E. Hasselbeck, *The G-Free Diet: A Gluten-Free Survival Guide* (New York: Center Street, 2009).

5. "Celiac Disease," Canadian Diabetes Association, accessed October 20, 2013, http://www.diabetes.ca/diabetes-and-you/complications/celiac-disease.

6. H. Cornell, "Coeliac Disease: A Review of the Causative Agents and Their Possible Mechanisms of Action," *Amino Acids* 10, no. 1 (1996): 1–19.

7. "Coeliac Disease: Causes," May 2, 2012, accessed October 20, 2013, http://www.nhs.uk.

8. "Celiac Disease," Mayo Clinic, accessed October 20, 2013, http://www.mayoclinic.org.

9. Shepard, *The First Year.*

10. Dennis and Leffler, *Real Life with Celiac Disease.*

11. Dennis and Leffler, *Real Life with Celiac Disease.*

12. R. Gibbons, "Everyday Tips for Living with Celiac Disease," Yahoo! Health, May 8, 2013, accessed December 13, 2013, www.http://health.yahoo.net.

13. Shepard, *The First Year.*

14. "Celiac Disease," National Library of Medicine, accessed January 3, 2014, http://www.nlm.nih.gov.

15. S. Plogsted, "Medications and Celiac Disease-Tips from a Pharmacist," *Practical Gastroenterology* 5 (2007): 58–64.

16. S. Adams, "Celiac Disease Common in Patients with Lactose Intolerance," Celiac.com, March 30, 2005, accessed October 23, 2013, http://www.celiac.com/articles/891/1/Celiac-Disease-Common-in-Patients-with-Lactose-Intolerance/Page1.html.

17. Adams, "Celiac Disease Common in Patients with Lactose Intolerance."

18. Adams, "Celiac Disease Common in Patients with Lactose Intolerance."

19. D. Mann, "New Treatment for Celiac Disease?" WebMD Health News, http://www.webmd.com/digestive-disorders/celiac-disease/news/20110208/new-treatment-for-celiac-disease.

20. Hasselbeck, *The G-Free Diet*.

21. A. Fasano, M. Araya, S. Bhatnagar, D. Cameron, C. Catassi, M. Dirks, M. Mearin, L. Ottigosa, and A. Phillips, "Federation of International Societies of Pediatric Gastroenterology, Hepatology, and Nutrition Consensus Report on Celiac Disease," *Journal of Pediatric Gastroenterology and Nutrition* 47, no. 2 (2008): 214–19.

22. J. Feinmann, *Living with Gluten Intolerance* (London: Sheldon Press, 2009).

23. Hasselbeck, *The G-Free Diet*.

24. Hasselbeck, *The G-Free Diet*.

25. Hasselbeck, *The G-Free Diet*.

26. Hasselbeck, *The G-Free Diet*.

27. Dennis and Leffler, *Real Life with Celiac Disease*.

28. Dennis and Leffler, *Real Life with Celiac Disease*.

29. Cornell, "Coeliac Disease."

30. Dennis and Leffler, *Real Life with Celiac Disease*.

31. L. Sollid and E. Thorsby, "HLA Susceptibility Genes in Celiac Disease: Genetic Mapping and Role in Pathogenesis," *Gastroenterology* 105, no. 3 (1993): 910–22.

32. N. Bizzaro, D. Villalta, E. Tonutti, A. Doria, M. Tampoia, D. Bassetti, R. Tozzoli, "IgA and IgG Tissue Transglutaminase Antibody Prevalence and Clinical Significance in Connective Tissue Diseases, Inflammatory Bowel Disease, and Primary Biliary Cirrhosis," *Digestive Diseases and Sciences* 48, no. 12 (2003): 2360–65; M. Clemente, M. Musu, F. Frau, C. Lucia, and S. De Virgiliis, "Antitissue Transglutaminase Antibodies Outside Celiac Disease," *Journal of Pediatric Gastroenterology and Nutrition* 34, no. 1 (2002): 31–34.

33. Dennis and Leffler, *Real Life with Celiac Disease*.

34. Shepard, *The First Year*.

35. L. Sollid, "Coeliac Disease: Dissecting a Complex Inflammatory Disorder," *Nature Reviews Immunology* 2, no. 9 (2002): 647–55.

36. F. Hausch, L. Shan, N. Santiago, G. Gray, and C. Khosla, "Intestinal Digestive Resistance of Immunodominant Gliadin Peptides," *American Journal of Physiology: Gastrointestinal and Liver Physiology* 283, no. 4 (2002): G996–1003.

37. F. Koning, D. Schuppan, N. Cerf-Bensussan, and L. Sollid, "Pathome-chanisms in Celiac Disease," *Best Practice & Research Clinical Gastroenterology* 19, no. 3 (2005): 373–87.

38. F. Leon, E. Roldan, L. Sanchez, C. Camarero, A. Bootello, and G. Roy, "Human Small-Intestinal Epithelium Contains Functional Natural Killer Lymphocytes," *Gastroenterology* 125, no. 2 (2003): 345–56.

39. F. Leon et al., "Human Small-Intestinal Epithelium Contains Functional Natural Killer Lymphocytes."

40. M. Zarkadas, A. Cranney, M. Molloy, et al., "The Impact of a Gluten-Free Diet on Adults with Celiac Disease: Results of a National Survey," *Journal of Human Nutrition and Dietetics* 19, no. 1 (2006): 41–49.

41. D. Schuppan, M. Dennis, and C. P. Kelly, "Celiac Disease: Epidemiology, Pathogenesis, Diagnosis, and Nutritional Management," *Nutrition in Clinical Care* 8, no. 2 (2005): 54–69.

42. P. Green and B. Jabri, "Coeliac Disease," *Lancet* 362, no. 9381 (2003): 383.

43. P. Green and R. Jones, *Celiac Disease: A Hidden Epidemic* (New York: HarperCollins, 2006).

44. J. Mention, M. Ben-Ahmed, B. Begue, U. Barbe, V. Verkarre, V. Asnafi, J. Colombel, P. Cugnenc, F. Ruemmele, E. McIntyre, N. Brousse, C. Cellier, and N. Cerf-Bensussan, "Interleukin 15: A Key to Disrupted Intraepithelial Lymphocyte Homeostasis and Lymphomagenesis in Celiac Disease," *Gastroenterology* 125, no. 3 (2003): 730–45; L. Maiuri, C. Ciacci, S. Auricchio, V. Brown, S. Quaratino, and M. Londei, "Interleukin 15 Mediates Epithelial Changes in Celiac Disease," *Gastroenterology* 119, no. 4 (2000): 996–1006.

45. D. Schuppan and W. Dieterich, "Pathogenesis, Epidemiology, and Clinical Manifestations of Celiac Disease in Adults," accessed December 12, 2013, http://www.uptodate.com/contents/pathogenesis-epidemiology-and-clinical-manifestations-of-celiac-disease-in-adults.

46. Hasselbeck, *The G-Free Diet*; Shepard, *The First Year*.

47. Shepard, *The First Year*.

48. J. Murray, "The Widening Spectrum of Celiac Disease," *American Journal of Clinical Nutrition* 69, no. 3 (1999): 354–65.

49. E. Decker, G. Engelmann, A. Findeisen, P. Gerner, M. Laass, D. Ney, C. Posovszky, L. Hoy, and M. Hornef, "Cesarean Delivery Is Associated with Celiac Disease but Not Inflammatory Bowel Disease in Children," *Pediatrics* 125, no. 6 (2010): e1433–40.

50. E. Decker, M. Hornef, and S. Stockinger, "Cesarean Delivery Is Associated with Celiac Disease but Not Inflammatory Bowel Disease in Children," *Gut Microbes* 2, no. 2 (2011): 91–98.

51. Shepard, *The First Year*.

52. J. Bach, "Infections and Autoimmune Diseases," *Journal of Autoimmunity* 25 (2005): 74–80.

4. PATHOLOGY OF CELIAC DISEASE

1. B. Dickson, C. Streutker, and R. Chetty, "Coeliac Disease: An Update for Pathologists," *Journal of Clinical Pathology* 59, no. 10 (2006): 1008–16.

2. D. Antonioli, "Celiac Disease: A Progress Report," *Modern Pathology* 16, no. 4 (2003): 342–46.

3. Dickson, Streutker, and Chetty, "Coeliac Disease: An Update for Pathologists."

4. Antonioli, "Celiac Disease: A Progress Report."

5. Antonioli, "Celiac Disease: A Progress Report."

6. P. Green and B. Jabri, "Celiac Disease," *Annual Review of Medicine* 57 (2006): 207–21; D. Dewar, S. Pereira, and P. Ciclitira, "The Pathogenesis of Coeliac Disease," *International Journal of Biochemistry & Cell Biology* 36, no. 1 (2004): 17–24.

7. C. Hardman, J. Garioch, J. Leonard, et al., "Absence of Toxicity of Oats in Patients with Dermatitis Herpetiformis," *New England Journal of Medicine* 337, no. 26 (1997): 1884–87.

8. H. Arentz-Hansen, B. Fleckenstein, O. Molberg, et al., "The Molecular Basis for Oat Intolerance in Patients with Celiac Disease," *Public Library of Science (PLOS)* 1, no. 1 (2004): e1.

9. Dickson, Streutker, and Chetty, "Coeliac Disease: An Update for Pathologists."

10. R. Farrell and C. Kelly, "Celiac Sprue," *New England Journal of Medicine* 346, no. 3 (2002): 180–88.

11. P. Green and C. Cellier, "Celiac Disease," *New England Journal of Medicine* 357, no. 17 (2007): 1731–43.

12. Green and Cellier, "Celiac Disease."

13. E. Hoffenberg, L. Emery, K. Barriga, et al., "Clinical Features of Children with Screening-Identified Evidence of Celiac Disease," *Pediatrics* 113, no. 5 (2004): 1254–59.

14. P. Bucci, F. Carile, A. Sangianantoni, F. D'Angiò, A. Santarelli, and L. Lo Muzio, "Oral Aphthous Ulcers and Dental Enamel Defects in Children with Coeliac Disease," *Acta Paediatrica* 95, no. 2 (2006): 203–7.

15. A. Rubio-Tapia and J. Murray, "The Liver in Celiac Disease," *Hepatology* 46, no. 5 (2007): 1650–58.

16. A. Fasano, "Clinical Presentation of Celiac Disease in the Pediatric Population," *Gastroenterology* 128, no. 4 (2005): S68–S73; A. Fasano, I. Berti,

T. Gerarduzzi, T. Not, R. Colletti, S. Drago, Y. Elitsur, P. Green, S. Guandalini, I. Hill, M. Pietzak, A. Ventura, M. Thorpe, D. Kryszak, F. Fornaroli, S. Wasserman, J. Murray, and K. Horvath, "Prevalence of Celiac Disease in At-Risk and Not-at-Risk Groups in the United States: A Large Multicenter Study," *Archives of Internal Medicine* 163, no. 3 (2003): 286–92; Farrell and Kelly, "Celiac Sprue"; Green and Cellier, "Celiac Disease."

17. J. Barker and E. Liu, "Celiac Disease: Pathophysiology, Clinical Manifestations and Associated Autoimmune Conditions," *Advances in Pediatrics* 55 (2008): 349–65.

18. Fasano, "Clinical Presentation of Celiac Disease in the Pediatric Population"; NIH Consensus Development Conference on Celiac Disease, *NIH Consensus and State-of-the-Science Statements* 21, no. 1 (2004): 1–23; Farrell and Kelly, "Celiac Sprue"; Green and Cellier, "Celiac Disease."

19. C. Catassi and E. Fabiani, "The Spectrum of Celiac Disease in Children," *Baillière's Clinical Gastroenterology* 11, no. 3 (1997): 485–507.

20. K. Fine, "The Prevalence of Occult Gastrointestinal Bleeding in Celiac Sprue," *New England Journal of Medicine* 334, no. 18 (1996): 1163–67.

21. A. Rubio-Tapia, I. Hill, C. Kelly, A. Calderwood, and J. Murray, "ACG Clinical Guidelines: Diagnosis and Management of Celiac Disease," *American Journal of Gastroenterology* 108, no. 5 (2013): 656–76.

22. Rubio-Tapia, Hill, Kelly, Calderwood, and Murray, "ACG Clinical Guidelines."

23. Rubio-Tapia, Hill, Kelly, Calderwood, and Murray, "ACG Clinical Guidelines."

24. J. Bai, M. Fried, G. Corazza, D. Schuppan, M. Farthing, C. Catassi, L. Greco, H. Cohen, C. Ciacci, R. Eliakim, A. Fasano, A. González, J. Krabshuis, and A. LeMair, "World Gastroenterology Organisation Global Guidelines on Celiac Disease," *Journal of Clinical Gastroenterology* 47, no. 2 (2013): 121–26.

25. Rubio-Tapia, Hill, Kelly, Calderwood, and Murray, "ACG Clinical Guidelines."

26. Bai, Fried, et al., "World Gastroenterology Organisation Global Guidelines on Celiac Disease."

27. Bai, Fried, et al., "World Gastroenterology Organisation Global Guidelines on Celiac Disease."

28. J. Barker and E. Liu, "Celiac Disease: Pathophysiology, Clinical Manifestations and Associated Autoimmune Conditions," *Advances in Pediatrics* 55 (2008): 349–65.

29. Barker and Liu, "Celiac Disease: Pathophysiology, Clinical Manifestations and Associated Autoimmune Conditions."

30. Dickson, Streutker, and Chetty, "Coeliac Disease."

31. Dickson, Streutker, and Chetty, "Coeliac Disease."

32. N. Goldstein, "Proximal Small-Bowel Mucosal Villous Intraepithelial Lymphocytes," *Histopathology* 44, no. 3 (2004): 199–205.

33. A. Ravelli, S. Bolognini, M. Gambarotti, and V. Villanacci, "Variability of Histologic Lesions in Relation to Biopsy Site in Gluten-Sensitive Enteropathy," *American Journal of Gastroenterology* 100, no. 1 (2005): 177–85.

34. Dickson, Streutker, and Chetty, "Coeliac Disease."

35. D. Darlington and A. Rogers, "Epithelial Lymphocytes in the Small Intestine of the Mouse," *Journal of Anatomy* 100, no. 4 (1966): 813–30.

36. G. Oberhuber, "Histopathology of Celiac Disease," *Biomedicine & Pharmacotherapy* 54, no. 7 (2000): 368–72.

37. Oberhuber, "Histopathology of Celiac Disease."

38. Dickson, Streutker, and Chetty, "Coeliac Disease."

39. Antonioli, "Celiac Disease: A Progress Report."

40. Dickson, Streutker, and Chetty, "Coeliac Disease."

41. Dickson, Streutker, and Chetty, "Coeliac Disease."

42. M. Rashid, M. Zarkadas, A. Anca, and H. Limeback, "Oral Manifestations of Celiac Disease: A Clinical Guide for Dentists," *Journal of the Michigan Dental Association* 93, no. 10 (2011): 42–46.

43. Rashid, Zarkadas, Anca, and Limeback, "Oral Manifestations of Celiac Disease."

44. Rashid, Zarkadas, Anca, and Limeback, "Oral Manifestations of Celiac Disease."

45. D. Martinelli, F. Fortunato, S. Tafuri, C. Germinario, and R. Prato, "Reproductive Life Disorders in Italian Celiac Women: A Case-Control Study," *BMC Gastroenterology* 10 (2010): 89.

46. Martinelli, Fortunato, Tafuri, Germinario, and Prato, "Reproductive Life Disorders in Italian Celiac Women."

47. I. Blumer and S. Crowe, *Celiac Disease for Dummies* (Ontario, Canada: John Wiley & Sons Canada, 2010).

48. S. Landaw and S. Schrier, "Approach to the Adult Patient with Splenomegaly and Other Splenic Disorders," UptoDate.com, accessed January 28, 2014, http://www.uptodate.com/contents/approach-to-the-adult-patient-with-splenomegaly-and-other-splenic-disorders.

49. "Lactose Intolerance," Coeliac Organization UK, accessed January 29, 2014, http://www.coeliac.org.uk.

5. DIAGNOSIS OF CELIAC DISEASE

1. N. Colledge, B. Walker, and S. Ralston, *Davidson's Principles and Practice of Medicine*, 21st ed. (Beijing: Elsevier Limited, 2010).

2. "Celiac Disease Facts and Figures," University of Chicago Celiac Disease Center, accessed October 22, 2013, http://www.uchospitals.edu.

3. J. Bai, M. Fried, G. Corazza, D. Schuppan, M. Farthing, C. Catassi, L. Greco, H. Cohen, C. Ciacci, R. Eliakim, A. Fasano, A. González, J. Krabshuis, and A. LeMair, "World Gastroenterology Organisation Global Guidelines on Celiac Disease," *Journal of Clinical Gastroenterology* 47, no. 2 (2013): 121–26.

4. A. Rubio-Tapia, I. Hill, C. Kelly, A. Calderwood, and J. Murray, "ACG Clinical Guidelines: Diagnosis and Management of Celiac Disease," *American Journal of Gastroenterology* 108, no. 5 (2013): 656–76.

5. Rubio-Tapia, Hill, Kelly, Calderwood, and Murray, "ACG Clinical Guidelines."

6. C. Goddard and H. Gillet, "Complications of Celiac Disease: Are All Patients at Risk?" *Postgraduate Medical Journal* 82, no. 973 (2006): 705–12.

7. Rubio-Tapia, Hill, Kelly, Calderwood, and Murray, "ACG Clinical Guidelines."

8. Rubio-Tapia, Hill, Kelly, Calderwood, and Murray, "ACG Clinical Guidelines."

9. Rubio-Tapia, Hill, Kelly, Calderwood, and Murray, "ACG Clinical Guidelines."

10. Bai, Fried, et al., "World Gastroenterology Organisation Global Guidelines on Celiac Disease."

11. Rubio-Tapia, Hill, Kelly, Calderwood, and Murray, "ACG Clinical Guidelines."

12. Rubio-Tapia, Hill, Kelly, Calderwood, and Murray, "ACG Clinical Guidelines."

13. Bai, Fried, et al., "World Gastroenterology Organisation Global Guidelines on Celiac Disease."

14. Bai, Fried, et al., "World Gastroenterology Organisation Global Guidelines on Celiac Disease."

15. Bai, Fried, et al., "World Gastroenterology Organisation Global Guidelines on Celiac Disease."

16. Bai, Fried, et al., "World Gastroenterology Organisation Global Guidelines on Celiac Disease."

17. Bai, Fried, et al., "World Gastroenterology Organisation Global Guidelines on Celiac Disease."

18. Bai, Fried, et al., "World Gastroenterology Organisation Global Guidelines on Celiac Disease."

19. Bai, Fried, et al., "World Gastroenterology Organisation Global Guidelines on Celiac Disease."

20. Bai, Fried, et al., "World Gastroenterology Organisation Global Guidelines on Celiac Disease."

21. Bai, Fried, et al., "World Gastroenterology Organisation Global Guidelines on Celiac Disease."

22. Rubio-Tapia, Hill, Kelly, Calderwood, and Murray, "ACG Clinical Guidelines."

23. Rubio-Tapia, Hill, Kelly, Calderwood, and Murray, "ACG Clinical Guidelines."

24. Rubio-Tapia, Hill, Kelly, Calderwood, and Murray, "ACG Clinical Guidelines."

25. Bai, Fried, et al., "World Gastroenterology Organisation Global Guidelines on Celiac Disease."

26. G. Douglas, F. Nicol, and C. Robertson, *Macleod's Clinical Examination*, 12th ed. (Beijing: Elsevier Limited, 2009).

27. Douglas, Nicol, and Robertson, *Macleod's Clinical Examination*.

28. Douglas, Nicol, and Robertson, *Macleod's Clinical Examination*.

29. Douglas, Nicol, and Robertson, *Macleod's Clinical Examination*; "How Is Celiac Disease Diagnosed?" Celiac Sprue Association, accessed October 28, 2013, http://www.csaceliacs.info.

30. Douglas, Nicol, and Robertson, *Macleod's Clinical Examination*; "How Is Celiac Disease Diagnosed?"

31. Douglas, Nicol, and Robertson, *Macleod's Clinical Examination*.

32. Colledge, Walker, and Ralston, *Davidson's Principles and Practice of Medicine*.

33. Colledge, Walker, and Ralston, *Davidson's Principles and Practice of Medicine*.

34. Bai, Fried, et al., "World Gastroenterology Organisation Global Guidelines on Celiac Disease."

35. Rubio-Tapia, Hill, Kelly, Calderwood, and Murray, "ACG Clinical Guidelines."

36. Bai, Fried, et al., "World Gastroenterology Organisation Global Guidelines on Celiac Disease."

37. Rubio-Tapia, Hill, Kelly, Calderwood, and Murray, "ACG Clinical Guidelines."

38. Rubio-Tapia, Hill, Kelly, Calderwood, and Murray, "ACG Clinical Guidelines."

39. Rubio-Tapia, Hill, Kelly, Calderwood, and Murray, "ACG Clinical Guidelines."

40. Rubio-Tapia, Hill, Kelly, Calderwood, and Murray, "ACG Clinical Guidelines."

41. Rubio-Tapia, Hill, Kelly, Calderwood, and Murray, "ACG Clinical Guidelines."

42. Rubio-Tapia, Hill, Kelly, Calderwood, and Murray, "ACG Clinical Guidelines."

43. Bai, Fried, et al., "World Gastroenterology Organisation Global Guidelines on Celiac Disease."

44. Bai, Fried, et al., "World Gastroenterology Organisation Global Guidelines on Celiac Disease."

45. M. Babron, S. Nilsson, S. Adamovic, A. Naluai, J. Wahlstrom, H. Ascher, P. Ciclitira, L. Sollid, J. Partanen, L. Greco, and F. Clerget-Darpoux, "European Genetics Cluster on Coeliac Disease. Meta and Pooled Analysis of European Coeliac Disease Data," *European Journal of Human Genetics* 11, no. 11 (2003): 828–34.

46. M. Piacentini, C. Rodolfo, M. Farrace, and F. Autuori, "'Tissue' Transglutaminase in Animal Development," *International Journal of Developmental Biology* 44, no. 6 (2000): 655–62; D. Aeschlimann and V. Thomazy, "Protein Crosslinking in Assembly and Remodelling of Extracellular Matrices: The Role of Transglutaminases," *Connective Tissue Research* 41, no. 1 (2000): 1–27; L. Lorand and R. Graham, "Transglutaminases: Crosslinking Enzymes with Pleiotropic Functions," *Nature Reviews Molecular Cell Biology* 4, no. 2 (2003): 140–56.

47. D. Leffler, S. Saha, and R. Farrell, "Celiac Disease," *American Journal of Managed Care* 9, no. 12 (2003): 825–31.

48. Bai, Fried, et al., "World Gastroenterology Organisation Global Guidelines on Celiac Disease."

49. Rubio-Tapia, Hill, Kelly, Calderwood, and Murray, "ACG Clinical Guidelines."

50. Bai, Fried, et al., "World Gastroenterology Organisation Global Guidelines on Celiac Disease."

51. Rubio-Tapia, Hill, Kelly, Calderwood, and Murray, "ACG Clinical Guidelines."

52. Rubio-Tapia, Hill, Kelly, Calderwood, and Murray, "ACG Clinical Guidelines."

53. Bai, Fried, et al., "World Gastroenterology Organisation Global Guidelines on Celiac Disease."

54. Bai, Fried, et al., "World Gastroenterology Organisation Global Guidelines on Celiac Disease."

55. Bai, Fried, et al., "World Gastroenterology Organisation Global Guidelines on Celiac Disease."

56. Rubio-Tapia, Hill, Kelly, Calderwood, and Murray, "ACG Clinical Guidelines."

57. Bai, Fried, et al., "World Gastroenterology Organisation Global Guidelines on Celiac Disease."

58. Bai, Fried, et al., "World Gastroenterology Organisation Global Guidelines on Celiac Disease."

59. Rubio-Tapia, Hill, Kelly, Calderwood, and Murray, "ACG Clinical Guidelines."

60. Rubio-Tapia, Hill, Kelly, Calderwood, and Murray, "ACG Clinical Guidelines."

61. Rubio-Tapia, Hill, Kelly, Calderwood, and Murray, "ACG Clinical Guidelines."

62. Bai, Fried, et al., "World Gastroenterology Organisation Global Guidelines on Celiac Disease."

63. Bai, Fried, et al., "World Gastroenterology Organisation Global Guidelines on Celiac Disease."

64. Bai, Fried, et al., "World Gastroenterology Organisation Global Guidelines on Celiac Disease."

65. Rubio-Tapia, Hill, Kelly, Calderwood, and Murray, "ACG Clinical Guidelines."

66. Rubio-Tapia, Hill, Kelly, Calderwood, and Murray, "ACG Clinical Guidelines."

67. Rubio-Tapia, Hill, Kelly, Calderwood, and Murray, "ACG Clinical Guidelines."

68. Rubio-Tapia, Hill, Kelly, Calderwood, and Murray, "ACG Clinical Guidelines."

69. Rubio-Tapia, Hill, Kelly, Calderwood, and Murray, "ACG Clinical Guidelines."

70. Rubio-Tapia, Hill, Kelly, Calderwood, and Murray, "ACG Clinical Guidelines."

71. Rubio-Tapia, Hill, Kelly, Calderwood, and Murray, "ACG Clinical Guidelines."

72. Rubio-Tapia, Hill, Kelly, Calderwood, and Murray, "ACG Clinical Guidelines."

73. Rubio-Tapia, Hill, Kelly, Calderwood, and Murray, "ACG Clinical Guidelines."

74. Colledge, Walker, and Ralston, *Davidson's Principles and Practice of Medicine*.

75. Rubio-Tapia, Hill, Kelly, Calderwood, and Murray, "ACG Clinical Guidelines."

76. Colledge, Walker, and Ralston, *Davidson's Principles and Practice of Medicine*.

77. "Serum Magnesium—Test," National Library of Medicine-National Institutes of Health, accessed November 2, 2013, http://www.nlm.nih.gov/medlineplus/ency/article/003487.htm.

78. "Calcium—Blood Test," National Library of Medicine-National Institutes of Health, accessed November 2, 2013, http://www.nlm.nih.gov/medlineplus/ency/article/003477.htm.

79. Rubio-Tapia, Hill, Kelly, Calderwood, and Murray, "ACG Clinical Guidelines."

80. Bai, Fried, et al., "World Gastroenterology Organisation Global Guidelines on Celiac Disease."

81. Rubio-Tapia, Hill, Kelly, Calderwood, and Murray, "ACG Clinical Guidelines."

82. Rubio-Tapia, Hill, Kelly, Calderwood, and Murray, "ACG Clinical Guidelines."

83. Rubio-Tapia, Hill, Kelly, Calderwood, and Murray, "ACG Clinical Guidelines."

84. Colledge, Walker, and Ralston, *Davidson's Principles and Practice of Medicine.*

85. "Bone Density Test," Mayo Clinic, accessed November 2, 2013, http://www.mayoclinic.org/tests-procedures/bone-density-test/basics/what-you-can-expect/prc-20020254; "Osteoporosis—Bone Density," National Osteoporosis Foundation, accessed November 2, 2013, http://nof.org/learn.

86. R. Small, "Uses and Limitation of Bone Mineral Density Measurements in the Management of Osteoporosis," *Medscape General Medicine* 7, no. 2 (2005): 3.

87. Rubio-Tapia, Hill, Kelly, Calderwood, and Murray, "ACG Clinical Guidelines."

88. J. Shepard, *The First Year: Celiac Disease and Living Gluten-Free: An Essential Guide for the Newly Diagnosed* (Cambridge, MA: Da Capo Press, 2008).

89. Shepard, *The First Year*; "Coeliac Disease: Causes," National Health Service United Kingdom, accessed October 20, 2013, www.nhs.uk/Conditions/Coeliac-disease/Pages/Causes.aspx.

90. Shepard, *The First Year.*

91. M. Sharrett, *Celiac Disease: A Guide to Living with Gluten Intolerance* (New York: Demos Health, 2006).

92. R. Gibbons, "Everyday Tips for Living with Celiac Disease," Yahoo! Health, May 8, 2013, accessed December 13, 2013, http://health.yahoo.net/experts/eatbetterlivebetter/everday-tips-living-with-celiac-disease.

93. S. Guandalini, "Celiac Disease Does Not Cause Infertility in the U.S. or Does It?" *Impact: University of Chicago Celiac Disease Center* 8, no. 1 (2008): 1–2; J. Norris, K. Barriga, E. Hoffenberg, I. Taki, D. Miao, J. Haas, L. Emery, R. Sokol, H. Erlich, G. Eisenbarth, and M. Rewers, "Risk of Celiac Disease Autoimmunity and Timing of Gluten Introduction in the Diet of Infants at Increased

Risk of Disease," *Journal of the American Medical Association* 293, no. 19 (2005): 2343–51.

94. M. Dennis and D. Leffler, *Real Life with Celiac Disease: Troubleshooting and Thriving Gluten Free* (Bethesda, MD: American Gastroenterological Association [AGA] Press, 2010); S. Plogsted, "Medications and Celiac Disease—Tips from a Pharmacist," *Practical Gastroenterology* 5 (2007): 58–64.

6. NEW ADVANCES IN CLINICAL RESEARCH

1. H. Freeman, A. Chopra, M. Clandinin, and A. Thomson, "Recent Advances in Celiac Disease," *World Journal of Gastroenterology* 17, no. 18 (2011): 2259–72; D. van Heel and J. West, "Recent Advances in Coeliac Disease," *Gut* 55, no. 7 (2006): 1037–46.

2. A. Akobeng, A. Ramanan, I. Buchan, and R. Heller, "Effect of Breast Feeding on Risk of Coeliac Disease: A Systematic Review and Meta-Analysis of Observational Studies," *Archives of Disease in Childhood* 91, no. 1 (2006): 39–43; A. Ivarsson, O. Hernell, H. Stenlund, and L. Persson, "Breast-Feeding Protects against Celiac Disease," *American Journal of Clinical Nutrition* 75, no. 5 (2002): 914–21; U. Peters, S. Schneeweiss, E. Trautwein, and H. Erbersdobler, "A Case-Control Study of the Effect of Infant Feeding on Celiac Disease," *Annals of Nutrition and Metabolism* 45, no. 4 (2001): 135–42; K. Fälth-Magnusson, L. Franzén, G. Jansson, P. Laurin, and L. Stenhammar, "Infant Feeding History Shows Distinct Differences between Swedish Celiac and Reference Children," *Pediatric Allergy and Immunology* 7, no. 1 (1996): 1–5; M. Pinier, G. Fuhrmann, E. Verdu, and J. Leroux, "Prevention Measures and Exploratory Pharmacological Treatments of Celiac Disease," *American Journal of Gastroenterology* 105, no. 12 (2010): 2551–61; J. Norris, K. Barriga, E. Hoffenberg, I. Taki, D. Miao, J. Haas, L. Emery, R. Sokol, H. Erlich, G. Eisenbarth, and M. Rewers, "Risk of Celiac Disease Autoimmunity and Timing of Gluten Introduction in the Diet of Infants at Increased Risk of Disease," *Journal of the American Medical* 293, no. 19 (2005): 2343–51.

3. Akobeng, Ramanan, Buchan, and Heller, "Effect of Breast Feeding on Risk of Coeliac Disease"; M. Silano, C. Agostoni, and S. Guandalini, "Effect of Timing of Gluten Introduction on the Development of Celiac Disease," *World Journal of Gastroenterology* 16, no. 16 (2010): 1939–42; Pinier, Fuhrmann, Verdu, and Leroux, "Prevention Measures and Exploratory Pharmacological Treatments of Celiac Disease."

4. Norris, Barriga, et al., "Risk of Celiac Disease Autoimmunity and Timing of Gluten Introduction"; Pinier, Fuhrmann, Verdu, and Leroux, "Prevention

Measures and Exploratory Pharmacological Treatments of Celiac Disease"; Sila-no, Agostoni, and Guandalini, "Effect of Timing of Gluten Introduction."

5. Norris, Barriga, et al., "Risk of Celiac Disease Autoimmunity."

6. Silano, Agostoni, and Guandalini, "Effect of Timing of Gluten Introduction on the Development of Celiac Disease"; Pinier et al., "Prevention Measures and Exploratory Pharmacological Treatments of Celiac Disease."

7. F. Ferrara, S. Quaglia, I. Caputo, C. Esposito, M. Lepretti, S. Pastore, R. Giorgi, S. Martelossi, G. Dal Molin, N. Di Toro, A. Ventura, and T. Not, "Anti-Transglutaminase Antibodies in Non-Coeliac Children Suffering from Infectious Diseases," *Clinical & Experimental Immunology* 159, no. 2 (2010): 217–23; Pinier et al., "Prevention Measures and Exploratory Pharmacological Treatments of Celiac Disease."

8. S. Rashtak and J. Murray, "Review Article: Coeliac Disease, New Approaches to Therapy," *Alimentary Pharmacology & Therapeutics* 35, no. 7 (2012): 768–81; Freeman, Chopra, Clandinin, and Thomson, "Recent Advances in Celiac Disease"; van Heel and West, "Recent Advances in Coeliac Disease."

9. J. Leeds, A. Hopper, and D. Sanders, "Coeliac Disease," *British Medical Bulletin* 88, no. 1 (2008): 157–70.

10. I. Hill, "What Are the Sensitivity and Specificity of Serologic Tests for Celiac Disease? Do Sensitivity and Specificity Vary in Different Populations?" *Gastroenterology* 128, no. 4 (2005): S25–S32; Leeds, Hopper, and Sanders, "Coeliac Disease"; van Heel and West, "Recent Advances in Coeliac Disease."

11. T. Boenisch, C. Taylor, A. Farmilo, R. Stead, J. Happel, R. Saxena, M. Key, J. Robinson, J. Sturgis, L. Rudbeck, H. Winther, S. Jensen, S. Müller, S. Matthiesen, K. Nielsen, U. Henriksen, A. Schönau, N. Christensen, H. Wendel-boe, O. Rasmussen, L. Winther, D. Osborn, R. Zucker, K. Bisgaard, G. Kumar, D. Spaulding, and K. Atwood, *Immunohistochemical Staining Methods*, 5th ed. (Carpinteria, CA: Dako North America, 2009).

12. Freeman, Chopra, Clandinin, and Thomson, "Recent Advances in Celiac Disease"; van Heel and West, "Recent Advances in Coeliac Disease"; Leeds, Hopper, and Sanders, "Coeliac Disease."

13. F. Cataldo, V. Marino, A. Ventura, G. Bottaro, and G. Corazza, "Working Groups on Coeliac Disease. Prevalance and Clinical Features of Selective Immunoglobulin A Deficiency in Coeliac Disease: An Italian Multicentre Study," *Gut* 42, no. 3 (1998): 362–65; Hill, "What Are the Sensitivity and Specificity of Serologic Tests for Celiac Disease?"; Ferrara et al., "Anti-Transglutaminase Antibodies in Non-Coeliac Children Suffering from Infectious Diseases"; V. Kumar, M. Jarzabek-Chorzelska, J. Sulej, K. Karnewska, T. Farell, and S. Jablonska, "Celiac Disease and Immunoglobulin A Deficiency: How Effective Are the Serological Methods of Diagnosis?" *Clinical and Diagnostic Laboratory*

Immunology 9, no. 6 (2002): 1295; Leeds, Hopper, and Sanders, "Coeliac Disease"; Cataldo et al., "Working Groups on Coeliac Disease."

14. N. Lewis and B. Scott, "Meta-Analysis: Deamidated Gliadin Peptide Antibody and Tissue Transglutaminase Antibody Compared as Screening Tests for Coeliac Disease," *Alimentary Pharmacology & Therapeutics* 31, no. 1 (2010): 73–81; E. Liu, M. Li, L. Emery, I. Taki, K. Barriga, C. Tiberti, G. Eisenbarth, M. Rewers, and E. Hoffenberg, "Natural History of Antibodies to Deamidated Gliadin Peptides and Transglutaminase in Early Childhood Celiac Disease," *Journal of Pediatric Gastroenterology & Nutrition* 45, no. 3 (2007): 293–300.

15. N. R. Lewis and B. B. Scott, "Meta-Analysis: Deamidated Gliadin Peptide Antibody and Tissue Transglutaminase Antibody Compared as Screening Tests for Coeliac Disease," *Alimentary Pharmacology & Therapeutics* 31 (2010): 73–81.

16. Liu et al., "Natural History of Antibodies to Deamidated Gliadin Peptides."

17. R. Anderson, M. Henry, R. Taylor, E. Duncan, P. Danoy, M. Costa, K. Addison, J. Tye-Din, M. Kotowicz, R. Knight, W. Pollock, G. Nicholson, B. Toh, M. Brown, and J. Pasco, "A Novel Serogenetic Approach Determines the Community Prevalence of Celiac Disease and Informs Improved Diagnostic Pathways," *BMC Medicine* 11, no. 1 (2013): 188; M. Hadithi, B. von Blomberg, J. Crusius, E. Bloemena, P. Kostense, J. Meijer, C. Mulder, C. Stehouwer, and A. Pena, "Accuracy of Serologic Tests and HLA-DQ Typing for Diagnosing Celiac Disease," *Annals of Internal Medicine* 147, no. 5 (2007): 294–302; L. Medrano, B. Dema, A. López-Larios, C. Maluenda, A. Bodas, N. López-Palacios, M. Figueredo, M. Fernández-Arquero, and C. Nuñez, "HLA and Celiac Disease Susceptibility: New Genetic Factors Bring Open Questions about the HLA Influence and Gene-Dosage Effects," *Public Library of Science (PLOS) One* 7, no. 10 (2012): e48403; F. Megiorni and A. Pizzuti, "HLA-DQA1 and HLA-DQB1 in Celiac Disease Predisposition: Practical Implications of the HLA Molecular Typing," *Journal of Biomedical Science* 19, no. 1 (2012): 88.

18. Leeds, Hopper, and Sanders, "Coeliac Disease"; A. Kapitány, L. Tóth, J. Tumpek, I. Csípot, E. Sipos, N. Woolley, J. Partanen, G. Szegedi, E. Oláh, S. Sipla, and I. Korponay-Szabó, "Diagnostic Significance of HLA-DQ Typing in Patients with Previous Coeliac Disease Diagnosis Based on Histology Alone," *Alimentary Pharmacology & Therapeutics* 24, no. 9 (2006): 1395–1402.

19. Pinier, Fuhrmann, Verdu, and Leroux, "Prevention Measures and Exploratory Pharmacological Treatments of Celiac Disease"; Rashtak and Murray, "Review Article: Coeliac Disease, New Approaches to Therapy"; C. Tennyson, S. Simpson, B. Lebwohl, S. Lewis, and P. Green, "Interest in Medical Therapy for

Celiac Disease," *Therapeutic Advances in Gastroenterology* 6, no. 5 (2013): 358–64.

20. Leeds, Hopper, and Sanders, "Coeliac Disease"; Freeman et al., "Recent Advances in Celiac Disease"; van Heel and West, "Recent Advances in Coeliac Disease."

21. Pinier, Fuhrmann, Verdu, and Leroux, "Prevention Measures and Exploratory Pharmacological Treatments of Celiac Disease"; Rashtak and Murray, "Review Article: Coeliac Disease, New Approaches to Therapy"; van Heel and West, "Recent Advances in Coeliac Disease."

22. Pinier, Fuhrmann, Verdu, and Leroux, "Prevention Measures and Exploratory Pharmacological Treatments of Celiac Disease"; Freeman et al., "Recent Advances in Celiac Disease."

23. C. Gianfrani, R. Siciliano, A. Facchiano, A. Camarca, M. Mazzeo, S. Costantini, V. Salvati, F. Maurano, G. Mazzarella, G. Laguinto, P. Bergamo, M. Rossi, "Transamidation of Wheat Flour Inhibits the Response to Gliadin of Intestinal T cells in Celiac Disease," *Gastroenterology* 133, no. 3 (2007): 780–89.

24. Freeman et al., "Recent Advances in Celiac Disease"; Rashtak and Murray, "Review Article: Coeliac Disease, New Approaches to Therapy"; Pinier, Fuhrmann, Verdu, and Leroux, "Prevention Measures and Exploratory Pharmacological Treatments of Celiac Disease."

25. Pinier, Fuhrmann, Verdu, and Leroux, "Prevention Measures and Exploratory Pharmacological Treatments of Celiac Disease."

26. Freeman et al., "Recent Advances in Celiac Disease"; Pinier, Fuhrmann, Verdu, and Leroux, "Prevention Measures and Exploratory Pharmacological Treatments of Celiac Disease."

27. Rashtak and Murray, "Review Article: Coeliac Disease, New Approaches to Therapy"; Freeman et al., "Recent Advances in Celiac Disease"; Pinier, Fuhrmann, Verdu, and Leroux, "Prevention Measures and Exploratory Pharmacological Treatments of Celiac Disease."

28. B. Zanini, B. Petroboni, T. Not, N. Di Toro, V. Villanacci, F. Lanzarotto, N. Pogna, C. Ricci, and A. Lanzini, "Search for Atoxic Cereals: A Single Blind, Cross-Over Study on the Safety of a Single Dose of Triticummonococcum in Patients with Celiac Disease," *BMC Gastroenterology* 13, no. 1 (2013): 92.

29. R. Zandonadi, R. Botelho, and W. Araujo, "Psyllium as a Substitute for Gluten in Bread," *Journal of the American Dietetic Association* 109, no. 10 (2009): 1781–84; Rashtak and Murray, "Review Article: Coeliac Disease, New Approaches to Therapy."

30. C. Kelly, P. Green, J. Murray, A. DiMarino, A. Colatrella, D. Leffler, T. Alexander, R. Arsenescu, F. Leon, J. Jiang, L. Arterburn, B. Paterson, and R. Fedorak, "Larazotide Acetate in Patients with Coeliac Disease Undergoing a Gluten Challenge: A Randomised Placebo-Controlled Study," *Alimentary Phar-*

macology & Therapeutics 37, no. 2 (2013): 252–62; Pinier, Fuhrmann, Verdu, and Leroux, "Prevention Measures and Exploratory Pharmacological Treatments of Celiac Disease"; Rashtak and Murray, "Review Article: Coeliac Disease, New Approaches to Therapy"; Freeman, Chopra, Clandinin, and Thomson, "Recent Advances in Celiac Disease."

31. Rashtak and Murray, "Review Article: Coeliac Disease, New Approaches to Therapy."

32. A. Fasano, "Intestinal Permeability and Its Regulation by Zonulin: Diagnostic and Therapeutic Implications," *Clinical Gastroenterology and Hepatology* 10, no. 10 (2012): 1096–1100.

33. J. Anderson, "Cephalon Acquires Rights to Potential Celiac Disease Treatment," About.com, accessed February 9, 2014, http://celiacdisease.about.com/b/2011/02/15/cephalon-acquires-rights-to-potential-celiac-disease-treatment.htm.

34. Pinier, Fuhrmann, Verdu, and Leroux, "Prevention Measures and Exploratory Pharmacological Treatments of Celiac Disease"; Rashtak and Murray, "Review Article: Coeliac Disease, New Approaches to Therapy."

35. Pinier, Fuhrmann, Verdu, and Leroux, "Prevention Measures and Exploratory Pharmacological Treatments of Celiac Disease."

36. Pinier, Fuhrmann, Verdu, and Leroux, "Prevention Measures and Exploratory Pharmacological Treatments of Celiac Disease."

37. Rashtak and Murray, "Review Article: Coeliac Disease, New Approaches to Therapy."

38. G. Mariappan, N. Bhuyan, J. Mohanty, S. Ganguli, and D. Dhachinamoorthi, "An Overview of the Method of Positional Scanning Synthetic Combinatorial Libraries," *Indian Journal of Pharmaceutical Sciences* 68, no. 4 (2006): 420–24.

39. Freeman, Chopra, Clandinin, and Thomson, "Recent Advances in Celiac Disease."

40. Rashtak and Murray, "Review Article: Coeliac Disease, New Approaches to Therapy"; Freeman, Chopra, Clandinin, and Thomson, "Recent Advances in Celiac Disease."

41. Freeman, Chopra, Clandinin, and Thomson, "Recent Advances in Celiac Disease."

42. Rashtak and Murray, "Review Article: Coeliac Disease, New Approaches to Therapy."

43. Pinier, Fuhrmann, Verdu, and Leroux, "Prevention Measures and Exploratory Pharmacological Treatments of Celiac Disease"; Rashtak and Murray, "Review Article: Coeliac Disease, New Approaches to Therapy"; Freeman, Chopra, Clandinin, and Thomson, "Recent Advances in Celiac Disease."

44. D. Mann, "New Treatment for Celiac Disease?" WebMD Health News, accessed January 13, 2014, http://www.webmd.com/digestive-disorders/celiac-disease/news/20110208/new-treatment-for-celiac-disease.

45. "Alvine's Lead Drug Candidate: ALV003," Alvine Pharma, accessed January 13, 2014, http://www.alvinepharma.com/alv003.

46. L. Benet, "Pharmacokinetics: Basic Principles and Its Use as a Tool in Drug Metabolism," in *Drug Metabolism and Drug Toxicity*, M. Horning and J. Mitchell (New York: Raven Press, 1984).

47. "Alvine's Lead Drug Candidate: ALV003."

48. M. Lähdeaho, K. Kaukinen, K. Laurila, P. Vuotikka, O. Koivurova, T. Kärjä-Lahdensuu, A. Marcantonio, D. Adelman, and M. Mäki, "The Glutenase ALV003 Attenuates Gluten-Induced Mucosal Injury in Patients with Celiac Disease," *Gastroenterology* (2014).

49. M. Pinier, G. Fuhrmann, H. Galipeau, N. Rivard, J. Murray, C. David, H. Drasarova, L. Tuckova, J. Leroux, and E. Verdu, "The Copolymer P(HEMA-co-SS) Binds Gluten and Reduces Immune Response in Gluten-Sensitized Mice and Human Tissues," *Gastroenterology* 142, no. 2 (2012): 316–25.

50. V. Georgiev, "Necatoriasis: Treatment and Developmental Therapeutics," *Expert Opinion in Investigational Drugs* 9, no. 5 (2005): 1065–78.

51. J. Croese, S. Gaze, and A. Loukas, "Changed Gluten Immunity in Celiac Disease by Necator Americanus Provides New Insights into Autoimmunity," *International Journal for Parasitology* 43, nos. 3–4 (2013): 275–82.

52. L. Crespo Pérez, G. Castillejo de Villasante, A. Cano Ruiz, and F. León, "Non-Dietary Therapeutic Clinical Trials in Coeliac Disease," *European Journal of Internal Medicine* 23, no. 1 (2011).

53. A. Zaballos, J. Gutierrez, R. Varona, C. Ardavin, and G. Marquez, "Cutting Edge: Identification of the Orphan Chemokine Receptor GPR-9-6 as CCR9, the Receptor for the Chemokine TECK," *Journal of Immunology* 162, no. 10 (1999): 5671–75.

54. Phase II Trial in Celiac Disease, ChemoCentryx, accessed February 4, 2014, http://www.chemocentryx.com/product/phaseII.html.

55. G. J. Tack, W. H. Verbeek, A. Al-Toma, D. J. Kuik, M. W. Schreurs, O. Visser, and C. J. Mulder, "Evaluation of Cladribine Treatment in Refractory Celiac Disease Type II," *World Journal of Gastroenterology* 17, no. 4 (2011): 506–13.

56. G. Tack, M. Wondergem, A. Al-Toma, W. Verbeek, A. Schmittel, M. Machado, F. Perri, G. Ossenkoppele, P. Huijgens, M. Schreurs, C. Mulder, and O. Visser, "Auto-SCT in Refractory Celiac Disease Type II Patients Unresponsive to Cladribine Therapy," *Bone Marrow Transplantation* 46, no. 6 (2011): 840–46.

57. C. Keech, J. Dromey, Z. Chen, R. Anderson, and J. McCluskey, "355 Immune Tolerance Induced by Peptide Immunotherapy in an HLA Dq2-dependent Mouse Model of Gluten Immunity," *Gastroenterology* 136, no. 5 (2009): A57.

58. "The Technology," ImmusanT, accessed January 10, 2010, http://www.immusant.com.

59. Rashtak and Murray, "Review Article: Coeliac Disease, New Approaches to Therapy."

7. MENTAL OUTCOMES OF CELIAC DISEASE

1. "Mental Health: A State of Well-Being," World Health Organization, December 2013, accessed January 5, 2014, http://www.who.int/features/factfiles/mental_health/en.

2. A. Isaacs, *Mental Health and Psychiatric Nursing*, 4th ed. (Philadelphia: Lippincott Williams & Wilkins, 2005).

3. P. Pynnönen, E. Isometsä, E. Aronen, M. Verkasalo, E. Savilahti, and V. Aalberg, "Mental Disorders in Adolescents with Celiac Disease," *Psychosomatics* 45, no. 4 (2004): 325–35; E. Waszczuk, L. Michalski, A. Suslo, M. Koszewicz, T. Adamowski, and L. Paradowski, "The Connection between Celiac Disease and Nervous System and Mental Disorders," *Advances in Clinical and Experimental Medicine* 17, no. 5 (2008): 495–502.

4. C. Gentile, "Celiac Disease and Mental Health," National Foundation for Celiac Awareness, accessed October 30, 2013, http://www.celiaccentral.org/mental-health.

5. Y. Shoenfeld, G. Zandman-Goddard, L. Stojanovich, M. Cutolo, H. Amital, Y. Levy, M. Abu-Shakra, O. Barzilai, Y. Berkun, M. Blank, J. Freire de Carvalho, A. Doria, B. Gilburd, U. Katz, I. Krause, P. Langevitz, H. Orbach, V. Pordeus, M. Ram, E. Toubi, and Y. Sherer, "The Mosaic of Autoimmunity: Hormonal and Environmental Factors Involved in Autoimmune Diseases," *IMAJ: The Israel Medical Association Journal* 10, no. 1 (2008): 8–12.

6. S. Videbeck, *Psychiatric-Mental Health Nursing*, 5th ed. (Philadelphia: Lippincott Williams & Wilkins, 2011).

7. G. Cicarelli, G. Della Rocca, M. Amboni, C. Ciacci, G. Mazzaca, A. Filla, and P. Barone, "Clinical and Neurological Abnormalities in Adult Celiac Disease," *Journal of Neurological Sciences* 24, no. 5 (2003): 311–17.

8. K. Bushara, "Neurologic Presentation of Celiac Disease," *Gastroenterology* 128, no. 4 (2005): S92–S97.

9. C. Rose and R. Howard, "Living with Celiac Disease: A Grounded Theory Study," *Journal of Human Nutrition and Dietetics* 27, no. 1 (2014): 30–40.

10. Videbeck, *Psychiatric-Mental Health Nursing*.

11. W. Hu, J. Murray, M. Greenaway, J. Parisi, and K. Josephs, "Cognitive Impairment and Celiac Disease," *Archives of Neurology* 63, no. 10 (2006): 1440–46.

12. C. Whitehead, "Obesity and Celiac Disease: Possible Effects of the Gluten-Free Diet," *Gastrointestinal Nursing* 11, no. 3 (2013): 31–36.

13. D. Leffler, M. Dennis, J. Edwards-George, and C. Kelly, "The Interaction between Eating Disorders and Celiac Disease: An Exploration of 10 Cases," *European Journal of Gastroenterology & Hepatology* 19, no. 3 (2007): 251–55.

14. A. Mathur, M. Law, T. Hamzelhoei, I. Megson, and J. Wei, "A Study of Genetic Association between Schizophrenia and Type-2 Diabetes," *Prostaglandins, Leukotrienes and Essential Fatty Acids* 81, no. 4 (2009): 273–77.

15. Mathur et al., "A Study of Genetic Association between Schizophrenia and Type-2 Diabetes."

16. Mathur et al., "A Study of Genetic Association between Schizophrenia and Type-2 Diabetes."

17. Mathur et al., "A Study of Genetic Association between Schizophrenia and Type-2 Diabetes."

18. Mathur et al., "A Study of Genetic Association between Schizophrenia and Type-2 Diabetes."

19. K. Merikangas, "Anxiety Disorders: Epidemiology," in *Comprehensive Textbook of Psychiatry*, 8th ed., edited by B. Sadock and V. Sadock (Philadelphia: Lippincott Williams & Wilkins, 2005).

20. Videbeck, *Psychiatric-Mental Health Nursing*.

21. Videbeck, *Psychiatric-Mental Health Nursing*.

22. S. Adams, "First Epidemiological Study of Gluten Intolerance in the US," accessed January 12, 2014, http://www.celiac.com.

23. E. Benveniste, "Inflammatory Cytokines within the Central Nervous System: Sources, Function, and Mechanism of Action," *American Journal of Physiology* 263, no. 1 (1992): C1–16; Videbeck, *Psychiatric-Mental Health Nursing*.

24. Isaacs, *Mental Health and Psychiatric Nursing*.

25. Videbeck, *Psychiatric-Mental Health Nursing*.

26. Isaacs, *Mental Health and Psychiatric Nursing*.

27. Videbeck, *Psychiatric-Mental Health Nursing*.

28. Isaacs, *Mental Health and Psychiatric Nursing*.

29. Videbeck, *Psychiatric-Mental Health Nursing*.

30. Isaacs, *Mental Health and Psychiatric Nursing*.

31. Videbeck, *Psychiatric-Mental Health Nursing*.

32. C. Padovan, "Serotonin in Anxiety and Depression," *Journal of Psychopharmacology* 27, no. 12 (2013): 1083.

33. Isaacs, *Mental Health and Psychiatric Nursing*.

34. Isaacs, *Mental Health and Psychiatric Nursing*.

35. R. Leyse-Wallace, *Linking Nutrition to Mental Health: A Scientific Exploration* (Lincoln, NE: iUniverse, Inc., 2008).

36. A. Hernanz and I. Polanco, "Plasma Precursor Amino Acids of Central Nervous System Monoamines in Children with Celiac Disease," *Gut* 32 (1991): 1478–81.

37. P. Whiteley, D. Haracopos, A. Knivsberg, K. Ludwig-Reichelt, S. Parlar, J. Jacobsen, A. Seim, L. Pedersen, M. Schondel, and P. Shattock, "The Scan Brit Randomized, Controlled, Single-Blind Study of a Gluten- and Casein-Free Dietary Intervention for Children with Autism Spectrum Disorders," *Nutritional Neuroscience* 13, no. 2 (2010): 87–100.

38. A. Diamanti, T. Capriati, C. Bizzarri, F. Panetta, F. Ferretti, M. Ancinelli, F. Romano, and M. Locatelli, "Celiac Disease and Endocrine Autoimmune Disorders in Children: An Update," *Expert Review of Clinical Immunology* 9, no. 12 (2013): 1289–1301.

39. W. Hauser, K. Janke, B. Klump, M. Gregor, and A. Hinz, "Anxiety and Depression in Adult Patients with Celiac Disease on a Gluten-Free Diet," *World Journal of Gastroenterology* 16, no. 22 (2010): 2780; S. Ford, R. Howard, and J. Oyebode, "Psychosocial Aspects of Coeliac Disease: a Cross-Sectional Survey of a UK Population," *British Journal of Health Psychology* 17, no. 4 (2012): 743–57.

40. Hauser et al., "Anxiety and Depression in Adult Patients with Celiac Disease on a Gluten-Free Diet."

41. L. Mazzone, L. Reale, M. Spina, M. Guarnera, E. Lionetti, S. Martorana, and D. Mazzone, "Compliant Gluten-Free Children with Celiac Disease: An Evaluation of Psychological Distress," *BMC Pediatrics* 11 (2011): 46.

42. Videbeck, *Psychiatric-Mental Health Nursing*.

43. Videbeck, *Psychiatric-Mental Health Nursing*.

44. "What Is Dementia?" Alzheimer's Association, accessed December 12, 2013, http://www.alz.org/what-is-dementia.asp.

45. "Celiac Disease Linked to Dementia," WebMD, accessed December 12, 2013, http://www.webmd.com/digestive-disorders/celiac-disease/news/20061013/celiac-disease-linked-dementia.

46. "Celiac Disease Linked to Dementia."

47. "Celiac Disease Linked to Dementia."

48. D. Wolfgang, "Preventative Concerns on Neurological Aspects of Celiac Disease Exposure to Heavy Metals in Relation to Alzheimer's Disease," Celiac Support Association, accessed December 12, 2013, http://www.csaceliacs.info.

49. Videbeck, *Psychiatric-Mental Health Nursing*.

50. Cicarelli, Della Rocca, Amboni, Ciacci, Mazzaca, Filla, and Barone, "Clinical and Neurological Abnormalities in Adult Celiac Disease"; A. Saleem, H. Connor, and P. Regan, "Adult Celiac Disease in Ireland: A Case Series," *Irish Journal of Medical Sciences* 181, no. 2 (2012): 225–29; F. Dickerson, C. Stallings, A. Origoni, C. Vaughan, S. Khushalani, A. Alaedini, and R. Yolken, "Markers of Gluten Sensitivity and Celiac Disease in Bipolar Disorder," *Bipolar Disorders* 13, no. 1 (2011): 52–58.

51. M. Bhatia, A. Jhanjee, and A. Oberoi, "Celiac Disease and Depression," *Delhi Psychiatry Journal* 15, no. 1 (2012): 223–24; C. Ciacci, A. Iavarone, G. Mazzacca, and A. De Rosa, "Depressive Symptoms in Adult Coeliac Disease," *Scandinavian Journal of Gastroenterology* 33, no. 3 (1998): 247–50.

52. "Depression," World Health Organization, accessed January 21, 2014, http://www.who.int/topics/depression/en/.

53. Isaacs, *Mental Health and Psychiatric Nursing*.

54. R. Caruso, F. Pallone, E. Stasi, S. Romeo, and G. Monteleone, "Appropriate Nutrient Supplementation in Celiac Disease," *Annals of Medicine* 45, no. 8 (2013): 522–31.

55. Hernanz and Polanco, "Plasma Precursor Amino Acids."

56. Videbeck, *Psychiatric-Mental Health Nursing*.

57. Videbeck, *Psychiatric-Mental Health Nursing*.

58. Isaacs, *Mental Health and Psychiatric Nursing*.

59. Isaacs, *Mental Health and Psychiatric Nursing*.

60. P. Delgado and F. Moreno, "Role of Norepinephrine in Depression," *Journal of Clinical Psychology* 61, no. 1 (Suppl. 1) (2000): 5–12.

61. Isaacs, *Mental Health and Psychiatric Nursing*.

62. M. Carta, M. Hardoy, P. Usai, B. Carpiniello, and J. Angst, "Recurrent Brief Depression in Celiac Disease," *Journal of Psychosomatic Research* 55, no. 6 (2003): 573–74; Hernanz and Polanco, "Plasma Precursor Amino Acids."

63. P. Lucassen, P. Meerlo, A. Naylor, A. van Dam, A. Dayer, E. Fuchs, C. Oomen, and B. Czech, "Regulation of Adult Neurogenesis by Stress, Sleep Disruption, Exercise and Inflammation: Implications for Depression and Antidepressant Action," *European Neuropsychopharmacology* 20, no. 1 (2010): 1–17.

64. O. Schiepers, W. Wichers, and M. Maes, "Cytokines and Major Depression," *Progress in Neuro-Psychopharmacology & Biological Psychiatry* 29, no. 2 (2005): 201–17.

65. Lucassen et al., "Regulation of Adult Neurogenesis by Stress, Sleep Disruption, Exercise and Inflammation."

66. American Psychiatric Association, *Diagnostic and Statistical Manual of Mental Disorders*, 4th ed. (Arlington, VA: American Psychiatric Publications, 2000).

67. Isaacs, *Mental Health and Psychiatric Nursing*; Videbeck, *Psychiatric-Mental Health Nursing*; American Psychiatric Association, *Diagnostic and Statistical Manual of Mental Disorders*.

68. Videbeck, *Psychiatric-Mental Health Nursing*.

69. Videbeck, *Psychiatric-Mental Health Nursing*.

70. Videbeck, *Psychiatric-Mental Health Nursing*.

71. American Psychiatric Association, *Diagnostic and Statistical Manual of Mental Disorders*.

72. Isaacs, *Mental Health and Psychiatric Nursing*.

73. Carta et al., "Recurrent Brief Depression in Celiac Disease."

74. D. Arigo, A. Anskis, and J. Smyth, "Psychiatric Comorbidities in Women with Celiac Disease," *Chronic Illness* 8, no. 1 (2012): 45–55.

75. Videbeck, *Psychiatric-Mental Health Nursing*.

76. Videbeck, *Psychiatric-Mental Health Nursing*.

77. Videbeck, *Psychiatric-Mental Health Nursing*.

78. Videbeck, *Psychiatric-Mental Health Nursing*.

79. Videbeck, *Psychiatric-Mental Health Nursing*.

80. R. Eitan and B. Lere, "Nonpharmacological, Somatic Treatments of Depression: Electroconvulsive Therapy and Novel Brain Stimulation Modalities," *Dialogues in Clinical NeuroSciences* 8, no. 2 (2006): 241–58.

81. M. Bond, "Psychodynamic Psychotherapy in the Treatment of Mood Disorders," *Current Opinion in Psychiatry* 19, no. 1 (2006): 40–43.

82. H. Niederhofer, "Association of Attention-Deficit/Hyperactivity Disorder and Celiac Disease: A Brief Report," *Primary Care Companion for CNS Disorders* 13, no. 3 (2011): ii.

83. Adams, "First Epidemiological Study of Gluten Intolerance in the US."

84. L. Hechtman, "Attention Deficit Disorders," in *Comprehensive Textbook of Psychiatry*, 8th ed., edited by B. Sadock and V. Sadock (Philadelphia: Lippincott Williams & Wilkins, 2005).

85. Hu, Murray, Greenaway, Parisi, and Josephs, "Cognitive Impairment and Celiac Disease."

86. Hechtman, "Attention Deficit Disorders."

87. M. T. Dang, D. Warrington, T. Tung, D. Baker, and R. Pan, "A School-Based Approach to Early Identification and Management of Students with ADHD," *Journal of School Nursing* 23, no. 1 (2007): 2–12.

88. Videbeck, *Psychiatric-Mental Health Nursing*.

89. D. Antai-Otong, "The Art of Prescribing Pharmacological Management of Adult ADHD: Implications for Care," *Perspectives in Psychiatric Care* 44, no. 3 (2008): 196–201.

90. D. Rowe and D. Hermens, "Attention-Deficit/Hyperactivity Disorder: Neurophysiology, Information Processing, Arousal, and Drug Development," *Expert Review of Neurotherapeutics* 6, no. 11 (2006): 1721–34.

91. Hechtman, "Attention Deficit Disorders."

92. Hechtman, "Attention Deficit Disorders."

93. R. Seeley, T. Stephens, and P. Tate, *Essentials of Anatomy and Physiology*, 6th ed. (New York: McGraw-Hill, 2007).

94. Hechtman, "Attention Deficit Disorders."

95. American Psychiatric Association, *Diagnostic and Statistical Manual of Mental Disorders*.

96. Isaacs, *Mental Health and Psychiatric Nursing*; Videbeck, *Psychiatric-Mental Health Nursing*.

97. Isaacs, *Mental Health and Psychiatric Nursing*; Videbeck, *Psychiatric-Mental Health Nursing*.

98. Isaacs, *Mental Health and Psychiatric Nursing*.

99. Antai-Otong, "The Art of Prescribing Pharmacological Management of Adult ADHD."

100. H. Searight, J. Burke, and F. Rottnek, "Adult ADHD: Evaluation and Treatment in Family Medicine, *American Family Physician* 62, no. 9 (2000): 2077–86, accessed January 29, 2014, http://www.aafp.org/afp/2000/1101/p2077.html; Antai-Otong, "The Art of Prescribing Pharmacological Management of Adult ADHD."

101. Videbeck, *Psychiatric-Mental Health Nursing*.

102. Hechtman, "Attention Deficit Disorders."

103. R. Lehne, *Pharmacology for Nursing Care*, 6th ed. (Philadelphia: W. B. Saunders, 2006).

104. Lehne, *Pharmacology for Nursing Care*.

105. J. Cheng, R. Chen, J. Ko, and E. Ng, "Efficacy and Safety of Atomoxetine for Attention-Deficit/Hyperactivity Disorder in Children and Adolescents—A Meta-Analysis and Meta-Regression Analysis," *Psychopharmacology* 194, no. 4 (2007): 197–209.

106. H. Niederhofer and K. Pittschieler, "A Preliminary Investigation of ADHD Symptoms in Persons with Celiac Disease," *Journal of Attention Disorders* 10, no. 2 (2006): 200–204.

107. Niederhofer and Pittschieler, "A Preliminary Investigation of ADHD Symptoms in Persons with Celiac Disease."

108. Videbeck, *Psychiatric-Mental Health Nursing*.

109. Isaacs, *Mental Health and Psychiatric Nursing*.

110. Videbeck, *Psychiatric-Mental Health Nursing*.

111. Centers for Disease Control, "Prevalence of Autism Spectrum Disorders—Autism and Developmental Disabilities Monitoring Network, 2006," *Morbidity and Mortality Weekly Report* 56, no. 1 (2007).

112. "Vaccines Didn't Cause Autism, Court Rules," Cable News Network (CNN), accessed January 31, 2014, http://edition.cnn.com/2009/HEALTH/02/12/autism.vaccines/index.html?eref=rss.

113. T. Buie, "The Relationship of Autism and Gluten," *Clinical Therapeutics* 35, no. 5 (2013): 578–83; N. Lau, P. Green, A. Taylor, D. Hellberg, M. Ajamian, C. Tan, B. Kosofsky, J. Higgins, A. Rajadhyaksha, and A. Alaedini, "Markers of Celiac Disease and Gluten Sensitivity in Children with Autism," *Public Library of Science (PLOS) ONE* 8, no. 6 (2013): 1–6.

114. Whiteley et al., "The Scan Brit Randomized, Controlled, Single-Blind Study of a Gluten- and Casein-Free Dietary Intervention for Children with Autism Spectrum Disorders."

115. Whiteley et al., "The Scan Brit Randomized, Controlled, Single-Blind Study of a Gluten- and Casein-Free Dietary Intervention for Children with Autism Spectrum Disorders."

116. Videbeck, *Psychiatric-Mental Health Nursing*.

117. F. Volkmar, C. Lord, A. Bailey, A. Klin, and R. Schultz, "Pervasive Developmental Disorders," in *Comprehensive Textbook of Psychiatry*, 8th ed., edited by B. Sadock and V. Sadock (Philadelphia: Lippincott Williams & Wilkins, 2005).

118. Isaacs, *Mental Health and Psychiatric Nursing*.

119. Videbeck, *Psychiatric-Mental Health Nursing*.

120. S. Myers and C. Johnson, "Management of Children with Autism Spectrum Disorders," *Pediatrics* 120, no. 5 (2007): 1162–82.

121. Volkmar et al., "Pervasive Developmental Disorders."

122. S. Hurwitz, "The Gluten-Free, Casein-Free Diet and Autism: Limited Return on Family Investment," *Journal of Early Intervention* 35, no. 1 (2013): 3–19.

123. Eating Disorders, "American Psychological Association," accessed January 29, 2014, http://www.apa.org/topics/eating.

124. American Psychiatric Association, *Diagnostic and Statistical Manual of Mental Disorders*.

125. T. de Toni, M. Casamassima, R. Gastaldi, and R. Franchini, "Celiac Disease and Anorexia Nervosa [Article in Italian]," *Minerva Pediatrica* 38, no. 10 (1986): 409–12.

126. Isaacs, *Mental Health and Psychiatric Nursing*.

127. Isaacs, *Mental Health and Psychiatric Nursing*; Videbeck, *Psychiatric-Mental Health Nursing*.

128. J. Lyke and J. Matsen, "Family Functioning and Risk Factors for Disordered Eating," *Eating Behaviors* 14, no. 4 (2013): 497–99.

129. Isaacs, *Mental Health and Psychiatric Nursing.*

130. "Body Image and Your Kids," accessed January 29, 2014, http://www.womenshealth.gov/body-image/kids/.

131. Leffler, Dennis, Edwards-George, and Kelly, "The Interaction between Eating Disorders and Celiac Disease."

132. V. Passananti, M. Siniscalchi, F. Zingone, C. Bucci, R. Tortora, P. Iovino, and C. Ciacci, "Prevalence of Eating Disorders in Adults with Celiac Disease," *Gastroenterology Research and Practice* (2013): 1–7.

133. Whitehead, "Obesity and Celiac Disease."

134. Isaacs, *Mental Health and Psychiatric Nursing*; Videbeck, *Psychiatric-Mental Health Nursing*; American Psychiatric Association, *Diagnostic and Statistical Manual of Mental Disorders.*

135. V. Ricca, E. Mannucci, A. Calabro, M. Bernardo, P. Cabras, and C. Rotella, "Anorexia Nervosa and Celiac Disease: Two Case Reports," *International Journal of Eating Disorders* 27, no. 1 (2000): 119–22.

136. "Anorexia Nervosa," A.D.A.M., *New York Times* online, accessed February 1, 2014, http://www.nytimes.com/health/guides/disease/anorexia-nervosa/diagnosis.html.

137. American Psychiatric Association, *Diagnostic and Statistical Manual of Mental Disorders.*

138. "Anorexia Nervosa," A.D.A.M., *New York Times.*

139. F. Connan and J. Treasure, "Working with Adults with Anorexia Nervosa in an Out-Patient Setting," *Advances in Psychiatric Treatment* 6, no. 2 (2000): 135–44.

140. American Psychiatric Association, "Treatment of Patients with Eating Disorders," *American Journal of Psychiatry* 163 (7 Suppl.) (2006): 4–54.

141. Videbeck, *Psychiatric-Mental Health Nursing.*

142. P. Mehler and K. Weiner, "Use of Total Parenteral Nutrition in the Refeeding of Selected Patients with Severe Anorexia Nervosa," *International Journal of Eating Disorders* 40, no. 3 (2007): 285–87.

143. Videbeck, *Psychiatric-Mental Health Nursing.*

144. N. Andreasen and D. Black, *Introductory Textbook of Psychiatry*, 4th ed. (Washington, DC: American Psychiatric Publishing, 2006).

145. Isaacs, *Mental Health and Psychiatric Nursing*; Videbeck, *Psychiatric-Mental Health Nursing.*

146. American Psychiatric Association, *Diagnostic and Statistical Manual of Mental Disorders.*

147. Isaacs, *Mental Health and Psychiatric Nursing.*

148. Leffler, Dennis, Edwards-George, and Kelly, "The Interaction between Eating Disorders and Celiac Disease"; Whitehead, "Obesity and Celiac Disease."

149. Leffler, Dennis, Edwards-George, and Kelly, "The Interaction between Eating Disorders and Celiac Disease."

150. A. Anderson and J. Yager, "Eating Disorders," in *Comprehensive Textbook of Psychiatry*, 8th ed., edited by B. Sadock and V. Sadock (Philadelphia: Lippincott Williams & Wilkins, 2005).

151. Videbeck, *Psychiatric-Mental Health Nursing*.

152. Isaacs, *Mental Health and Psychiatric Nursing*.

153. American Psychiatric Association, *Diagnostic and Statistical Manual of Mental Disorders*.

154. C. Corega, L. Vaida, D. Festila, G. Rigoni, M. Albanese, A. D'Agostino, A. Pardo, A. Rossetto, P. Nocini, and D. Bertossi, "Dental White Spots Associated with Bulimia Nervosa in Orthodontic Patients," *Minerva Stomatologica* (2014).

155. A. Karwautz, G. Wagner, G. Berger, U. Sinnreich, V. Grylli, and W. Huber, "Eating Pathology in Adolescents with Celiac Disease," *Psychosomatics* 49, no. 5 (2008): 399–406.

156. S. Wonderlich, C. Peterson, R. Crosby, T. Smith, M. Klein, J. Mitchell, and S. Crow, "A Randomized Controlled Comparison of Integrative Cognitive-Affective Therapy (ICAT) and Enhanced Cognitive-Behavioral Therapy (CBT-E) for Bulimia Nervosa," *Psychological Medicine* 44, no. 3 (2014): 543–53.

157. U. Schmidt, S. Lee, J. Beecham, S. Perkins, J. Treasure, I. Yi, S. Winn, P. Robinson, R. Murphy, S. Keville, E. Johnson-Sabine, M. Jenkins, S. Frost, L. Dodge, M. Berelowitz, and I. Eisler, "A Randomized Controlled Trial of Family Therapy and Cognitive Behaviour Therapy Guided Self-Care for Adolescents with Bulimia Nervosa and Related Disorders," *American Journal of Psychiatry* 164, no. 4 (2007): 591–98.

158. S. McElroy, A. Guerdjikova, N. Mori, and A. O'Melia, "Current Pharmacotherapy Options for Bulimia Nervosa and Binge Eating Disorder," *Expert Opinion on Pharmacotherapy* 13, no. 14 (2012): 2015–26.

159. W. Agras, "Treatment of Eating Disorders," in *Essentials of Clinical Psychopharmacology*, 2nd ed., edited by A. Schatzberg and C. Nemeroff (Washington, DC: American Psychiatric Association, 2006).

160. D. Schuppan, M. Dennis, and C. Kelly, "Celiac Disease: Epidemiology, Pathogenesis, Diagnosis, and Nutritional Management," *Nutrition in Clinical Care* 8, no. 2 (2005): 54–69.

161. Arigo, Anskis, and Smyth, "Psychiatric Comorbidities in Women with Celiac Disease."

162. S. Telles, N. Singh, A. Bhardwaj, A. Kumar, and A. Balkrishna, "Effect of Yoga or Physical Exercise on Physical, Cognitive and Emotional Measures in

Children: A Randomized Controlled Trial," *Child and Adolescent Psychiatry and Mental Health* 7, no. 1 (2013): 1–28.

163. M. Zarkadas, S. Dubois, K. MacIsaac, I. Cantin, M. Rashid, K. Roberts, S. La Vieille, S. Godefroy, and O. Pulido, "Living with Celiac Disease and a Gluten-Free Diet: A Canadian Perspective," *Journal of Human Nutrition and Dietetics* 26, no. 1 (2013): 10–23.

164. Zarkadas et al., "Living with Celiac Disease and a Gluten-Free Diet."

8. PHYSICAL DISORDERS ASSOCIATED WITH CELIAC DISEASE

1. X. McFarlane, A. Bhalla, D. Reeves, L. Morgan, and D. Robertson, "Osteoporosis in Treated Adult Celiac Disease," *Gut* 36 (1995): 710–14.

2. "What People with Celiac Disease Need to Know About Osteoporosis," National Institute for Arthritis and Musculoskeletal and Skin Diseases, accessed December 14, 2013, http://www.niams.nih.gov/Health_Info/Bone/Osteoporosis/Conditions_Behaviors/celiac.asp.

3. "What People with Celiac Disease Need to Know About Osteoporosis."

4. "What People with Celiac Disease Need to Know About Osteoporosis."

5. "What People with Celiac Disease Need to Know About Osteoporosis."

6. N. Molteni, M. Caraceni, M. Bardella, S. Ortolani, G. Gandolini, and P. Bianchi, "Bone-Mineral Density in Adult Celiac Patients and the Effect of Gluten-Free Diet from Childhood," *American Journal of Gastroenterology* 85, no. 1 (1990): 51–53.

7. P. L. Riches, E. McRorie, W. Fraser, C. Determann, R. van't Hof, and S. Ralston, "Osteoporosis Associated with Neutralizing Autoantibodies against Osteoprotegerin," *New England Journal of Medicine* 361, no. 15 (2009): 1459–65.

8. M. Sahebari, S. Sigari, H. Heidari, and O. Biglarian, "Osteomalacia Can Still Be a Point of Attention to Celiac Disease," *Clinical Cases in Mineral and Bone Metabolism* 8, no. 3 (2011): 14–15.

9. E. Lubrano, C. Ciacci, P. Ames, G. Mazzacca, P. Oriente, and R. Scarpa, "The Arthritis of Coeliac Disease: Prevalence and Pattern in 200 Adult Patients," *British Journal of Rheumatology* 35, no. 12 (1996): 1314–18.

10. "Celiac and Arthritis," LoveToKnow.com, accessed December 14, 2013, http://gluten.lovetoknow.com/celiac-arthritis.

11. "Rheumatoid Arthritis," Arthritis Foundation, accessed December 14, 2013, http://www.arthritis.org/conditions-treatments/disease-center/rheumatoid-arthritis.

12. "Rheumatoid Arthritis."

13. "Rheumatoid Arthritis."

14. "Arthritis and Celiac Disease," Celiac.com, accessed December 15, 2013, http://www.celiac.com/articles/85/1/Arthritis-and-Celiac-Disease/Page1.html.

15. "Rheumatoid Arthritis."

16. J. T. Bourne, P. Kumar, E. Huskisson, R. Mageed, D. Unsworth, and J. Wojtulewski, "Arthritis and Coeliac Disease," *Annals of the Rheumatic Diseases* 44, no. 9 (1995): 5592–98.

17. "Arthritis and Celiac Disease."

18. Bourne et al., "Arthritis and Coeliac Disease."

19. "Arthritis and Celiac Disease."

20. "Celiac Disease," Children's National, http://www.childrensnational.org, accessed December 16, 2013.

21. D. Nemet, A. Raz, E. Zifman, H. Morag, and A. Eliakim, "Short Stature, Celiac Disease and Growth Hormone Deficiency," *Journal of Pediatric Endocrinology and Metabolism* 22, no. 10 (2009): 979–83.

22. M. Bozzola, D. Giovenale, E. Bozzola, E. Meazza, M. Martinetti, C. Tinelli, and G. Corazza, "Growth Hormone Deficiency and Coeliac Disease: An Unusual Association?" *Clinical Endocrinology (Oxford)* 62, no. 3 (2005): 372–75.

23. Bozzola et al., "Growth Hormone Deficiency and Coeliac Disease."

24. Bozzola et al., "Growth Hormone Deficiency and Coeliac Disease."

25. Bozzola et al., "Growth Hormone Deficiency and Coeliac Disease."

26. Bozzola et al., "Growth Hormone Deficiency and Coeliac Disease."

27. C. Keller, E. Gamboa, A. Hays, J. Karlitz, G. Lowe, P. Green, and G. Bhagat, "Fatal CNS Vasculopathy in a Patient with Refractory Celiac Disease and Lymph Node Cavitation," *Virchows Archive* 448, no. 2 (2006): 209–13.

28. G. Holmes, "Mesenteric Lymph Node Cavitation in Coeliac Disease," *Gut* 27, no. 6 (1986): 728–33.

29. Holmes, "Mesenteric Lymph Node Cavitation in Coeliac Disease."

30. H. Freeman, "Mesenteric Lymph Node Cavitation Syndrome," *World Journal of Gastroenterology* 16, no. 24 (2010): 2991–93.

31. D. O'Donoghue, "Fatal Pneumococcal Septicaemia in Coeliac Disease," *Postgraduate Medical Journal* 62, no. 725 (1986): 229–30.

32. B. William and G. Corazza, "Hyposplenism: A Comprehensive Review. Part I: Basic Concepts and Causes," *Hematology* 12, no. 1 (2007): 1–13.

33. William and Corazza, "Hyposplenism."

34. B. Huppert, M. Farrell, A. Kawashima, and J. Murray, "Diagnosis of Cavitating Mesenteric Lymph Node Syndrome in Celiac Disease Using MRI," *American Journal of Roentgenology* 183, no. 5 (2004): 1375–77.

35. Huppert et al., "Diagnosis of Cavitating Mesenteric Lymph Node Syndrome in Celiac Disease Using MRI."

36. J. O'Grady, F. Stevens, B. Harding, T. O'Gorman, B. McNicholl, and C. McCarthy, "Hyposplenism and Gluten-Sensitive Enteropathy. Natural History, Incidence, and Relationship to Diet and Small Bowel Morphology," *Gastroenterology* 87, no. 6 (1984): 1326–31.

37. A. Howat, J. McPhie, D. Smith, N. Agel, A. Taylor, S. Cairns, W. Thomas, and J. Underwood, "Cavitation of Mesenteric Lymph Nodes: A Rare Complication of Coeliac Disease Associated with a Poor Outcome," *Histopathology* 27, no. 4 (1995): 349–54; R. Arotçarena, P. Hammel, T. Terris, A. Guth, P. Bernades, and P. Ruszniewski, "Regression of Mesenteric Lymph Node Cavitation Syndrome Complicating Celiac Disease after a Gluten Free Diet," *Gastroentérologie Clinique et Biologique* 24, no. 5 (2000): 579–81.

38. B. Lebwohl, F. Granath, A. Ekbom, K. Smedby, J. Murray, A. Neugut, P. Green, and J. Ludvigsson, "Mucosal Healing and Risk for Lymphoproliferative Malignancy in Celiac Disease: A Population-Based Cohort Study," *Annals of Internal Medicine* 159, no. 3 (2013): 169–75.

39. Lebwohl et al., "Mucosal Healing and Risk for Lymphoproliferative Malignancy in Celiac Disease."

40. Lebwohl et al., "Mucosal Healing and Risk for Lymphoproliferative Malignancy in Celiac Disease."

41. Halfdanarson, Litzow, and Murray, "Hematologic Manifestations of Celiac Disease."

42. S. Saibeni, A. Lecchi, G. Meucci, M. Cattaneo, L. Tagliabue, E. Rondonotti, S. Formenti, R. de Franchis, and M. Vecchi, "Prevalence of Hyperhomocysteinemia in Adult Gluten-Sensitive Enteropathy at Diagnosis: Role of B12, Folate and Genetics," *Journal of Clinical Gastroenterology Hepatology* 3, no. 6 (2005): 574–80.

43. Saibeni et al., "Prevalence of Hyperhomocysteinemia in Adult Gluten-Sensitive Enteropathy at Diagnosis."

44. C. Chen, E. Cumbler, and A. Triebling, "Coagulopathy Due to Celiac Disease Presenting as Intramuscular Hemorrhage," *Journal of General Internal Medicine* 22, no. 11 (2007): 1608–12.

45. Chen, Cumbler, and Triebling, "Coagulopathy Due to Celiac Disease Presenting as Intramuscular Hemorrhage."

46. Chen, Cumbler, and Triebling, "Coagulopathy Due to Celiac Disease Presenting as Intramuscular Hemorrhage."

47. R. Waldo, "Iron-Deficiency Anemia Due to Silent Celiac Sprue," *Baylor University Medical Center Proceedings (BUMC Proceedings)* 15, no. 1 (2002): 16–17.

48. Halfdanarson, Litzow, and Murray, "Hematologic Manifestations of Celiac Disease."

49. A. Hoffbrand, "Anaemia and Coeliac Disease," *Journal of Clinical Gastroenterology* 3 (1974): 71–89.

50. R. Mody, P. Brown, and D. Wechsler, "Refractory Iron Deficiency Anemia as the Primary Clinical Manifestation of Celiac Disease," *Journal of Pediatric Hematology/Oncology* 25, no. 2 (2003): 169–72.

51. G. Bottaro, F. Cataldo, N. Rotolo, M. Spina, and G. Corazza, "The Clinical Pattern of Subclinical/Silent Celiac Disease: An Analysis on 1026 Consecutive Cases," *American Journal of Gastroenterology* 94, no. 3 (1999): 691–96.

52. I. Kosnai, P. Kuitunen, and M. Siimes, "Iron Deficiency in Children with Coeliac Disease on Treatment with Gluten-Free Diet: Role of Intestinal Blood Loss," *Archives of Disease in Childhood* 54, no. 5 (1979): 375–78.

53. M. Mant, V. Bain, C. Maguire, K. Murland, and B. Yacyshyn, "Prevalence of Occult Gastrointestinal Bleeding in Celiac Disease," *Journal of Clinical Gastroenterology and Hepatology* 4, no. 4 (2006): 451–54.

54. R. Shamir, A. Levine, and M. Yalon-Hacohen, "Faecal Occult Blood in Children with Celiac Disease," *European Journal of Pediatrics* 159 (2000): 832–934.

55. Halfdanarson, Litzow, and Murray, "Hematologic Manifestations of Celiac Disease."

56. Halfdanarson, Litzow, and Murray, "Hematologic Manifestations of Celiac Disease."

57. J. Gregory III and E. Quinlivan, "In Vivo Kinetics of Folic Metabolism," *Annual Review of Nutrition* (2002): 199–220.

58. Halfdanarson, Litzow, and Murray, "Hematologic Manifestations of Celiac Disease."

59. Gregory III and Quinlivan, "In Vivo Kinetics of Folic Metabolism."

60. Halfdanarson, Litzow, and Murray, "Hematologic Manifestations of Celiac Disease."

61. Halfdanarson, Litzow, and Murray, "Hematologic Manifestations of Celiac Disease."

62. Hoffbrand, "Anaemia and Coeliac Disease."

63. D. Stevens, "Nutritional Anemia in Childhood Coeliac Disease," *Proceedings of the Nutrition Society* 38, no. 3 (1979): 102A.

64. Halfdanarson, Litzow, and Murray, "Hematologic Manifestations of Celiac Disease."

65. A. M. Kuzminski, E. J. Del Giacco, R. H. Allen, S. P. Stabler, and J. Lindembaum, "Effective Treatment of Cobalamin Deficiency with Oral Cobalamin," *Blood* 92 (1998): 1191–98.

66. Halfdanarson, Litzow, and Murray, "Hematologic Manifestations of Celiac Disease."

67. W. Dickey and D. F. Hughes, "Histology of the Terminal Ileum in Coeliac Disease," *Scandinavian Journal of Gastroenterology* 39, no. 7 (2004): 665–67.

68. Halfdanarson, Litzow, and Murray, "Hematologic Manifestations of Celiac Disease."

69. Halfdanarson, Litzow, and Murray, "Hematologic Manifestations of Celiac Disease."

70. "Dermatitis Herpetiformis: Skin Manifestation of Celiac Disease," National Digestive Diseases Information Clearinghouse (NDDIC), accessed November 9, 2013, http://www.digestive.niddk.nih.gov/ddiseases/pubs/dh.

71. K. Campbell, "Five Common Skin Conditions Associated with Celiac Disease," Celiac.com, February 16, 2010, accessed November 9, 2013, http://www.celiac.com/articles/22021/1/Five-Common-Skin-Conditions-Associated-With-Celiac-Disease/Page1.html.

72. B. Scott, S. Young, S. Rajah, J. Marks, and M. Losowsky, "Celiac Disease and Dermatitis Herpetiformis: Further Studies of their Relationship," *Gut* 17, no. 10 (1976): 759–62.

73. V. Petronic-Rosic, "Dermatitis Herpetiformis and Celiac Disease," *Impact: A Publication of the University of Chicago Celiac Disease Center*, 1st Quarter (2011): 1–3, accessed November 9, 2013, http://www.cureceliacdisease.org.

74. M. Caproni, E. Antiga, L. Melani, and P. Fabbri, "Guidelines for the Diagnosis and Treatment of Dermatitis Herpetiformis," *Journal of the European Academy of Dermatology and Venereology* 23, no. 6 (2009): 633–38.

75. J. Hall and B. Hall, *Hall's Manual of Skin as a Marker of Underlying Disease* (Shelton, CT: People's Medical Publishing House-USA, 2011).

76. G. Corazza, M. Andreani, N. Venturo, M. Bernardi, A. Tosti, G. Gasbarrini, "Celiac Disease and Alopecia Areata: Report of a New Association," *Gastroenterology* 109, no. 4 (1995): 1333–37.

77. H. Pruessner, "Detecting Celiac Disease in Your Patients," *American Family Physician* 57, no. 5 (1998): 1023–34.

78. M. Hautekeete, L. De Clerck, and W. Stevens, "Chronic Urticaria Associated with Celiac Disease," *Lancet* 1, no. 8525 (1987): 157; C. Gallo, G. Vighi, J. Schroeder, et al., "Chronic Urticaria Atopic Dermatitis and Celiac Disease," *American Journal of Gastroenterology* 87, no. 11 (1992): 1684; M. Liutu, K. Kalimo, J. Uksila, and H. Kalimo, "Etiologic Aspects of Chronic Urticaria," *International Journal of Dermatology* 37 (1998): 515–19; E. Scala, M. Giani, L. Pirrotta, E. Guerra, O. De Pita, and P. Puddu, "Urticaria and Adult Celiac Disease," *Allergy* 54 (1999): 1008–9; A. Levine, I. Dalal, and Y. Bujanover, "Celiac Disease Associated with Familial Chronic Urticaria and Thyroid Autoimmunity in a Child," *Pediatrics* 104, no. 2 (1999): e25.

79. M. Gabrielli, M. Candelli, F. Cremonini, V. Ojetti, L. Santarelli, E. Nista, E. Nucera, D. Schiavino, G. Patriarca, G. Gasbarrini, P. Pola, and A. Gasbarrini, "Idiopathic Chronic Urticaria and Celiac Disease," *Digestive Diseases and Sciences* 50, no. 9 (2005): 1702–4.

80. L. Abenavoli, I. Proietti, L. Leggio, A. Ferrulli, L. Vonghia, R. Capizzi, M. Rotoli, P. Amerio, G. Gasbarrini, and G. Addolorato, "Cutaneous Manifestations in Celiac Disease," *World Journal of Gastroenterology* 12, no. 6 (2006): 843–52.

81. L. Guenther and W. Gulliver, "Psoriasis Comorbidities," *Journal of Cutaneous Medicine and Surgery* 13 (Suppl. 2) (2009): S77–87.

82. S. Birkenfeld, J. Dreiher, D. Weitzman, and A. Cohen, "Celiac Disease Associated with Psoriasis," *British Journal of Dermatology* 161, no. 6 (2009): 1331–34.

83. S. Singh, G. Sonkar, and S. Usha, "Celiac Disease-Associated Antibodies in Patients with Psoriasis and Correlation with HLA Cw6," *Journal of Clinical Laboratory Analysis* 24, no. 4 (2010): 269–72.

84. Singh, Sonkar, and Usha, "Celiac Disease-Associated Antibodies in Patients with Psoriasis and Correlation with HLA Cw6."

85. Campbell, "Five Common Skin Conditions Associated with Celiac Disease."

86. J. Anderson, "Can Eating Gluten-Free Help with Your Eczema Treatment?" About.com, accessed November 9, 2013, http://celiacdisease.about.com/od/commoncomplicationsofcd/a/Can-Eating-Gluten-Free-Help-With-Your-Eczema-Treatment.htm.

87. Campbell, "Five Common Skin Conditions Associated with Celiac Disease."

88. Campbell, "Five Common Skin Conditions Associated with Celiac Disease."

89. G. Cicarelli, G. Della Rocca, M. Amboni, C. Ciacci, G. Mazzacca, A. Filla, and P. Barone, "Clinical and Neurological Abnormalities in Adult Celiac Disease," *Journal of the Neurological Sciences* 24, no. 5 (2003): 311–17.

90. "Peripheral Neuropathy," National Foundation for Celiac Awareness, accessed December 5, 2013, www.celiaccentral.org.

91. J. Kaplan, D. Pack, D. Horoupian, T. DeSouza, M. Brin, and H. Schaumburg, "Distal Axonopathy Associated with Chronic Gluten Enteropathy: A Treatable Disorder," *Neurology* 38, no. 4 (1988): 642–45; L. Luostarinen, S. Himanen, M. Luostarinen, P. Collin, and T. Pirttilä, "Neuromuscular and Sensory Disturbances in Patients with Well Treated Celiac Disease," *Journal of Neurology, Neurosurgery & Psychiatry* 74, no. 4 (2003): 490–94.

92. W. Cooke and W. Smith, "Neurological Disorders Associated with Adult Celiac Disease," *Brain* 89, no. 4 (1966): 683–722.

93. M. Hadjivassiliou, D. Sanders, N. Woodroofe, C. Williamson, and R. Grünewald, "Gluten Ataxia," *Cerebellum* 7, no. 3 (2008): 494–98.

94. Hadjivassiliou et al., "Gluten Ataxia."

95. H. Freeman, "Neurological Disorders in Adult Celiac Disease," *Canadian Journal of Gastroenterology & Hepatology* 22, no. 11 (2008): 909–11.

96. "The Increased Risk of Epilepsy in Individuals with Celiac Disease," accessed December 13, 2013, http://www.epilepsy.com/newsletter/jul12/epilepsy_celiac_disease.

97. "The Increased Risk of Epilepsy in Individuals with Celiac Disease."

98. "Gluten Intolerance & Seizures," Health Now Medical Center, accessed December 13, 2013, http://www.healthnowmedical.com.

99. A. Cernibori and G. Gobbi, "Partial Seizures, Cerebral Calcifications and Celiac Disease," *Italian Journal of Neurological Sciences* 16, no. 3 (1995): 187–91.

100. Cernibori and Gobbi, "Partial Seizures, Cerebral Calcifications and Celiac Disease."

101. M. Emami, H. Taheri, S. Kohestani, A. Chitsaz, M. Etemadifar, S. Karimi, M. Eshaghi, and M. Hashemi, "How Frequent Is Celiac Disease among Epileptic Patients?" *Journal of Gastrointestinal and Liver Diseases* 17, no. 4 (2008): 379–82.

102. M. Collado, M. Calabuig, and Y. Sanz, "Differences between the Fecal Microbiota of Celiac Infants and Healthy Controls," *Current Issues in Intestinal Microbiology* 8, no. 1 (2007): 9–14.

103. Collado, Calabuig, and Sanz, "Differences between the Fecal Microbiota of Celiac Infants and Healthy Controls."

104. I. Nadal, E. Donat, C. Ribes-Koninckx, M. Calabuig, and Y. Sanz, "Imbalance in the Composition of the Duodenal Microbiota of Children with Celiac Disease," *Journal of Medical Microbiology* 56, no. 12 (2007): 1669–74.

105. M. Kagnoff, R. K. Austin, J. Hubert, J. Bernardin, and D. Kasarda, "Possible Role for a Human Adenovirus in the Pathogenesis of Celiac Disease," *Journal of Experimental Medicine* 160, no. 5 (1984): 1544–57.

106. G. Corazza, "Complicated Adult Celiac Disease," Associazone Italiana Caliachia, accessed November 5, 2013, www.celiachia.it.

107. "Celiac Disease: Oral and Dental Manifestations," Canadian Celiac Association, accessed October 27, 2013, http://www.celiac.ca.

108. L. Aine, M. Maki, P. Collin, and O. Keyrilainen, "Dental Enamel Effects in Celiac Disease," *Journal of Oral Pathology & Medicine* 19, no. 6 (1990): 241–45.

109. "Celiac Disease: Oral and Dental Manifestations."

110. Aine, Maki, Collin, and Keyrilainen, "Dental Enamel Effects in Celiac Disease."

111. "Dental Enamel Defects and Celiac Disease," National Institute of Health, accessed December 16, 2013, http://www.celiac.nih.gov/DentalEnamel.aspx.

112. "Dental Enamel Defects and Celiac Disease."

113. "Dental Enamel Defects and Celiac Disease."

114. "Dental Enamel Defects and Celiac Disease."

115. M. Vanderpump and W. Tunbridge, *Thyroid Disease: The Facts* (New York: Oxford University Press, 2008).

116. P. Collin, J. Salmi, O. Hallstrom, T. Reunala, and A. Pasternack, "Autoimmune Thyroid Disorders and Celiac Disease," *European Journal of Endocrinology* 130 (1994): 137–40; K. Kaukinen, P. Collin, A. Mykkanen, J. Partanen, M. Maki, and J. Salmi, "Celiac Disease and Autoimmune Endocrinologic Disorders," *Digestive Diseases and Sciences* 44, no. 7 (1999): 1428–33; C. Ch'ng, M. Jones, and J. Kingham, "Celiac Disease and Autoimmune Thyroid Disease," *Clinical Medicine & Research* 5, no. 3 (2007): 184–92; P. Elfstrom, S. Montgomery, O. Kampe, A. Ekbom, and J. Ludvigsson, "Risk of Thyroid Disease in Individuals with Celiac Disease," *Journal of Clinical Endocrinology and Metabolism* 93, no. 10 (2008): 3915–21.

117. Elfstrom et al., "Risk of Thyroid Disease in Individuals with Celiac Disease."

118. Ch'ng, Jones, and Kingham, "Celiac Disease and Autoimmune Thyroid Disease"; D. Larizza, V. Calcaterra, C. De Giacomo, A. De Silvestri, M. Asti, C. Badulli, M. Autelli, E. Coslovich, and M. Martinetti, "Celiac Disease in Children with Autoimmune Thyroid Disease," *Journal of Pediatrics* 139, no. 5 (2001): 738–40.

119. C. Harris and G. Kaplan, "Two of a Kind–Research Connects Celiac and Thyroid Diseases and Suggests a Gluten-Free Diet Benefits Both," *Today's Dietitian* 12, no. 11 (2010): 52.

120. A. Abdo, J. Meddings, and M. Swain, "Liver Abnormalities in Celiac Disease," *Clinical Gastroenterology & Hepatology* 2, no. 2 (2004): 107–12.

121. U. Volta, L. De Franceschi, F. Lari, N. Molinaro, M. Zoli, and F. Bianchi, "Celiac Disease Hidden by Cryptogenic Hypertransaminasaemia," *Lancet* 352, no. 9121 (1998): 26–29.

122. S. Lindgren, K. Sjoberg, and S. Eriksson, "Unsuspected Celiac Disease in Chronic 'Cryptogenic' Liver Disease," *Scandinavian Journal of Gastroenterology* 29, no. 7 (1994): 661–64.

123. M. Bardella, M. Vecchi, D. Conte, E. Del Ninno, M. Fraquelli, S. Pacchetti, E. Minola, M. Landoni, B. Cesana, and R. DeFranchis, "Chronic Unexplained Hypertransaminasemia May Be Caused by Occult Celiac Disease," *Hepatology* 29, no. 3 (1999): 654–57.

124. B. Hagander, N. Berg, L. Brandt, A. Norden, K. Sjolund, and M. Stenstam, "Hepatic Injury in Adult Celiac Disease," *Lancet* 2, no. 8032 (1977): 270–72.

125. M. Bonamico, G. Pitzalis, and F. Culasso, "Hepatic damage During Celiac Disease in Childhood," *Minerva Pediatrica* 38, no. 21 (1986): 959–62.

126. M. Jacobsen, O. Fausa, K. Elgjo, and E. Schrumpf, "Hepatic Lesions in Adult Celiac Disease," *Scandinavian Journal of Gastroenterology* 25, no. 7 (1990): 656–62; M. Bardella, M. Fraquelli, M. Quatrini, N. Molteni, P. Bianchi, and D. Conte, "Prevalence of Hypertransaminasemia in Adult Celiac Patients and Effect of Gluten-Free Diet," *Hepatology* 22, no. 3 (1995): 833–36.

127. G. Novacek, W. Miehsler, F. Wrba, P. Ferenci, E. Penner, and H. Vogelsang, "Prevalence and Clinical Importance of Hypertransaminasaemia in Celiac Disease," *European Journal of Gastroenterology and Hepatology* 11, no. 3 (1999): 283–88.

128. J. Kingham and D. Parker, "The Association between Primary Biliary Cirrhosis and Celiac Disease: A Study of Relative Prevalences," *Gut* 42, no. 1 (1998): 120–22.

129. H. Sorensen, A. Thulstrup, P. Blomqvist, B. Norgaard, K. Fonager, and A. Ekbom, "Risk of Primary Biliary Liver Cirrhosis in Patients with Celiac Disease: Danish and Swedish Cohort Data," *Gut* 44, no. 5 (1999): 736–38; W. Dickey, S. McMillan, and M. Callender, "High Prevalence of Celiac Sprue among Patients with Primary Biliary Cirrhosis," *Journal of Clinical Gastroenterology* 25, no. 1 (1997): 328–29.

130. M. Bardella, M. Quatrini, M. Zuin, M. Podda, L. Cesarini, P. Velio, P. Bianchi, and D. Conte, "Screening Patients with Celiac Disease for Primary Biliary Cirrhosis and Vice Versa," *American Journal of Gastroenterology* 92, no. 9 (1997): 1524–26; U. Volta, L. De Franceschi, N. Molinaro, F. Cassani, L. Muratori, M. Lenzi, F. Bianchi, and A. Czaja, "Frequency and Significance of Anti-Gliadin and Anti-Endomysial Antibodies in Autoimmune Hepatitis," *Digestive Diseases and Sciences* 43, no. 10 (1998): 2190–95.

131. E. Schrumpf, M. Abdelnoor, and O. Fausa, "Risk Factors in Primary Sclerosing Cholangitis," *Journal of Hepatology* 21, no. 6 (1994): 1061–66.

132. U. Volta, L. Rodrigo, A. Granito, N. Petrolini, P. Muratori, L. Muratori, A. Linares, L. Veronesi, D. Fuentes, D. Zauli, and F. Bianchi, "Celiac Disease in Autoimmune Cholestatic Liver Disorders," *American Journal of Gastroenterology* 97, no. 10 (2002): 2609–13.

133. Volta et al., "Frequency and Significance of Anti-Gliadin and Anti-Endomysial Antibodies in Autoimmune Hepatitis."

134. Jacobsen et al., "Hepatic Lesions in Adult Celiac Disease"; Novacek et al., "Prevalence and Clinical Importance of Hypertransaminasaemia in Celiac Disease."

135. Abdo, Meddings, and Swain, "Liver Abnormalities in Celiac Disease."

136. R. Saalman and S. Fällström, "High Incidence of Urinary Tract Infection in Patients with Coeliac Disease," *Archives of Diseases in Childhood* 74, no. 2 (1996): 170–71.

137. Saalman and Fällström, "High Incidence of Urinary Tract Infection in Patients with Coeliac Disease."

138. E. Coli Infection, WebMD, accessed December 18, 2013, http://www.webmd.com.

139. R. Gama and F. Schweitzer, "Renal Calculus: A Unique Presentation of Celiac Disease," *British Journal of Urology International* 84, no. 4 (1999): 304–6.

140. E. Yarnell, "A Child with Atypical Celiac Disease and Recurrent Urolithiasis," *Italian Journal of Kidney Diseases* 6, no. 2 (2012): 146–48.

141. K. Jhaveri, V. D'Agati, R. Pursell, and D. Serur, "Celiac Sprue-Associated Membranoproliferative Glomerulonephritis (MPGN)," *Nephrology Dialysis Transplantation* 24, no. 11 (2009): 3545–48.

142. T. Gardner and A. Warner, *Questions and Answers about the Diseases of the Pancreas* (Burlington, MA: Jones & Bartlett Learning, 2012).

143. D. Dreiling, "The Pancreatic Secretion in the Malabsorption Syndrome and Related Malnutrition States," *Journal of the Mount Sinai Hospital* 24, no. 3 (1957): 243–50.

144. E. DiMagno, W. Go, and W. Summerskill, "Impaired Cholecystokinin-pancreozymin Secretion, Intraluminal Dilution, and Maldigestion of Fat in Sprue," *Gastroenterology* 63, no. 1 (1972): 25–32; P. Regan and E. DiMagno, "Exocrine Pancreatic Insufficiency in Celiac Sprue: A Cause of Treatment Failure," *Gastroenterology* 78, no. 3 (1980): 484–87; Z. Weizman, J. Hamilton, H. Kopelman, G. Cleghorn, and P. Durie, "Treatment Failure in Celiac Disease Due to Coexistent Exocrine Pancreatic Insufficiency," *Pediatrics* 80, no. 6 (1987): 924–26; H. Freeman, "Hepatobiliary Tract and Pancreatic Disorders in Celiac Disease," *Canadian Journal of Gastroenterology* 11, no. 1 (1997): 77–81.

145. J. Leeds, A. Hopper, D. Hurlstone, S. Edwards, M. McAlindon, A. Lobo, M. Donnelly, S. Morley, and D. Sanders, "Is Exocrine Pancreatic Insufficiency in Adult Celiac Disease a Cause of Persisting Symptoms?" *Alimentary Pharmacology & Therapeutics* 25, no. 3 (2007): 265–71.

146. K. Evans, J. Leeds, S. Morley, and D. Sanders, "Pancreatic Insufficiency in Adult Celiac Disease: Do Patients Require Long-Term Enzyme Supplementation?" *Digestive Diseases and Sciences* 55, no. 10 (2010): 2999–3004.

147. F. Farraye, *Questions & Answers about Ulcerative Colitis* (Sudbury, MA: Jones & Bartlett Learning, 2011).

148. A. Yang, Y. Chen, E. Scherl, A. Neugut, G. Bhagat, and P. Green, "Inflammatory Bowel Disease in Patients with Celiac Disease," *Inflammatory Bowel Diseases* 11, no. 6 (2005): 528–32.

149. J. Leeds, B. Horoldt, R. Sidhu, A. Hopper, K. Robinson, B. Toulson, L. Dixon, A. Lobo, M. E. McAlindon, D. Hurlston, and D. Sanders, "Is There an Association between Celiac Disease and Inflammatory Bowel Diseases? A Study of Relative Prevalence in Comparison with Population Controls," *Scandinavian Journal of Gastroenterology* 42, no. 10 (2007): 1214–20.

150. G. Casella, R. D'Inca, L. Oliva, M. Daperno, V. Saladino, G. Zoli, V. Annese, W. Fries, and C. Cortellezi, "Prevalence of Celiac Disease in Inflammatory Bowel Diseases: An IG-IBD Multicenter Study," *Digestive and Liver Disease* 42, no. 3 (2010): 175–78.

151. E. Magee, *Tell Me What to Eat If I Have Irritable Bowel Syndrome* (New York: Rosen Publishing Group, 2009).

152. D. Sanders, "Celiac Disease and IBS-Type Symptoms: The Relationship Exists in Both Directions," *American Journal of Gastroenterology* 98, no. 3 (2003): 707–8; Z. Mehdi, E. Sakineh, F. Mohammad, R. Mansour, and A. Alireza, "Celiac Disease: Serologic Prevalence in Patients with Irritable Bowel Syndrome," *Journal of Research in Medical Sciences* 17, no. 9 (2012): 839–42.

153. D. Sanders, M. Carter, D. Hurlstone, A. Pearce, A. Ward, M. McAlindon, and A. Lobo, "Association of Adult Celiac Disease with Irritable Bowel Syndrome: A Case-Control Study in Patients Fulfilling ROME II Criteria Referred to Secondary Care," *Lancet* 358, no. 9292 (2001): 1504–8.

154. B. Shahbazkhani, M. Forootan, S. Merat, M. Akbari, S. Nasserimoghadam, H. Vahedi, and R. Malekzadeh, "Celiac Disease Presenting with Symptoms of Irritable Bowel Syndrome," *Alimentary Pharmacology & Therapeutics* 18, no. 2 (2003): 231–35.

155. A. Ford, W. Chey, N. Talley, A. Malhotra, B. Spiegel, and P. Moayyedi, "Yield of Diagnostic Tests for Celiac Disease in Individuals with Symptoms Suggestive of Irritable Bowel Syndrome: A Systematic Review and Meta-Analysis," *Archives of Internal Medicine* 169, no. 7 (2009): 651–58.

156. S. Mein and U. Ladabaum, "Serological Testing for Celiac Disease in Patients with Symptoms of Irritable Bowel Syndrome: A Cost-Effectiveness Analysis," *Alimentary Pharmacology & Therapeutics* 19, no. 11 (2004): 1199–1210.

157. M. Galsky, *Everything You Need to Know about Cancer* (Sudbury, MA: Jones and Bartlett, 2010).

158. A. Adrouny, *Understanding Colon Cancer* (Jackson: University Press of Mississippi, 2002).

159. C. Swinson, G. Slavin, E. Coles, and C. Booth, "Celiac Disease and Malignancy," *Lancet* 1, no. 8316 (1983): 111–15.

160. J. Askling, M. Linet, G. Gridley, T. Halstensen, K. Ekstrom, and A. Ekbom, "Cancer Incidence in a Population-Based Cohort of Individuals Hospitalized with Celiac Disease or Dermatitis Herpetiformis," *Gastroenterology* 123, no. 5 (2002): 1428–35.

161. C. Catassi, I. Bearzi, and G. Holmes, "Association of Celiac Disease and Intestinal Lymphomas and Other Cancers," *Gastroenterology* 128, no. 4 (2005): S79–86.

162. H. Freeman, "Malignancy in Adult Celiac Disease," *World Journal of Gastroenterology* 15, no. 13 (2009): 1581–83.

163. B. Lebwohl, E. Stavsky, A. Neugut, and P. Green, "Risk of Colorectal Adenomas in Patients with Celiac Disease," *Alimentary Pharmacology and Therapeutics* 32 (2010): 1037–43.

164. R. Warren, "Infertility and Celiac Disease," *Creating Families* 4, no. 2 (2008): 55–56.

165. Warren, "Infertility and Celiac Disease."

166. G. Meloni, S. Dessole, N. Vargiu, P. Tomasi, and S. Musumeci, "The Prevalence of Celiac Disease in Infertility," *Human Reproduction* 14, no. 11 (1999): 2759–61.

167. M. Brill, *Diabetes* (Minneapolis, MN: Twenty-First Century Books, 2011).

168. G. Holmes, "Celiac Disease and Type 1 Diabetes Mellitus: The Case for Screening," *Diabetic Medicine* 18, no. 13 (2001): 169–77.

169. U. Volta, F. Tovoli, and G. Caio, "Clinical and Immunological Features of Celiac Disease in Patients with Type 1 Diabetes Mellitus," *Expert Review of Gastroenterology and Hepatology* 5, no. 4 (2011): 479–87.

170. D. Smyth, V. Plagnol, N. Walker, J. Cooper, K. Downes, J. Yang, J. Howson, H. Stevens, R. McManus, C. Wijmenga, G. Heap, P. Dubois, D. Clayton, K. Hunt, D. van Heel, and J. Todd, "Shared and Distinct Genetic Variants in Type 1 Diabetes and Celiac Disease," *New England Journal of Medicine* 359, no. 26 (2008): 2767–77.

171. Smyth et al., "Shared and Distinct Genetic Variants in Type 1 Diabetes and Celiac Disease."

172. L. Philipson and J. Martin, "Celiac Disease and Type 1 Diabetes: Autoimmune Disorders with Common Roots," *Impact: A Publication of the University of Chicago Celiac Disease Center*, 4th Quarter (2011).

9. PAIN AND CELIAC DISEASE

1. P. Green, H. Peter, and R. Jones, *Celiac Disease: A Hidden Epidemic* (New York: William Morrow, 2009).

2. J. Murray, T. Watson, B. Clearman, and F. Mitros, "Effect of a Gluten-Free Diet on Gastrointestinal Symptoms in Celiac Disease," *American Journal of Clinical Nutrition* 79, no. 4 (2004): 669–73.

3. Green, Peter, and Jones, *Celiac Disease*.

4. J. Anderson, "Celiac Disease and Joint Pain: Gluten-Free Diet Should Help You Improve Celiac Disease," About.com, March 29, 2014, http://celiacdisease.about.com.

5. G. Diaconu, M. Burlea, I. Grigore, D. Anton, and M. Trandafir, "Celiac Disease with Neurologic Manifestations in Children," *Revista Medico-Chirurgicala a Societatii de Medici si Naturalisti din Iasi's* 117, no. 1 (2013): 88–94.

6. "Celiac Disease and Neurological Conditions," National Foundation for Celiac Awareness, accessed November 19, 2013, http://www.celiaccentral.org/neurological-conditions.

7. H. Freeman, "Neurological Disorders in Adult Celiac Disease," *Canadian Journal of Gastroenterology* 22, no. 11 (2008): 909–91.

8. R. Collins, ed., *Differential Diagnosis in Primary Care*, 5th ed. (Philadelphia: Lippincott Williams & Wilkins, 2008).

9. N. Enattah, T. Sahi, E. Savilahti, J. Terwilliger, L. Peltonen, and I. Järvelä, "Identification of a Variant Associated with Adult-Type Hypolactasia," *Nature Genetics* 30, no. 2 (2002): 233–37.

10. Green, Peter, and Jones, *Celiac Disease: A Hidden Epidemic*.

11. M. Melin-Rogovin, "Refractory Sprue," Celiac.com, accessed November 26, 2013, http://www.celiac.com/articles/710/1/Refractory-Sprue-by-Michelle-Melin-Rogovin-University-of-Chicago-Celiac-Disease-Program/Page1.html.

12. D. Martin, "Prednisone and Other Corticosteroids," Mayo Clinic.com, accessed November 20, 2013, http://www.mayoclinic.org/steroids/art-20045692.

13. V. Conte and M. Greco, "The Indications and Controversies for the Use of Corticosteroids in Respiratory Deficits in the Multiple-Trauma Patient," *Minerva Chirurgica* 54, no. 9 (1999): 607–25.

14. "Side Effects of Corticosteroids," NHS Choices.com, accessed November 20, 2013, www.nhs.uk/Conditions/Corticosteroid-(drugs)/Pages/Sideeffects.aspx.

15. Martin, "Prednisone and other Corticosteroids."

16. "Dermatitis Herpetiformis," American Osteopathic College of Dermatology, accessed February 2, 2014, http://www.aocd.org/?page=DermatitisHerpetifo.

17. J. Smith, J. Fowler, and J. Zone, "The Effect of Ibuprofen on Serum Dapsone Levels and Disease Activity in Dermatitis Herpetiformis," *Archives of Dermatology* 130, no. 2 (1994): 257–59.

10. NATURAL TREATMENTS AND DIET

1. "Celiac Disease Facts and Figures," National Foundation for Celiac Awareness, accessed December 13, 2013, http://www.celiaccentral.org/celiac-disease/facts-and-figures.

2. "Facts and Figures 2012, The Pharmaceutical Industry and Global Health," International Federation of Pharamaceutical Managers & Associations, accessed December 3, 2013, http://www.ifpma.org.

3. S. Bower and M. Sharrett, *Celiac Disease: A Guide to Living with Gluten Intolerance* (New York: Demos Health, 2006).

4. J. Shepard, *The First Year: Celiac Disease and Living Gluten-Free: An Essential Guide for the Newly Diagnosed* (Cambridge, MA: Da Capo Press, 2008).

5. Shepard, *The First Year.*

6. Bower and Sharrett, *Celiac Disease.*

7. L. Dawn, "Top 12 Benefits of Aloe Vera," Sacred Source Nutrition, accessed December 9, 2013, http://www.sacredsourcenutrition.com/top-12-benefits-of-aloe-vera.

8. A. Bhupinder, "Abdominal Pain," Medicine Net, September 30, 2013, accessed November 25, 2013, http://www.medicinenet.com/abdominal_pain_causes_remedies_treatment/article.htm.

9. Bhupinder, "Abdominal Pain."

10. L. Keir, B. Wise, and C. Krebs, *Medical Assisting: Essentials of Administrative and Clinical Competencies*, 1st ed. (Columbus, OH: Cengage Learning, 2002).

11. Keir, Wise, and Krebs, *Medical Assisting.*

12. J. Heller, "Abdominal Pain," U.S. National Library of Medicine, accessed November 30, 2013, www.nlm.nih.gov.

13. B. Bolen, "Eating Tips for When You Have Irritable Bowel Syndrome Pain," About.com, accessed on November 30, 2013, http://ibs.about.com/od/ibs-food/qt/EatforPain.htm.

14. T. Bommarito, *The Beginning to a Gluten Free Lifestyle* (Nashville: Thomas Nelson, 2012).

15. S. Biradar, S. Bahagvati, and B. Shegunshi, "Probiotics and Antibiotics: A Brief Overview," *Internet Journal of Nutrition and Wellness* 2, no. 1 (2005).

16. G. Reid, J. Jass, M. Sebulsky, and J. McCormick, "Potential Uses of Probiotics in Clinical Practice," *Clinical Microbiology Reviews* 16, no. 4 (2003): 658–72.

17. C. Lutter and K. Dewey, "Proposed Nutrient Composition for Fortified Complementary Foods," *Journal of Nutrition* 133, no. 9 (2003): 3011S–20S.

18. M. Zamakhchari, G. Wei, F. Dewhirst, J. Lee, D. Schuppan, F. Oppenheim, and E. Helmerhorst, "Identification of Rothia Bacteria as Gluten-Degrading Natural Colonizers of the Upper Gastro-Intestinal Tract," *PLoS One* 6, no. 9 (2011): e24455.

19. Bommarito, *The Beginning to a Gluten Free Lifestyle.*

20. Bommarito, *The Beginning to a Gluten Free Lifestyle.*

21. Bommarito, *The Beginning to a Gluten Free Lifestyle.*

22. S. Devkota, Y. Wang, and E. Chang, "Dietary Fat-Induced Taurocholic Acid Promotes Pathobiont and Colitis in IL-10$^{-/-}$ Mice," *Nature* 487, no. 7405 (2012): 104–8.

23. Devkota, Wang, and Chang, "Dietary Fat-Induced Taurocholic Acid Promotes Pathobiont and Colitis in IL-10$^{-/-}$ Mice."

24. V. Padler-Karavani, H. Yu, H. Cao, H. Chokhawala, F. Karp, N. Varki, X. Chen, and A. Varki, "Diversity in Specificity, Abundance, and Composition of Anti-Neu5Gc Antibodies in Normal Humans: Potential Implications for Disease," *Glycobiology* 18, no. 10 (2008): 818–30.

I I. SURGERY FOR CELIAC DISEASE

1. I. Blumer and S. Crowe, *Celiac Disease for Dummies* (Mississauga, ON: John Wiley and Sons Canada, 2010).

2. J. Norton, P. Barie, R. Bollinger, A. Chang, S. Lowry, S. Mulvihill, H. Pass, and R. Thompsom, *Surgery: Basic Science and Clinical Evidence* (New York: Springer, 2008).

3. D. Sanders, A. Hopper, I. Azmy, N. Rahman, D. Hurlstone, J. Leeds, R. George, and N. Bhala, "Association of Adult Celiac Disease with Surgical Abdominal Pain: A Case-Control Study in Patients Referred to Secondary Care," *Annals of Surgery* 242, no. 2 (2005): 201–7.

4. "Testing for Celiac Disease in Patients with Surgical Abdominal Pain," accessed January 27, 2014, Celiac.com, http://www.celiac.com.

5. M. Grade, M. Quintel, and B. Ghadimi, "Standard Perioperative Management in Gastrointestinal Surgery," *Langenbeck's Archives of Surgery* 396, no. 5 (2011): 591–606.

6. A. Ghaferi, J. Birkmeyer, and J. Dimick, "Variation in Hospital Mortality Associated with Inpatient Surgery," *New England Journal of Medicine* 361, no. 14 (2009): 1368–75.

7. J. Fielding and M. Hallissey, *Upper Gastrointestinal Surgery*, 1st ed. (Birmingham, UK: Springer-Verlag London, 2005).

8. "What Is Enteral Nutrition?" American Society for Parenteral and Enteral Nutrition, accessed January 28, 2014, https://www.nutritioncare.org/uploadedfiles/information_for_patients/ii_a1_enteral_nutrition.pdf.

9. Fielding and Hallissey, *Upper Gastrointestinal Surgery*.

10. Grade, Quintel, and Ghadimi, "Standard Perioperative Management in Gastrointestinal Surgery."

11. A. Urologe, "Preoperative Evaluation of Adult Patients Prior to Elective, Non-Cardiac Surgery: Joint Recommendations of German Society of Anesthesiology and Intensive Care Medicine, German Society of Surgery and German Society of Internal Medicine," *U.S. National Library of Medicine Institute of Health* 50, no. 9 (2011): 1169–82.

12. A. Ryding, S. Kumar, A. Worthington, and D. Burgess, "Prognostic Value of Brain Natriuretic Peptide in Noncardiac Surgery: A Meta-Analysis," *Anesthesiology* 111, no. 2 (2009): 311–19; H. Feringa, O. Schouten, M. Dunkelgrun, J. Bax, E. Boersma, A. Elhendy, R. Jonge, S. Karagiannis, R. Vidakovic, and D. Poldermans, "Plasma N-Terminal Pro-B-Type Natriuretic Peptide as Long-Term Prognostic Marker after Major Vascular Surgery," *Heart and Education in Heart* 93, no. 2 (2007): 226–31.

13. Grade, Quintel, and Ghadimi, "Standard Perioperative Management in Gastrointestinal Surgery."

14. G. Ackland and M. Edwards, "Defining Higher-Risk Surgery," *Current Opinion in Critical Care* 16, no. 4 (2010): 339–46.

15. G. Copeland, D. Jones, and M. Walters, "POSSUM: A Scoring System for Surgical Audit," *British Journal of Surgery* 78, no. 3 (1991): 355–60; Y. Haga, S. Ikei, and M. Ogawa, "Estimation of Physiologic Ability and Surgical Stress (E-PASS) as a New Prediction Scoring System for Postoperative Morbidity and Mortality following Elective Gastrointestinal Surgery," *Surgery Today* 29, no. 3 (1999): 219–25.

16. P. Markus, J. Martell, I. Leister, O. Horstmann, J. Brinker, and H. Becker, "Predicting Postoperative Morbidity by Clinical Assessment," *British Journal of Surgery* 92, no. 1 (2005): 101–6.

17. K. Fleischmann, J. Beckman, K. Brown, E. Chaikof, H. Calkins, L. Fleisher, W. Freeman, J. Froehlich, E. Kasper, J. Kersten, J. Robb, and B. Riegel, "ACCF/AHA Focused Update on Perioperative Beta Blockade: A Report of the American College of Cardiology Foundation/American Heart Association Task Force on Practice Guidelines," *Circulation* 120, no. 21 (2009): 2102–28.

18. A. Duncan, C. Koch, M. Xu, M. Manlapaz, B. Batdorf, G. Pitas, and N. Starr, "Recent Metformin Ingestion Does Not Increase In-Hospital Morbidity or Mortality after Cardiac Surgery," *Anesthesia Analgesia* 104, no. 1 (2007): 42–50.

19. D. Lindstrom, O. Sadr Azodi, A. Wladis, H. Tonnesen, S. Linder, H. Nasell, S. Ponzer, and J. Adami, "Effects of a Perioperative Smoking Cessation Intervention on Postoperative Complications: A Randomized Trial," *Annals of Surgery* 248, no. 5 (2008): 739–45.

20. F. Bozzetti, L. Gianotti, M. Braga, V. Di Carlo, and L. Mariani, "Postoperative Complications in Gastrointestinal Cancer Patients: The Joint Role of the Nutritional Status and the Nutritional Support," *Clinical Nutrition* 26, no. 6 (2007): 698–709.

21. R. Merkow, K. Bilimoria, M. McCarter, and D. Bentrem, "Effect of Body Mass Index on Short-Term Outcomes after Colectomy for Cancer," *Journal of the American College of Surgery* 208, no. 1 (2009): 53–61.

22. M. Tokunaga, N. Hiki, T. Fukunaga, T. Ogura, S. Miyata, and T. Yamaguchi, "Effect of Individual Fat Areas on Early Surgical Outcomes after Open Gastrectomy for Gastric Cancer," *British Journal of Surgery* 96, no. 5 (2009): 496–500.

23. S. Sahai, A. Zalpour, and M. Rozner, "Preoperative Evaluation of the Oncology Patient," *Medical Clinics of North America* 94, no. 2 (2010): 403–19.

24. "Bowel Diversion Surgeries: Ileostomy, Colostomy, Ileoanal Reservoir, and Continent Ileostomy," National Digestive Disease Information Clearinghouse (NDDIC), accessed February 5, 2014, http://digestive.niddk.nih.gov.

25. "Bowel Surgery," British United Provident Association (BUPA), accessed February 5, 2014, http://www.bupa.co.uk.

26. "Gastric Bypass Surgery Procedure," Johns Hopkins Medicine, accessed February 5, 2014, http://www.hopkinsmedicine.org.

27. N. Ward, "Nutrition Support to Patients Undergoing Gastrointestinal Surgery," *Nutritional Journal* 2 (2003): 18.

28. Grade, Quintel, and Ghadimi, "Standard Perioperative Management in Gastrointestinal Surgery."

29. P. White, H. Kehlet, J. Neal, T. Schricker, D. Carr, and F. Carli, "The Role of the Anesthesiologist in Fast-Track Surgery: From Multimodal Analgesia to Perioperative Medical Care," *Anesthesia and Analgesia* 104, no. 6 (2007): 1380–96.

30. S. Carey, R. Laws, S. Ferrie, J. Young, M. Allman-Farinelli, "Struggling with Food and Eating—Life After Major Upper Gastrointestinal Surgery," *National Center for Biotechnology Information (NCBI)* (2013): 2749–57.

31. B. Catchpole, "Smooth Muscle and the Surgeon," *Australian and New Zealand Journal of Surgery* 59, no. 3 (1989): 199–208.

32. K. Lassen, J. Kjaeve, T. Fetveit, G. Trano, H. Sigurdsson, A. Horn, and A. Revhaug, "Allowing Normal Food at Will after Major Upper Gastrointestinal Surgery Does Not Increase Morbidity: A Randomized Multicenter Trial," *National Center for Biotechnology Information (NCBI)* 247, no. 5 (2008): 721–29.

33. J. Kinney, J. Duke, C. Long, and F. Gump, "Tissue Fuel and Weight Loss after Injury," *Journal of Clinical Pathology Supplement-Royal College of Pathologists* 4 (1970): 65–72.

34. Ward, "Nutrition Support to Patients Undergoing Gastrointestinal Surgery."

12. PHARMACOLOGICAL APPROACHES
TO CELIAC DISEASE

1. "Learn More about a Gluten-Free Diet," University of Chicago Celiac Disease Center, http://www.cureceliacdisease.org/medical-professionals/guide/treatment.

2. A. Lanzini, F. Lanzarotto, V. Villanacci, A. Mora, S. Bertolazzi, D. Turini, G. Carella, A. Malagoli, G. Ferrante, B. Cesana, and C. Ricci, "Complete Recovery of Intestinal Mucosa Occurs Very Rarely in Adult Coeliac Patients Despite Adherence to Gluten-Free Diet," *Alimentary Pharmacology and Therapeutics* 29, no. 12 (2009): 1299–308.

3. G. Ou, M. Hedberg, P. Hörstedt, V. Baranov, G. Forsberg, M. Drobni, O. Sandström, S. Wai, I. Johansson, M. Hammarström, O. Hernell, and S. Hammarström, "Proximal Small Intestinal Microbiota and Identification of Rod-Shaped Bacteria Associated with Childhood Celiac Disease," *American Journal of Gastroenterology* 104, no. 12 (2009): 3058–67.

4. A. Rubio-Tapia, M. Rahim, J. See, B. Lahr, T. Wu, and J. Murray, "Mucosal Recovery and Mortality in Adults with Celiac Disease after Treatment with a Gluten-free Diet," *American Journal of Gastroenterology* 105, no. 6 (2010): 1412–20.

5. M. Medina, G. De Palma, C. Ribes-Koninckx, M. Calabuig, and Y. Sanz, "Bifidobacterium Strains Suppress in Vitro the Pro-Inflammatory Milieu Triggered by the Large Intestinal Microbiota of Coeliac Patients," *Journal of Inflammation* 5, no. 19 (2008).

6. S. Drago, R. El Asmar, M. Di Pierro, M. Grazia-Clemente, A. Tripathi, A. Sapone, M. Thakar, G. Iacono, A. Carroccio, C. D'Agate, T. Not, L. Zampini, C. Catassi, and A. Fasano, "Gliadin, Zonulin and Gut Permeability: Effects on Celiac and Non-Celiac Intestinal Mucosa and Intestinal Cell Lines," *Scandinavian Journal of Gastroenterology* 41, no. 4 (2006): 408–19.

7. E. Vilela, H. Torres, M. Ferrari, A. Lima, and A. Cunha, "Intestinal Permeability in Intestinal Diseases," *Brazilian Journal of Medical and Biological Research* 41, no. 12 (2008): 1105–9.

8. B. Toman, "Celiac Disease: On the Rise," *Discovery's Edge*: Mayo Clinic's Online Research Magazine, accessed January 12, 2014, http://www.mayo.edu/research/discoverys-edge/celiac-disease-rise.

9. Toman, "Celiac Disease: On the Rise."

10. P. Halloran, "Immunosuppressive Drugs for Kidney Transplantation," *New England Journal of Medicine* 351, no. 26 (2004): 2715–29.

11. J. Stone, P. Merkel, R. Spiera, P. Seo, C. Langford, G. Hoffman, C. Kallenberg, E. St. Clair, A. Turkiewicz, N. Tchao, L. Webber, L. Ding, L. Sejismundo, K. Mieras, D. Weitzenkamp, D. Ikle, V. Seyfert-Margolis, M. Mueller, P. Brunetta, N. Allen, F. Fervenza, D. Geetha, K. Keogh, E. Kissin, P. Monach, T. Peikert, C. Stegeman, S. Ytterberg, and U. Specks, "Rituximab versus Cyclophosphamide for ANCA-Associated Vasculitis," *New England Journal of Medicine* 363, no. 3 (2010): 221–32.

12. M. Dooley, D. Jayne, E. Ginzler, D. Isenberg, N. Olsen, D. Wofsy, F. Eitner, G. Appel, G. Contreras, L. Lisk, and N. Solomons, "Mycophenolate versus Azathioprine as Maintenance Therapy for Lupus Nephritis: A Meta-Analysis," *New England Journal of Medicine* 365, no. 20 (2011): 1886–95.

13. "Prograf Highlights of Prescribing Information," Astellas Pharma U.S., Inc., accessed February 13, 2014, http://www.astellas.us/docs/prograf.pdf.

13. CELIAC DISEASE AND EXERCISE

1. D. van Heel and J. West, "Recent Advances in Coeliac Disease," *Gut* 55, no. 7 (2006): 1037–46.

2. C. Atkin, "Celiac Disease and Physical Activity," Celiac.com, June 2, 2009, accessed January 14, 2014, http://www.celiac.com/articles/21826/1/Celiac-Disease-and-Physical-Activity/Page1.html.

3. S. Bower, M. Sharrett, and S. Plogsted, *Celiac Disease: A Guide to Living with Gluten Intolerance* (New York: Demos Health, 2006).

4. R. Taylor-Piliae, "Tai Chi as an Adjunct to Cardiac Rehabilitation Exercise Training," *Journal of Cardiopulmonary Rehabilitation* 23, no. 2 (2003): 90–96.

5. B. Lynn, "Cutaneous Nociceptors," in *The Neurobiology of Pain*, by W. Winlow and A. Holden (Manchester, UK: Manchester University Press, 1984).

6. H. Breivik, P. Borchgrevink, S. Allen, L. Rosseland, L. Romundstad, E. Hals, G. Kvarstein, and A. Stubhaug, "Assessment of Pain," *British Journal of Anaesthesia* 101, no. 1 (2008): 17–24.

7. S. Mior, "Exercise in the Treatment of Chronic Pain," *Clinical Journal of Pain* 17, no. 4 (2001): S77–85.

8. M. Buman, E. Hekler, D. Bliwise, and A. King, "Moderators and Mediators of Exercise-Induced Objective Sleep Improvements in Midlife and Older Adults with Sleep Complaints," *Health Psychology* 30, no. 5 (2011): 579–87.

9. "Health Benefits of Walking," Community Development Department, City of Cambridge, Massachusetts, accessed February 9, 2014, http://www.cambridgema.gov/cdd/transportation/gettingaroundcambridge/byfoot/healthbenefits.aspx.

10. K. Cooper, *Aerobics* (New York: Bantam Books, 1993).

11. J. Kloubec, "Pilates: How Does It Work and Who Needs It?" *Muscles Ligaments Tendons Journal* 1, no. 2 (2011): 61–66.

12. "Pilates for Beginners: Explore the Core of Pilates," Mayo Clinic, accessed February 19, 2014, http://www.mayoclinic.org/healthy-living/fitness/in-depth/pilates-for-beginners/art-20047673.

13. L. Ada, S. Dorsch, and C. Canning, "Strengthening Interventions Increase Strength and Improve Activity after Stroke: A Systematic Review," *Australian Journal of Physiotherapy* 52, no. 4 (2006): 241–48.

14. P. Weerapong, P. Hume, and G. Kolt, "Stretching: The Mechanisms and Benefits for Sport Performance and Injury Prevention," *Physical Therapy Reviews* 9, no. 4 (2004): 189–206.

15. G. Reynolds, "Stretching: The Truth," *New York Times*, October 31, 2008, accessed February 13, 2014, http://www.nytimes.com/2008/11/02/sports/playmagazine/112pewarm.html?_r=0.

16. M. Yessis, "Runners Need Active Stretching," *AMAA Journal* 18, no. 2 (2006): 8–18.

17. B. McFarlin, M. Flynn, M. Phillips, L. Stewart, and K. Timmerman, "Chronic Resistance Exercise Training Improves Natural Killer Cell Activity in Older Women," *Journals of Gerontology* 60, no. 10 (2005): 1315–18.

18. A. Peterson and B. Pedersen, "The Anti-Inflammatory Effect of Exercise," *Journal of Applied Physiology* 98, no. 4 (2005): 1154–62.

19. H. Ploeger, T. Takken, M. de Greef, and B. Timmons, "The Effects of Acute and Chronic Exercise on Inflammatory Markers in Children and Adults with a Chronic Inflammatory Disease: A Systematic Review," *Exercise Immunology Review* 15 (2009): 6–41; K. Timmerman, M. Flynn, P. Coen, M. Markofski, and B. Pence, "Exercise Training-Induced Lowering of Inflammatory (CD14+CD16+) Monocytes: A Role in the Anti-Inflammatory Influence of Exercise?" *Journal of Leukocyte Biology* 84, no. 5 (2008): 1271–78.

14. MOTIVATION AND CELIAC DISEASE

1. N. Hall, G. Rubin, and A. Charnock, "Intentional and Inadvertent Non-Adherence in Adult Coeliac Disease: A Cross-Sectional Survey," *Appetite* 68 (2013): 56–62.

2. Hall, Rubin, and Charnock, "Intentional and Inadvertent Non-Adherence in Adult Coeliac Disease."

3. M. Pietzak, "Follow-Up of Patients with Celiac Disease: Achieving Compliance with Treatment," *Gastroenterology* 128, no. 4 (2005): S135–41.

4. K. Sainsbury, B. Mullan, and L. Sharpe, "Gluten Free Diet Adherence in Coeliac Disease: The Role of Psychological Symptoms in Bridging the Intention-Behavior Gap," *Gastroenterology* 61, no. 1 (2013): 52–58.

5. P. Brar, A. Lee, S. Lewis, G. Bhagat, and P. Green, "Celiac Disease in African-Americans," *Digestive Diseases and Sciences* 51, no. 5 (2006): 1012–15.

6. S. Case, "The Gluten-Free Diet: How to Provide Effective Education and Resources," *Gastroenterology* 128, no. 4 (2005): S128–34.

7. K. Kurppa, O. Lauronen, P. Collin, A. Ukkola, K. Laurila, H. Huhtala, M. Mäki, and K. Kaukinen, "Factors Associated with Dietary Adherence in Celiac Disease: A Nationwide Study," *Digestion* 86, no. 4 (2012): 309–14.

8. Kurppa et al., "Factors Associated with Dietary Adherence in Celiac Disease."

9. A. Rubio-Tapia, I. Hill, C. Kelly, A. Calderwood, and J. Murray, "ACG Clinical Guidelines: Diagnosis and Management of Celiac Disease," *American Journal of Gastroenterology* 108, no. 5 (2013).

10. D. Falvo, *Effective Patient Education: A Guide to Increased Adherence*, 4th ed. (Burlington, MA: Jones and Bartlett Publishers, 2011).

11. Falvo, *Effective Patient Education.*

12. Falvo, *Effective Patient Education.*

13. Case, "The Gluten-Free Diet."

14. M. Sharrett and P. Cureton, "Kids and the Gluten-Free Diet," *Practical Gastroenterology* 6 (2007): 49–65.

15. Sharrett and Cureton, "Kids and the Gluten Free Diet."

16. M. Dennis and D. McKiernan, "Budgeting on the Gluten Free Diet," Beth Israel Deaconess Medical Center, accessed February 17, 2014, http://www.bidmc.org/CentersandDepartments/Departments/DigestiveDiseaseCenter/CeliacCenter/CeliacNow/THRVGF/BGTNGFD.aspx.

17. J. Murray, "The Widening Spectrum of Celiac Disease," *American Society for Clinical Nutrition* 69, no. 3 (1999): 354–65.

18. Sharrett and Cureton, "Kids and the Gluten Free Diet."

19. G. Addolorato, G. De Lorenzi, L. Abenavoli, L. Leggio, E. Capristo, and G. Gasbarrini, "Psychological Support Counselling Improves Gluten-Free Diet Compliance in Coeliac Patients with Affective Disorders," *Alimentary Pharmacology & Therapeutics* 20, no. 7 (2004): 777–82.

20. S. Errichiello, O. Esposito, R. Di Mase, M. Camarca, C. Natale, M. Limongelli, C. Marano, A. Coruzzo, M. Lombardo, P. Strisciuglio, and L. Greco, "Celiac Disease: Predictors of Compliance with a Gluten-Free Diet in Adolescents and Young Adults," *Journal of Pediatric Gastroenterology and Nutrition* 50, no. 1 (2010): 54–60.

21. Errichiello et al., "Celiac Disease: Predictors of Compliance with a Gluten-Free Diet in Adolescents and Young Adults."

22. Sharrett and Cureton, "Kids and the Gluten Free Diet"; O. Anson, Z. Weizman, and N. Zeevi, "Celiac Disease: Parental Knowledge and Attitudes of Dietary Compliance," *Pediatrics* 85, no. 1 (1990): 98–103.

23. Sharrett and Cureton, "Kids and the Gluten Free Diet."

24. Anson, Weizman, and Zeevi, "Celiac Disease: Parental Knowledge and Attitudes of Dietary Compliance."

25. Anson, Weizman, and Zeevi, "Celiac Disease: Parental Knowledge and Attitudes of Dietary Compliance."

26. Sharrett and Cureton, "Kids and the Gluten Free Diet."

27. Rubio-Tapia et al., "ACG Clinical Guidelines."

28. Rubio-Tapia et al., "ACG Clinical Guidelines."

29. Sharrett and Cureton, "Kids and the Gluten Free Diet."

30. Case, "The Gluten-Free Diet."

31. Falvo, *Effective Patient Education.*

32. V. Sdepanian, M. de Morais, and U. Fagundes-Neto, "Celiac Disease: Evaluation of Compliance to Gluten-Free Diet and Knowledge of Disease in Patients Registered at the Brazilian Celiac Association (ACA)," *Arquivos de Gastroenterologia* 38, no. 4 (2001): 232–39.

33. B. Redman, *The Practice of Patient Education: A Case Study Approach*, 10th ed. (New York: Elsevier Health Sciences, 2007).

34. Redman, *The Practice of Patient Education.*

35. Redman, *The Practice of Patient Education.*

36. Redman, *The Practice of Patient Education.*

37. Redman, *The Practice of Patient Education.*

38. Redman, *The Practice of Patient Education.*

39. J. Chauhan, P. Kumar, A. Dutta, S. Basu, and A. Kumar, "Assessment of Dietary Compliance to Gluten Free Diet and Psychosocial Problems in Indian Children with Celiac Disease," *Indian Journal of Pediatrics* 77, no. 6 (2010): 649–54.

40. Chauhan et al., "Assessment of Dietary Compliance to Gluten Free Diet and Psychosocial Problems in Indian Children with Celiac Disease."

41. Brar et al., "Celiac Disease in African-Americans."

15. CONCLUSION

1. "Celiac Disease–Sprue," MedLine Plus, accessed February 13, 2014, http://www.nlm.nih.gov/medlineplus/ency/article/000233.htm.

2. R. Kieffer, "The Role of Gluten Elasticity in the Baking Quality of Wheat," accessed November 11, 2013, http://www.muehlenchemie.de/downloads-future-of-flour/FoF_Kap_14.pdf.

3. "Gluten-Free Labeling of Foods," U.S. Food and Drug Administration (USFDA), accessed February 19, 2014, http://www.fda.gov/food/resourcesforyou/consumers/ucm367654.Htm.

4. C. Catassi, E. Fabiani, G. Iacono, C. D'Agate, R. Francavilla, F. Biagi, U. Volta, S. Accomando, A. Picarelli, I. De Vitis, P. Pianelli, R. Gesuita, F. Carle, A. Mandolesi, I. Bearzi, and A. Fasano, "A Prospective, Double-Blind, Placebo-Controlled Trial to Establish a Safe Gluten Threshold for Patients with Celiac Disease," *American Journal of Clinical Nutrition* 85, no. 1 (2007): 160–66.

5. "Chapter 2: Profiling Food Consumption in America," U.S. Department of Agriculture (USDA), accessed November 27, 2013, http://www.usda.gov/factbook/chapter2.pdf.

6. World Trade Organization (WHO), "Agreement on the Application of Sanitary and Phytosanitary Measures," accessed January 21, 2014, http://www.wto.org/english/tratop_e/sps_e/spsagr_e.htm.

7. Food and Agriculture Organization of the United Nations (FAO) and World Health Organization (WHO), *Understanding the Codex Alimentarious*, 3rd ed. (Rome: Food and Agriculture Organization of the United Nations, 2006).

8. Food and Agriculture Organization of the United Nations (FAO) and World Health Organization (WHO), "Codex Standard for Foods for Special Dietary Use for Persons Intolerant to Gluten," *Codex Standard* 118 (2008): 1–3.

9. Food and Agriculture Organization of the United Nations (FAO) and World Health Organization (WHO), "Codex Standard for Foods."

10. Food and Agriculture Organization of the United Nations (FAO) and World Health Organization (WHO), *Understanding the Codex Alimentarious*.

11. M. Maki, K. Mustalahti, J. Kokkonen, P. Kulmala, M. Haapalahti, T. Karttunen, J. Ilonen, K. Laurila, I. Dahlbom, T. Hansson, P. Hopfl, and M. Knip, "Prevalence of Celiac Disease among Children in Finland," *New England Journal of Medicine* 348, no. 25 (2003): 2517–24.

12. S. Bower, M. Sharrett, and S. Plogsted, *American Academy of Neurology: Celiac Disease: A Guide to Living with Gluten Intolerance* (New York: Demos Medical Publishing, 2007).

13. Walter and Eliza Hall Institute of Medical Research, "Biotech Raises $20 Million for Australian-Developed Coeliac Disease Vaccine," accessed February 2, 2014, http://www.wehi.edu.au/uploads/Coeliac_vaccine_ImmusanT_capital_raising_Dec2011_Final.pdf.

14. Walter and Eliza Hall, "Biotech Raises $20 Million for Australian-Developed Coeliac Disease Vaccine."

15. Bower, Sharrett, and Plogsted, *American Academy of Neurology.*

16. "Financial Support," Coeliac Society of Ireland, accessed October 27, 2013, http://www.coeliac.ie.

17. R. Benabou and J. Tirole, "Self-Confidence and Personal Motivation," *Quarterly Journal of Economics* 117, no. 3 (2002): 871–915.

18. B. Hansford and J. Hattie, "The Relationship between Self and Achievement/Performance Measures," *Review of Educational Research* 52 (1982): 123–42.

19. H. Cheng and A. Furnham, "Personality, Peer Relations, and Self-Confidence as Predictors of Happiness and Loneliness," *Journal of Adolescence* 25, no. 3 (2002): 327–39.

20. Bower, Sharrett, and Plogsted, *American Academy of Neurology.*

21. Spirituality and Medicine, University of Washington School of Medicine, accessed November 2, 2013, http://www.depts.washington.edu.

22. Bower, Sharrett, and Plogsted, *American Academy of Neurology.*

23. C. Laine and D. Weinberg, "How Can Physicians Keep Up-to-Date?" *Annual Review of Medicine* 50 (1999): 99–110.

24. M. Ruiz, "Risks of Self-Medication Practices," *Current Drug Safety* 5, no. 4 (2010): 315–23.

25. World Health Organization (WHO), "The Benefits and Risk of Self-Medication," *WHO Drug Information* 14 (2000): 1.

26. C. Hughes, J. McElnay, and G. Fleming, "Benefits and Risks of Self Medication," *Drug Safety* 24, no. 14 (2001): 1027–37.

BIBLIOGRAPHY

PREFACE

Eberman, L., H. Mata, and L. Kahanov. "Physical Examination of the Thorax and Abdomen." *International Journal of Athletic Therapy & Training* 18, no. 5 (2013): 32–37.

Fleckenstein, B., O. Molberg, S. Qiao, D. Schmid, F. von der Mülbe, K. Elgstoen, G. Jung, and L. Sollid. "Gliadin T Cell Epitope Selection by Tissue Transglutaminase in Celiac Disease. Role of Enzyme Specificity and Ph Influence on the Transamidation versus Deamidation Process." *Journal of Biological Chemistry* 277, no. 37 (2002): 34109–16.

CHAPTER I

Richards, M. "A Brief Review of the Archaeological Evidence for Palaeolithic and Neolithic Subsistence." *European Journal of Clinical Nutrition* 56, no. 12 (2002): 1262.

Tommasini, A., T. Not, and A. Ventura. "Ages of Celiac Disease: From Changing Environment to Improved Diagnostics." *World Journal of Gastroenterology* 17, no. 32 (2011): 3665–71.

Yan, D., and P. Holt. "Willem Dicke. Brilliant Clinical Observer and Translational Investigator. Discoverer of the Toxic Cause of Celiac Disease." *Clinical and Translational Science* 2, no. 6 (2009): 446–48.

CHAPTER 2

Khanal, T., H. Kim, S. Jin, E. Shim, H. Han, K. Noh, S. Park, D. Lee, W. Kang, H. K. Yeo, D. Kim, T. Jeong, and H. Jeong. "Protective Role of Metabolism by Intestinal Microflora in Butyl Paraben-Induced Toxicity in HepG2 Cell Cultures." *Toxicology Letters* 213, no. 2 (2012): 174–83.

Pedersen, A., A. Bardow, S. Jensen, and B. Nauntofte. "Saliva and Gastrointestinal Functions of Taste, Mastication, Swallowing and Digestion." *Oral Diseases* 8, no. 3 (2002): 117–29.

Synowiecki, J., B. Grzybowska, and A. Zdzieblo. "Sources, Properties and Suitability of New Thermostable Enzymes in Food Processing." *Critical Reviews in Food Science and Nutrition* 46, no. 3 (2006): 197–205.

CHAPTER 3

Di Stefano, M., G. Veneto, G. Corrao, and G. Corazza. "Role of Lifestyle Factors in the Pathogenesis of Osteopenia in Adult Coeliac Disease: A Multivariate Analysis." *European Journal of Gastroenterology and Hepatology* 12, no. 11 (2000): 1195–99.

Sams, A., and J. Hawks. "Patterns of Population Differentiation and Natural Selection on the Celiac Disease Background Risk Network." *Public Library of Science (PLOS) One* 8, no. 7 (2013): e70564.

Sollid, L., S. McAdam, O. Molberg, H. Quarsten, H. Arentz-Hansen, A. Louka, and K. Lundin. "Genes and Environment in Celiac Disease." *Acta Odontologica Scandinavica* 59, no. 3 (2001): 183–86.

CHAPTER 4

Hoffenberg, E., T. MacKenzie, K. Barriga, G. Eisenbarth, F. Bao, J. Haas, H. Erlich, T. Bugawan, R. Sokol, I. Taki, J. Norris, and M. Rewers. "A Prospective Study of the Incidence of Childhood Celiac Disease." *Journal of Pediatrics* 143, no. 3 (2003): 308–14.

León, F., E. Roldán, L. Sanchez, C. Camarero, A. Bootello, and G. Roy. "Human Small-Intestinal Epithelium Contains Functional Natural Killer Lymphocytes." *Gastroenterology* 125, no. 2 (2003): 345–56.

Ludvigsson, J. F., J. Ludvigsson, A. Ekbom, and S. Montgomery. "Celiac Disease and Risk of Subsequent Type 1 Diabetes: A General Population Cohort Study of Children and Adolescents." *Diabetes Care* 29, no. 11 (2006): 2483–88.

Rubin, C., L. Brandborg, P. Phelps, and H. Taylor Jr. "The Apparent Identical and Specific Nature of the Duodenal and Proximal Jejunal Lesion in Celiac Disease and Idiopathic Sprue." *Gastroenterology* 54, no. 4 (1968): 800–802.

Torre, P., S. Fusco, F. Quaglia, M. La Rotonda, F. Paparo, M. Maglio, R. Troncone, and L. Greco. "Immune Response of the Coeliac Nasal Mucosa to Locally-Instilled Gliadin." *Clinical & Experimental Immunology* 127, no. 3 (2002): 513–18.

CHAPTER 5

Cheng, J., P. Brar, A. Lee, and P. Green. "Body Mass Index in Celiac Disease: Beneficial Effect of a Gluten-Free Diet." *Journal of Clinical Gastroenterology* 44, no. 4 (2010): 267–71.

Health Quality Ontario. "Clinical Utility of Serologic Testing for Celiac Disease in Asymptomatic Patients: An Evidence-Based Analysis." *Ontario Health Technology Assessment Series* 11, no. 3 (2011): 1–63.

Husby, S., S. Koletzko, I. Korponay-Szabó, M. Mearin, A. Phillips, R. Shamir, R. Troncone, K. Giersiepen, D. Branski, C. Catassi, M. Lelgeman, M. Mäki, C. Ribes-Koninckx, A. Ventura, and K. Zimmer. "European Society for Pediatric Gastroenterology, Hepatology, and Nutrition Guidelines for the Diagnosis of Celiac Disease." *Journal of Pediatric Gastroenterology and Nutrition* 54, no. 1 (2012): 136–60.

Nachman, F., E. Sugai, H. Vázquez, A. González, P. Andrenacci, S. Niveloni, R. Mazure, E. Smecuol, M. Moreno, H. Hwang, M. Sánchez, E. Mauriño, and J. Bai. "Serological Tests for Celiac Disease as Indicators of Long-Term Compliance with the Gluten-Free Diet." *European Journal of Gastroenterology and Hepatology* 23, no. 6 (2011): 473–80.

Packer, S., V. Charlton, J. Keeling, R. Risdon, D. Ogilvie, R. Rowlatt, V. Larcher, and J. Harries. "Gluten Challenge in Treated Coeliac Disease." *Archives of Disease in Childhood* 53, no. 6 (1978): 449–55.

Reilly, N., and P. Green. "Epidemiology and Clinical Presentations of Celiac Disease." *Seminars in Immunopathology* 34, no. 4 (2012): 473–78.

CHAPTER 6

Hill, P., J. Forsyth, D. Semeraro, and G. Holmes. "IgA Antibodies to Human Tissue Transglutaminase: Audit of Routine Practice Confirms High Diagnostic Accuracy." *Scandinavian Journal of Gastroenterology* 39, no. 11 (2004): 1078–82.
Kaukinen, K., J. Partanen, M. Mäki, and P. Collin. "HLA-DQ Typing in the Diagnosis of Celiac Disease." *American Journal of Gastroenterology* 97, no. 3 (2002): 695–99.
Niewinski, M. "Advances in Celiac Disease and Gluten-Free Diet." *Journal of the American Dietetic Association* 108, no. 4 (2008): 661–72.
Sollid, L. "Molecular Basis of Celiac Disease." *Annual Review of Immunology* 18 (2000): 53–81.
Szajewska, H., A. Chmielewska, M. Pieścik-Lech, A. Ivarsson, S. Kolacek, S. Koletzko, M. Mearin, R. Shamir, R. Auricchio, and R. Troncone. "Systematic Review: Early Infant Feeding and the Prevention of Coeliac Disease." *Alimentary Pharmacology & Therapeutics* 36, no. 7 (2012): 607–18.
Tjellström, B., L. Högberg, L. Stenhammar, K. Fälth-Magnusson, K.-E. Magnusson, E. Norin, T. Sundqvist, and T. Midtvedt. "Faecal Short-Chain Fatty Acid Pattern in Childhood Coeliac Disease Is Normalised After More Than One Year's Gluten-Free Diet." *Microbial Ecology in Health and Disease* 24 (2013).

CHAPTER 7

Casella, S., B. Zanini, F. Lanzarotto, C. Ricci, A. Marengoni, G. Romanelli, and A. Lanzini. "Cognitive Performance Is Impaired in Coeliac Patients on Gluten-Free Diet: A Case-Control Study in Patients Older Than 65 Years of Age." *Digestive and Liver Disease* 44, no. 9 (2012): 729–35.
Genuis, S., and T. Bouchard. "Celiac Disease Presenting as Autism." *Journal of Child Neurology* 25, no. 1 (2010): 114–19.
Jackson, J., W. Eaton, N. Cascella, A. Fasano, and D. Kelly. "Neurologic and Psychiatric Manifestations of Celiac Disease and Gluten Sensitivity." *Psychiatric Quarterly* 83, no. 1 (2012): 91–102.
Ludvigsson, J., A. Reichenberg, C. Hultman, and J. Murray. "A Nationwide Study of the Association between Celiac Disease and the Risk of Autistic Spectrum Disorders." *JAMA Psychiatry* 70, no. 11 (2013): 1224–30.
Passananti, V., M. Siniscalchi, F. Zingone, C. Bucci, R. Tortora, P. Iovino, and C. Ciacci. "Prevalence of Eating Disorders in Adults with Celiac Disease." *Gastroenterology Research and Practice* (2013): 491–657.
Potocki, P., and K. Hozyasz. "Psychiatric Symptoms and Coeliac Disease." *Psychiatria Polska* 36, no. 4 (2002): 567–78.
Yucel, B., N. Ozbey, K. Demir, A. Polat, and J. Yager. "Eating Disorders and Celiac Disease: A Case Report." *International Journal of Eating Disorders* 39, no. 6 (2006): 530–32.

CHAPTER 8

Duerksen, D., and W. Leslie. "Positive Celiac Disease Serology and Reduced Bone Mineral Density in Adult Women." *Canadian Journal of Gastroenterology & Hepatology* 24, no. 2 (2010): 103–7.

Evron, E., J. Abarbanel, D. Branski, and Z. Sthoeger. "Polymyositis, Arthritis, and Proteinuria in a Patient with Adult Celiac Disease." *Journal of Rheumatology* 23, no. 4 (1996): 782–83.

Haussmann, J., and A. Sekar. "Chronic Urticaria: A Cutaneous Manifestation of Celiac Disease." *Canadian Journal of Gastroenterology & Hepatology* 20, no. 4 (2006): 291–93.

Kaukinen, K., L. Halme, P. Collin, M. Färkkilä, M. Mäki, P. Vehmanen, J. Partanen, and K. Höckerstedt. "Celiac Disease in Patients with Severe Liver Disease: Gluten-Free Diet May Reverse Hepatic Failure." *Gastroenterology* 122, no. 4 (2002): 881–88.

Sahebari, M., S. Sigari, H. Heidari, and O. Biglarian. "Osteomalacia Can Still Be a Point of Attention to Celiac Disease." *Clinical Cases in Mineral and Bone Metabolism* 8, no. 3 (2011): 14–15.

Zone, J. "Skin Manifestations of Celiac Disease." *Gastroenterology* 128, no. 4 (2005): S87–91.

CHAPTER 9

Marcoccia, A., M. Zippi, A. Bruni, F. Salvatori, D. Badiali, G. Donato, and A. Picarelli. "Chronic Abdominal Pain Associated with Intermittent Compression of the Celiac Artery." *Minerva Gastroenterologica e Dietologica* 53, no. 2 (2007): 209–13.

Porpora, M., A. Picarelli, R. Prosperi Porta, M. Di Tola, C. D'Elia, and E. Cosmi. "Celiac Disease as a Cause of Chronic Pelvic Pain, Dysmenorrhea, and Deep Dyspareunia." *Obstetrics & Gynecology* 99, no. 5 (2002): 937–39.

Sanders, D., A. Hopper, I. Azmy, N. Rahman, D. Hurlstone, J. Leeds, R. George, and N. Bhala. "Association of Adult Celiac Disease with Surgical Abdominal Pain." *Annals of Surgery* 242, no. 2 (2005): 201–7.

Saps, M., P. Adams, S. Bonilla, and D. Nichols-Vinueza. "Abdominal Pain and Functional Gastrointestinal Disorders in Children with Celiac Disease." *Journal of Pediatrics* 162, no. 3 (2013): 505–9.

CHAPTER 10

Dahele, A., and S. Ghosh. "Vitamin B12 Deficiency in Untreated Celiac Disease." *American Journal of Gastroenterology* 96, no. 3 (2001): 745–50.

Dickey, W., M. Ward, C. Whittle, M. Kelly, K. Pentieva, G. Horigan, S. Patton, and H. McNulty. "Homocysteine and Related B-Vitamin Status in Coeliac Disease: Effects of Gluten Exclusion and Histological Recovery." *Scandinavian Journal of Gastroenterology* 43, no. 6 (2008): 682–88.

Djuric, Z., S. Zivic, and V. Katic. "Celiac Disease with Diffuse Cutaneous Vitamin K-Deficiency Bleeding." *Advances in Therapy* 24, no. 6 (2007): 1286–89.

Fric, P., D. Gabrovska, and J. Nevoral. "Celiac Disease, Gluten-Free Diet, and Oats." *Nutrition Reviews* 69, no. 2 (2011): 107–15.

Pietzak, M. "Celiac Disease, Wheat Allergy, and Gluten Sensitivity: When Gluten Free Is Not a Fad." *Journal of Parenteral and Enteral Nutrition (JPEN)* 36, no. 1 (2012): 68S–75S.

Tavakkoli, A., D. DiGiacomo, P. Green, and B. Lebwohl. "Vitamin D Status and Concomitant Autoimmunity in Celiac Disease." *Journal of Clinical Gastroenterology* 47, no. 6 (2013): 515–19.

Thompson, T. "Wheat Starch, Gliadin, and the Gluten-Free Diet." *Journal of the American Dietetic Association* 101, no. 12 (2001): 1456–59.

CHAPTER 11

Absah, I., R. Grothe, D. Potter, T.-T. Wu, and J. Murray. "Duodenal Perforation as an Unusual Celiac Disease Presentation in Two Patients." *Journal of Medical Cases* 4, no. 2 (2013): 109–13.
Bai, J., C. Moran, C. Martinez, S. Niveloni, E. Crosetti, A. Sambuelli, and L. Boerr. "Celiac Sprue after Surgery of the Upper Gastrointestinal Tract. Report of 10 Patients with Special Attention to Diagnosis, Clinical Behavior, and Follow-Up." *Journal of Clinical Gastroenterology* 13, no. 5 (1991): 521–24.
Ciacci, C., R. Cavallaro, R. Romano, D. Galletta, F. Labanca, M. Marino, M. Donisi, and G. Mazzacca. "Increased Risk of Surgery in Undiagnosed Celiac Disease." *Digestive Diseases and Sciences* 46, no. 10 (2001): 2206–8.

CHAPTER 12

Freeman, H. "Non-Dietary Forms of Treatment for Adult Celiac Disease." *World Journal of Gastrointestinal Pharmacology and Therapeutics* 4, no. 4 (2013): 108–12.
Malamut, G., J. Murray, and C. Cellier. "Refractory Celiac Disease." *Gastrointestinal Endoscopy Clinics of North America* 22, no. 4 (2012): 759–72.
Pinier, M., G. Fuhrmann, E. Verdu, and J. Leroux. "Prevention Measures and Exploratory Pharmacological Treatments of Celiac Disease." *American Journal of Gastroenterology* 105, no. 12 (2010): 2551–61.
Wahab, P., J. Crusius, J. Meijer, J. Uil, and C. Mulder. "Cyclosporin in the Treatment of Adults with Refractory Coeliac Disease—An Open Pilot Study." *Alimentary Pharmacology & Therapeutics* 14, no. 6 (2000): 767–74.

CHAPTER 13

Black, K., P. Skidmore, and R. Brown. "Case Study: Nutritional Strategies of a Cyclist with Celiac Disease during an Ultraendurance Race." *International Journal of Sport Nutrition and Exercise Metabolism* 22, no. 4 (2012): 304–10.
Passananti, V., A. Santonicola, C. Bucci, P. Andreozzi, A. Ranaudo, D. Di Giacomo, and C. Ciacci. "Bone Mass in Women with Celiac Disease: Role of Exercise and Gluten-Free Diet." *Digestive and Liver Disease* 44, no. 5 (2012): 379–83.

CHAPTER 14

Barbero, E., S. McNally, M. Donohue, and M. Kagnoff. "Barriers Impeding Serologic Screening for Celiac Disease in Clinically High-Prevalence Populations." *BMC Gastroenterology* 5, no. 14 (2014): 42.

Valderas, J., B. Starfield, B. Sibbald, C. Salisbury, and M. Roland. "Defining Comorbidity: Implications for Understanding Health and Health Services." *Annals of Family Medicine* 7, no. 4 (2009): 357–63.

CHAPTER 15

Bakshi, A., S. Stephen, M. Borum, and D. Doman. "Emerging Therapeutic Options for Celiac Disease: Potential Alternatives to a Gluten-Free Diet." *Gastroenterology and Hepatology* 8, no. 9 (2012): 582–88.
Feasey, D. "The Patience of a Patient." *Journal of Critical Psychology Counseling and Psychotherapy* 6, no. 1 (2006): 1.
Liubarskiene, Z., L. Soliūniene, V. Kilius, and E. Peicius. "Patient Confidence in Health Care." *Medicina (Kaunas)* 40, no. 3 (2004): 278–85.
Noble, L., A. Kubacki, J. Martin, and M. Lloyd. "The Effect of Professional Skills Training on Patient-Centeredness and Confidence in Communicating with Patients." *Medical Education* 41, no. 5 (2007): 432–40.
Ogden, J., K. Fuks, M. Gardner, S. Johnson, M. McLean, P. Martin, and R. Shah. "Doctors' Expressions of Uncertainty and Patient Confidence." *Patient Education and Counseling* 48, no. 2 (2002): 171–76.

INDEX

ABOUT THE AUTHOR

Naheed Ali, MD, PhD, began writing professionally in 2005. For years, he taught at colleges where he lectured on various biomedical topics. Additional information is available at http://naheedali.com/.